Proceedings in Life Sciences

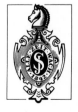

Hormonally Defined Media

A Tool in Cell Biology

Lectures and Posters Presented at the
First European Conference on Serum-Free Cell Culture
Heidelberg, October 7–9, 1982

Edited by
G. Fischer and R.J. Wieser

With 185 Figures

Springer-Verlag
Berlin Heidelberg New York Tokyo 1983

Dr. G. Fischer
Institut für Neurobiologie
der Universität Heidelberg
Im Neuenheimer Feld 504
6900 Heidelberg 1, FRG

Dr. R. J. Wieser
Institut für Pharmakologie
der Universität Mainz
Obere Zahlbacher Str. 67
6500 Mainz, FRG

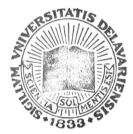

QP
571
.E87
1982

ISBN 3-540-12668-6 Springer-Verlag Berlin Heidelberg New York Tokyo
ISBN 0-387-12668-6 Springer-Verlag New York Heidelberg Berlin Tokyo

Typesetting, printing and bookbinding: Brühlsche Universitätsdruckerei, Giessen.
2131/3130-543210

Preface

Until some years ago serum or crude tissue extracts were used predominantly or exclusively as media supplements for the cultivation of cells. However, during this time evidence accumulated that these supplements could not provide in an optimal way most of the cultivated cells with all factors necessary for their survival, their proliferation and/or differentiation. Moreover, a variety of cells could not be cultivated at all under these conditions and often the composition of the cultures changed within rather short periods of time by overgrowth of initially present subpopulations of those cells which grow well in these supplements, as for example fibroblasts. Nevertheless, using these supplements (or fractions thereof), insight could be gained into some of the influences of serum or tissue extract constituents with regard to survival, proliferation and differentiation of cells in culture. It became obvious from these experiments that serum or tissue extracts did not only supply cells with nutrients or vitamins (which are now constituents of all basic media), but also with hormones as well as growth-, differentiation-, and attachment-factors.

In course of time experiments were performed in which serum enriched with hormones and other growth factors was used to successfully cultivate those cells which could not survive in serum-supplemented media alone. Under normal conditions in an organism, however, only a small population of cells has direct contact with serum. Serum combines plasma and platelet-derived molecules (among them growth factors) which are set free during injury and blood coagulation. Therefore, most of the cells in an organism will be exposed only to plasma or plasma filtrates. It is interesting also from this point of view that often high serum concentrations were used when proliferating cells were studied and low serum concentrations for quiescent cells.

The knowledge gained from these experiments led to the search for methods by which serum is replaced by mixtures of hormones, growth factors, transport proteins, and attachment factors. Inspiring experiments by G. Sato and colleagues made it soon possible not only to cultivate established cell lines under the new "defined" conditions - by adapting the cells from serum to serum-free, hormonally defined conditions - but also successfully to establish culture conditions for a variety of primary cell cultures. It was not surprising that now, under these "defined" conditions, even those cells could be cultivated that had failed to survive in serum-supplemented media.

The quickly expanding influence of this cultivation technique on different aspects of cell biology, including research on cell proliferation and differentiation, cell-cell interactions, tumor growth as well as endocrinological and pharmacological investigations, had made it desirable to organize a conference in Europe which concentrated on this new tool in cell biology and to provide a forum for direct exchange of experience.

Gerd Brunner was instrumental in the organization of this conference. He died a few months before the conference took place. We will always remember him as a good friend and enthusiastic scientist who has contributed his almost unlimited resources on ideas and energy to make this conference a success.

This conference was generously supported by Bethesda Research Laboratories. We are also grateful for the endorsement of the Gesellschaft für Biologische Chemie and the Gesellschaft für Zellbiologie.

We wish to thank our co-organizers T. Leenen and T. Wäli for their excellent cooperation, and J. Becker and I. Makowiecki for their help in preparing these proceedings.

July, 1983   G. FISCHER
                                                    R.J. WIESER

Contents

CELL-SUBSTRATUM INTERACTIONS

NEURAL CELLS

ENDOCRINE AND EXOCRINE CELLS

HEMOPOIETIC AND IMMUNE SYSTEM

LIVER- AND KIDNEY-DERIVED CELLS

MUSCLE CELLS, EPITHELIAL CELLS, FIBROADIPOGENIC CELLS, MELANOCYTES AND CHONDROCYTES

TUMOR CELLS

Contributors

You will find the addresses at the beginning of the respective contribution

Adolphe, M.   377
Albrecht, M.   446
Ambesi-Impiombato, F.S.   285
Andersen, B.   330
Antoniou, M.   234
Arnold, B.   314
Artur, M.   127
Avola, R.   215
Baffet, G.   344
Banerjee, M.R.   234
Barritault, D.   123,132
Basset, P.   219
Baulieu, E.E.   114
Bauriedel, G.   380
Belleville, F.   127
Berndt, J.   324
Betsholtz, C.   103
Borel, J.   127
Boss, B.   120
Brenner, M.K.   300
Breton-Gorius, J.   320
Briand, P.   436
Brunet, N.   132
Brunner, G.   162,222,250,294
Bürk, R.R.   57
Bunge, R.P.   178
Carey, D.J.   178
Casadevall, N.   320
Castell, J.V.   333,340
Chaintreuil, J.   387
Chambard, J.C.   88
Chapman, J.   320
Clark, J.   6
Clément, B.   344
Coloma, J.   333
Corvol, M.T.   377
Courtois, Y.   123
Courty, J.   123
Cupissol, D.   443
Curti, D.   215
Darmon, M.   143
Daune, G.   229
De Lavergne, E.   127
Dembinski, T.C.   439
Dollenmeier, P.   358
Don, P.   390
Ebendal, T.   393
Eldridge, C.   178
Eppenberger, H.M.   358
Erdmann, E.   380

Eschenbruch, M.   107
Farkash, Y.   274
Farrant, J.   300
Faure, T.   387
Ferber, E.   304
Fischer, G.   189
Flesch, I.   304
Fooij, M.   403
Forest, N.   377
Franchi, A.   88
Frati, L.   317
Froger, B.   377
Gebb, Ch.   393
Genetet, N.   127
Geschier, C.   127
Giesen, E.M.   337
Gillery, P.   127
Glaise, D.   344
Gómez-Lechón, M.J.   333,340
Gourdji, D.   132
Green, C.D.   439
Güntert, B.   203
Guguen-Guillouzo, C.   344
Guillouzo, A.   344
Ham, R.G.   16
Hamm, U.   324
Hatzfeld, A.   307
Hatzfeld, J.A.   307
Heath, J.K.   111
Heldin, C.-H.   103
Henry, P.-E.   403
Herman, A.   127
Heulin, M.H.   127
Higgins, D.   178
Hölzel, F.   446
Honegger, P.   203
Horster, M.   347
Hütter, J.F.   400
Imbs, J.L.   337
Isacke, C.M.   111
Jimenez de Asua, L.   46,107,120
Joshi, J.   234
Jungermann, K.   330,354
Jung-Testas, I.   114
Kaighn, M.E.   418
Kawamoto, T.   310
Kessler-Icekson, G.   383
Ketelsen, U.-P.   304
Krause, U.   250
Krawietz, W.   380

Opening Lecture

Divining the Role of Serum in Cell Culture

Gordon H. Sato

Cancer Center, Q-058, University of California, San Diego, La Jolla, CA 92093, USA

The use of biological fluids as a medium for cells outside the body is a natural and logical step to take.

The first to do so was Arnold, who in 1887, observed the migration of frog leukocytes from elder pith soaked in aqueous humor (1). Almost twenty years later, Ross Harrison observed the growth of nerve cell processes from fragments of spinal ganglia embedded in clotted lymph (2). These experiments were both the beginning of tissue culture and a dramatic reaffirmation of the cell as the fundamental, discrete and potentially autonomous unit of life. The use of serum and chick embryo extract was introduced shortly thereafter by Burrows (3) and Carrel (4).

What vital functions were these natural fluids providing for cells in culture? The universal approach to this question has been analytical. The logical premise has been that serum contains factors necessary for the growth and survival of cells in culture and that suitable fractionation should lead to the identification of these factors and to an understanding of their function. A few examples are instructive. In the 1930's Fritz Lipmann, working in the laboratory of Albert Fischer, made a brief attempt to isolate the active factor in embryo extract (5). He had the good sense to abandon this untimely project and to proceed to other more fruitful areas. In the 1950's Harold Fisher, T. T. Puck and I fractionated fetal calf serum and concluded that albumin and fetuin were the critical components (6). We later learned that Jacquez and Barry had essentially reached the same conclusion a few years earlier (7). Robert Pierson, working in the laboratory of Howard Temin, fractionated serum and correctly concluded that non-suppressible insulin-like activity (NSILA) was an important part of the activity of serum (8). The group of Robert Holley introduced some interesting modifications to the procedures of serum fractionation that enabled them to identify separable entities such as survival factor, migration factor, etc (9).

In retrospect, an analytical approach is awesomely difficult because of the complex synergistic interactions between factors and the minute quantities of hormones in blood. Our own approach was inspired by the pioneering work of Jacob Furth on hormone dependent tumors (10). Our efforts to develop hormone dependent cell lines (11,12,13) led to the hypothesis that the role of serum in culture is to provide complexes of hormones that are specific for a given cell type (14). Izumi Hayashi provided the first experimental evidence for this hypothesis (15). This hypothesis has since been expanded to include the role of transport proteins and biomatrix (16).

We can now state that the role of serum in culture could only be elucidated by knowing the answer before asking the question. I am not conscious of exerting any effort to realize the critical role of hormones in culture. It was suggested in an easy and natural way by the great mass of information in related fields.

Gerd Brunner would have been sympathetic. His attitude toward science was that of an imaginative free spirit. He inspired and nurtured these feelings in his students. Their respect and affection for him have been expressed in many ways throughout this meeting.

I wish to thank Gerd and his students: Elke and Klaus Lange, Tomas von Ruden, Bernd Nitzgen, Raimond Wieser, Georg Tschank, Dieter Kaufmann, Becker Udith, Martin Otter and Ingrid Mackowieki for a memorable symposium that will have a lasting effect on European cell biology.

REFERENCES

1. Arnold, J. (1887). Ueber Theilungsvorgänge and der Wanderzellen: ihre progressiven und regressiven Metamorphosen. Arch. Mikrosk. Anat. 30, 205-310.

2. Harrison, R. G. (1906). Observations on the living developing nerve fiber. Proc. Soc. Exp. Biol. Med. 7, 140-143.

3. Barrows, M. T. (1910). The cultivation of tissues of the chick embryo outside the body. J. Am. Med. Assoc. 55, 2057-2058.

4. Carrel, A. and Burrows, M. T. (1910). Le culture de tissus adultes en dehors de l'organisme. C. V. Soc. Biol. (Paris) 69, 293-294.

5. Lipmann, F. (1971) in Wanderings of a Biochemist, pp. 20-22, Wiley Interscience, New York, London, Sydney, Toronto.

6. Fisher, H. W., Puck, T. T. and Sato, G. (1958) Molecular growth requirements of single mammalian cells: The action of fetuin in promoting cell attachment to glass. Proc. Natl. Acad. Sci. 44: 4-10.

7. Jacquez, J. A. and Barry, E. (1951). Tissue culture media. J. Gen. Physiol. 34: 765-774.

8. Temin, H., Pierson, Jr., R. W. and Dulak, N. C. (1972). The role of serum in the control of multiplication of avian and mammalian cells in culture, in Growth, Nutrition and Metabolism of Cells in Culture, Vol. I, pp. 49-81, (Rothblat, G. H. and Cristafalo, V. J. eds.), Academic Press, New York and London.

9. Holley, R. w. and Kiernan, J. A. (1974). Control of the initiation of DNA synthesis in 3T3 cells: Serum Factors. Proc. Natl. Acad. Sci. USA 71: 2908-2911.

10. Furth, J. (968) in Thule International Symposium on Cancer and Aging, pp. 131-151, Nordiska Bokanoelun, Förlag, Stockholm.

11. Clark, J. L., Jones, K. L., Gospodarowicz, D. and Sato, G. H. (1972). Growth response to hormones by a new rat ovary cell line. Nature New Bio. 236: 180-181.

12. Armelin, H. A. (1973). Pituitary extracts and steroid hormones in the control of 3T3 cell growth. Proc. Nat. Acad. Sci. USA 70: 2702-2706.

13. Nishikawa, K., Armelin, H. A. and Sato, G. (1975). Control of ovarian cell growth in culture by serum and pituitary factors. Proc. Natl. Acad. Sci. USA 72: 483-487.

14. Sato, G. (975). The role of serum in cell culture, in: Biochemical Action of Hormones, Vol. III, pp. 391-396, (Litwak, G., ed.), Academic Press, Inc., New York, San Francisco, London.

15. Hayashi, I. and Sato, G. (1976). Replacement of serum by hormones permits the growth of cells in a defined medium. Nature 259: 132-134.

16. Barnes, D. and Sato, G. (1981). Serum-free cell culture: A unifying approach. Cell 22: 649-655.

Nutritional Requirements

Reducing the Requirement for Serum Supplements in High Yield Microcarrier Cell Culture

Julian Clark

Cell Biology Group, Pharmacia Fine Chemicals AB, Box 175, S-751 04 Uppsala, Sweden

ABSTRACT

Various methods of reducing the requirement and cost of serum supplements for the growth of MRC-5 and Vero cells on Cytodex^R microcarriers were examined. The base medium was DME/Medium 199 (50/50) and a supplement of 10% (v/v) foetal calf serum (FCS) was the control. Greater economy of serum could be achieved by selecting the types and concentration of serum on the basis of whether the serum was to support the attachment and growth of cells at low densities or at later stages in the culture cycle. The concept of using a fixed concentration of serum throughout the culture cycle is questioned.

Low-serum and serum-free media could support the growth of cells on Cytodex 1. Medium supplemented with 0.5% FCS, bovine serum albumin (BSA, 2 mg/ml) and either EGF (10 ng/ml), or insulin (1 µg/ml) and transferrin (25 µg/ml), proved to be satisfactory for stirred cultures and supported cell proliferation to nearly the same extent as the control. Various serum-free media were tested and maximum yields were obtained when the base medium was supplemented with fibronectin (2 µg/ml), BSA (2 mg/ml), insulin (1 µg/ml), transferrin (25 µg/ml), putrescine (100 µM), fetuin (1 mg/ml) and EGF (10 ng/ml). Replacement of fetuin by dexamethasone (50 ng/ml) and trace metals (Mo, Cd, Se) resulted in a small reduction in cell proliferation. Cell yield was approx. 40-50% of that obtained with 10% FCS. A possible protective effect of larger molecules in low-serum and serum-free media may be important for reproducible results with stirred microcarrier cultures.

INTRODUCTION

Low-serum or serum-free media provide important possibilities for production scale animal cell culture. Although the routine use of serum-free media for large scale production follows behind use at the research scale, such media have major potential advantages including:

- improved reproducibility between cultures
- reduced risk of contamination (e.g. virus and mycoplasma)
- reduced time spent screening batches of sera
- simpler purification of culture products
- improved economy
- possibility to culture a wider range of differentiated and functional cells

In order to realize these advantages, advances in methods for cell production need to be accompanied by a systematic attempt to reduce and eliminate the requirement for a serum supplement.

Recent developments in the microcarrier culture technique (4,10), provide one of the most efficient methods for immobilizing and growing primary, normal diploid and established cells in high yields. This method enables the culture of anchorage-dependent cells in homogeneous suspensions at concentrations greater than 10^6 cells/ml (3, 10) in routine production culture volumes of up to 1000 litres (8, 10, 15). Although microcarrier culture provides an advanced technique for cell production, widespread use of this technique for the production of large numbers of certain cell types may be restricted by the cost and limited supply of the serum supplements. Therefore, the possibility of using low-serum and serum-free media in the microcarrier system has been examined. Because of their widespread use in production, monkey kidney cells (Vero) and diploid human fibroblasts (MRC-5) were considered and subsequently proved to be capable of proliferating on Cytodex 1 microcarriers when cultured in certain formulations of low-serum and serum-free media. Some of these results have been presented previously (2).

MATERIALS AND METHODS

The techniques of microcarrier culture have been described elsewhere (10). Stock cultures of cells were maintained in DME containing 10% (v/v) foetal calf serum (FCS) and all inocula were harvested from exponentially growing cultures by trypsinization at low temperature (5 and see 7) and cell number was determined by counting extruded nuclei (12). Cultures in Petri dishes were grown in an atmosphere of 95% air/5% CO_2 and microcarrier cultures were contained in spinner vessels having a gas headspace volume equal to the culture volume (10). The spinner vessels were briefly flushed with this gas mixture every 24 h.

The base medium for all experiments was DME/Medium 199 (50/50, v/v) containing 10 mM HEPES but no antibiotics. All media were prepared and well mixed before contact with either the culture surface or cells. Inocula were washed in base medium containing soybean trypsin inhibitor (0.5 mg/ml) and then in base medium alone, before plating in the various formulations. Initial growth tests were conducted in Petri dishes and when a formulation resulted in growth to greater than 10% confluence, it was tested in microcarrier culture with Cytodex 1. The microcarriers were used at a concentration of 3 mg/ml final culture volume (up to 1 litre). Cultures were inoculated with 2×10^5 MRC-5 cells/ml final culture volume (11×10^3 cells/cm^2) or 9×10^4 Vero cells/ml final culture volume (5×10^3 cells/cm^2) and were initiated in 30% of final volume with a static attachment

period (3 h) before continuous stirring at 40 - 60 rpm. After 1 day the culture
was diluted with medium to 50% of the final volume and after 3 days the culture was
diluted to the final volume. On day 5, 50% of the culture medium was replaced by
fresh medium. Cytodex 1, Ficoll^R 70 and Dextran T-70 were from Pharmacia Fine
Chemicals, Uppsala; bovine serum albumin (BSA), putrescine, insulin, transferrin
and fetuin were supplied by Sigma; fibronectin and EGF were from Collaborative
Research, Waltham MA, USA.

RESULTS AND DISCUSSION

In initial attempts to reduce the cost of serum supplements, alternative types of
sera were examined for their ability to support the growth of cells on
microcarriers (2). Provided suitable batches of sera were used (selected for
maximum plating efficiency) it was observed that the total requirement and cost of
FCS could be reduced. The most effective procedure was to use 5% FCS in combination
with a reduced initial culture volume (10) and then to dilute the culture to the
final volume gradually during the culture cycle with medium containing 5% newborn
calf serum (NCS). This procedure could be used for both MRC-5 and Vero cells
growing on Cytodex 1 and provided a way of reducing the requirement for serum per
litre of confluent culture from 150 ml FCS to 15 ml FCS and 95 ml NCS with only
approx. a 20% reduction in cell yield. Alternatively, initiating the culture at
30% of final culture volume with 10% FCS and diluting to the final volume with
medium containing 5% FCS resulted in a reduction of FCS from 150 ml to 85 ml with
no reduction in cell yield. As a result of these observations, the concept of
using a constant serum concentration throughout the culture cycle is questioned and
it is apparent that reduced serum concentrations can be used during the later
stages of the culture cycle. The success of this method depends on selecting
batches of serum giving the maximum plating efficiency and growth of cells.

Low-serum media

The concentration of the serum supplement was reduced further by using 0.5% FCS in
combination with defined supplements (Table 1).

Table 1. Relative yields of cells grown on Cytodex 1 in the presence of various low-serum media. Cells were allowed to attach in 30% of the final culture volume in medium containing 5% FCS. After 24 h this medium was removed and replaced by low-serum medium to 50% of final volume. On day 3 fresh low-serum medium was added to give the final culture volume. Supplements: BSA, 2 mg/ml; fatty acid-free BSA (FAF. BSA), 2 mg/ml; Ficoll 70, 2 mg/ml; EGF, 10 ng/ml; insulin (IN), 1 µg/ml; transferrin (TR), 25 µg/ml. Absolute yield in 10% FCS: 2.2 x 10^6 MRC-5 cells/ml (day 10), 4.9 x 10^6 Vero cells/ml (day 8).

Supplement	Relative yield	
	MRC-5	Vero
no supplement	0	5
10% FCS	100	100
0.5% FCS + BSA + EGF	82	88
0.5% FCS + BSA + IN + TR	74	83
0.5% FCS + BSA + IN + TR + EGF	85	87
0.5% FCS + FAF. BSA + IN + TR	38	77
0.5% FCS + Ficoll 70 + IN + TR	30	65
0.5% FCS + IN + TR	14	42

The most effective and simple low-serum formulation was 0.5% FCS, 2 mg/ml BSA and 10 ng/ml EGF and cell morphology and population doubling time appeared unaltered in this medium. A BSA supplement was necessary for good growth and it is concluded that the less pure BSA contained contaminants which stimulated cell growth. Both fatty acid-free BSA and Ficoll 70 increased cell yield with respect to a basic supplement of 0.5% FCS, insulin and transferrin (Table 1). Preliminary experiments comparing cell growth in static and stirred microcarrier cultures (data not shown) indicate that fatty acid-free BSA and Ficoll 70 have the greatest effect in stirred microcarrier cultures. Therefore, it is suggested that these components of approx. MW 70,000 may also have a protective role in stirred cultures (6).

Serum free media

An essential component for successful microcarrier culture of Vero and MRC-5 cells in serum-free medium has previously been reported to be fibronectin and this attachment glycoprotein proved superior to Holme's protein (2). Fibronectin was an essential component for only the early stages of the culture cycle and omission at refeeding stages did not alter cell growth or yield. The combinations of supplements most effective in supporting cell growth in serum-free media are shown in Figure 1. The formulation resulting in maximum growth of Vero and MRC-5 cells was fibronectin (2 µg/ml), BSA (2 mg/ml), insulin (1 µg/ml), transferrin (25 µg/ml), putrescine (100 µM), fetuin (1 mg/ml) and EGF (10 ng/ml). The yield of cells in this medium was at least 65% of that observed in medium supplemented with 10% FCS.

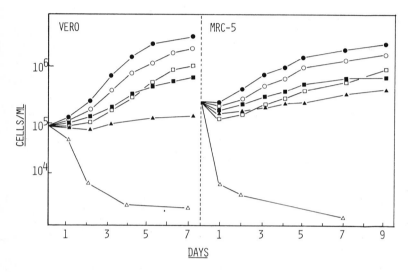

Fig. 1. The growth of Vero and MRC-5 cells on Cytodex 1 in the presence of serum-free media. The serum-free medium was base medium supplemented with fibronectin (2 µg/ml), BSA (2 mg/ml), insulin (1 µg/ml), transferrin (25 µg/ml), putrescine (100 µM), EGF (10 ng/ml) and fetuin (1 ng/ml). Base medium + 10% FCS (-●-), serum-free medium (-o-), serum-free medium without fetuin (-□-), serum-free medium without EGF (-■-), serum-free medium without insulin and transferrin (-▲-), base medium without supplements (-△-).

EGF was an important supplement and insulin and transferrin were essential for growth. Putrescine had a beneficial, but variable effect on cell growth in all formulations. However, we have yet to confirm that this component is essential for growth of MRC-5 and Vero cells in serum-free medium.

A supplement of MW 70,000 added to the serum-free medium improved cell yields in stirred microcarrier cultures (Fig. 2). This effect was more pronounced for MRC-5 cells and such a component could be BSA, Ficoll 70 or Dextran T-70. Since Ficoll 70 and Dextran T-70 are purified, biologically inert carbohydrate polymers, it is unlikely that these components have a nutritional role. It is suggested that these components have some protective (physical) effect in the stirred microcarrier cultures, possibly similar to that previously suggested for some suspension cultures (6). Part of the effect of BSA on the growth of MRC-5 cells is probably attributable to contaminants since the use of fatty acid-free BSA instead of BSA results in a 25% reduction in cell yield (Fig.2). The yield of cells grown in media supplemented with Ficoll 70 or Dextran T-70 instead of BSA was reduced by approximately 40%. It is not known whether the molecular weight of the polysaccharides is important and MW 70,000 was chosen only for the purpose of comparison with BSA. In the case of Vero cells (data not shown) it was noticed that Ficoll 70 and Dextran T-70 had no reproducible effect on cell yield in stirred microcarrier cultures and the effect of BSA was probably due to adsorbed contaminants.

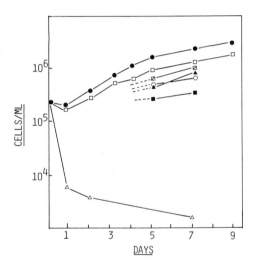

Fig.2 The effect of a MW 70,000 component in serum-free media on the growth of MRC-5 cells on Cytodex 1. The serum-free medium contained fibronectin, insulin, transferrin, putrescine, EGF and fetuin as described in Fig. 1. This medium was supplemented with BSA (-□-, 2 mg/ml); fatty acid-free BSA (-▨-, 2 mg/ml); Ficoll 70 (-○-, 2 mg/ml) or Dextran T-70 (-▲-, 2 mg/ml). The base medium was tested alone (-△-) or supplemented with 10% FCS(-●-).

Since fetuin is derived from FCS, attempts were made to replace this component by non-serum derived supplements previously shown to be beneficial in serum-free media (1). Table 2 presents the simplest formulations which resulted in maximum cell growth in the absence of fetuin.

Table 2. The effect of replacing fetuin in serum-free medium by dexamethasone and trace metals. The absolute yield of MRC-5 cells in base medium supplemented with 10% FCS was 1.1.x 10^6 cells/ml (day 7).

Supplement	Relative yield of MRC-5 cells
1. No supplement	0
2. 10% FCS	100
3. Serum-free medium: fibronectin (2 µg/ml), insulin (1 µg/ml), transferrin (25 µg/ml), putrescine (100 µM), EGF (10 ng/ml), BSA (2 mg/ml)	33
4. Serum-free medium + $(NH_4)_6$. $Mo_7O_{24}.4H_2O$ (0.5 nM), $CdSO_4$ (50nM), H_2SeO_3 (15 nM)	40
5. Serum-free medium + dexamethasone (50 ng/ml)	35
6. Serum-free medium + trace metals and dexamethasone (as above)	48

Replacement of fetuin by trace metals and dexamethasone resulted in a serum-free medium (Table 2, Medium 6) which could support growth of MRC-5 cells to give a yield almost 50% of that obtained when 10% FCS was used as a supplement. In three separate experiments 5.9, 5.4 and 4.5 x 10^5 cells/ml were obtained in this serum-free medium (c.f. 1.1 x 10^6 cells/ml in medium supplemented with 10% FCS).

Similar serum-free media for human fibroblasts have recently been reported (7, 11, 13). The reduction in yield of MRC-5 cells in the serum-free medium appeared to be partly due to a lower saturation density (2). Addition of platelet-derived growth factor (PDGF) to the media described here may improve saturation density and thus yield of MRC-5 cells (11). Kan and Yamane (7) used media similar to those reported here and noted a difference between BSA and delipidized BSA with respect to cell growth. The importance of BSA is likely to be as a carrier of lipids and certain metal ions rather than of growth factors (7). The results reported here confirm the importance of BSA in serum-free media of this nature.

The results also indicate an important role for insulin and transferrin in promoting the growth of cells in low-serum and serum-free media. Weinstein et al. (14) have recently demonstrated the strong growth promoting activity of insulin and transferrin in the presence of low-concentrations of FCS. Furthermore, they did not find PDGF was a major mitogen for human fibroblasts (14). Walthall and Ham (13) observed that supplements of EGF, insulin and dexamethasone were sufficient for growth of human fibroblasts. The fact that the studies presented here demonstrated an additional requirement for BSA and transferrin may be related to differences in the basal media and supply of iron (13).

Subculturing of cells on the microcarriers was possible with the serum-free medium (Table 2, Medium 6) provided that the residual trypsin remaining after harvesting was inactivated by soybean trypsin inhibitor (0.1%, w/v) rather than by medium containing serum. The effect of successive subcultivations in this serum-free medium has not been tested.

These experiments demonstrate that anchorage-dependent cells can be grown in low-serum and serum-free media in the microcarrier system. Although the growth of cells on microcarriers in the presence of serum-free medium was never as extensive as growth in medium supplemented with 10% FCS, these preliminary studies demonstrate that serum requirements can be reduced while still retaining the advantages of microcarrier culture. Importantly, such media provide a way of reducing or even eliminating a requirement for FCS whilst still exploiting the main advantage of microcarrier culture - high cell yields in a small culture volume. The approach we have used when formulating serum-free media is derived from that used by others working with traditional monolayer methods (1). While serum-free media are clearly compatible with microcarrier culture, the results indicate that there may be differences between media which are optimal for static monolayer or stirred microcarrier cultures. The beneficial effect of polymers in stirred microcarrier cultures will need to be examined with other cell types before the above observations can be generalized. Interestingly, Crespi et.al. (3) recently observed a difference in the requirements for the serum-free cultivation of MDCK cells in stationary and microcarrier cultures. Microcarrier culture of these cells in serum-free medium required the presence of dibutyryl-cAMP and an increased concentration of insulin (3).

Norrgren et. al. (9) from our group have reported that a serum-free medium supported the growth of chicken heart cells on microcarriers (Fig. 3). The yield in the serum-free medium was approximately 60% of that obtained with a supplement of 10% FCS and could be increased to 80-90% by replacing the dexamethasone by a dialysate (MW<10,000) of FCS (9).

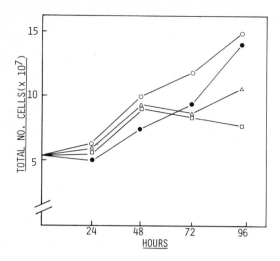

Fig. 3. The growth of primary chicken heart cells on Cytodex 3 in the presence of
serum-free media . Base medium (DME/F10, 50/50) was supplemented with a) 10% FCS
(-o-), b) insulin, transferrin, human serum albumin (HSA), fibronectin (-□-),
c) insulin, transferrin, HSA, fibronectin, dexamethasone (-△-) or d) insulin,
transferrin, HSA, fibronectin and a MW <10,000 dialysate of FCS (-●-).Supplements:
insulin, 1 μg/ml; transferrin, 25 μg/ml; HSA, 2 mg/ml; fibronectin, 10 μg/ml;
dexamethasone, 200 ng/ml. (Data from Norrgren et al.(8), reproduced by kind
permission).

Having demonstrated that it is possible to reduce the requirement for serum in
high-yield microcarrier culture, future experiments will be directed at examining
the long term effects of culturing cells in low-serum and serum-free media. We
anticipate that increases in the economy and efficiency of large scale microcarrier
culture are likely to result from a combination of the approaches discussed here.
Firstly, by having flexibility in selecting the type and concentration of a serum
supplement on the basis of the stage in the culture cycle, and secondly, by
changing to a low-serum or serum-free medium.

REFERENCES

1. Barnes, D., Sato, G. (1980) Methods for growth of cultured cells in serum-free
    medium. Anal. Biochem, 102: 255-270.

2. Clark, J., Gebb, Ch., Hirtenstein, M. (1982) Serum supplements and serum-free
    media: applicability for microcarrier culture of animal cells. Devel. Biol.
    Stand. 50: 81-91.

3. Crespi, C.L., Imamura, T., Leong, P., Fleischaker, R. Brunengraber, H., Thilly, W., Giard, D. (1981) Microcarrier culture: applications in biologicals production and cell biology. Biotechnol. Bioeng. 23: 2673-2689.

4. Gebb, Ch., Clark, J., Hirtenstein, M. et al. (1982) Alternative surfaces for microcarrier culture of animal cells. Devel. Biol. Stand. 50: 93-102.

5. Ham, R.G. (1980) Dermal fibroblasts. Methods Cell Biol. 21A: 255-276.

6. Healy, G.M., Parker, R.C. (1966) Cultivation of mammalian cells in defined media with protein and non-protein supplements. J. Cell Biol. 30: 539-553.

7. Kan, M., Yamane, I. (1982) In vitro proliferation and lifespan of human diploid fibroblasts in serum-free BSA-containing medium. J. Cell. Physiol. 111: 155-162.

8. Montagnon, B., Fanget, B. (1982) Thousand litres scale microcarrier culture of Vero cells for killed poliovirus vaccine: promising results. Devel. Biol. Stand. (in press).

9. Norrgren, G., Ebendal, T., Gebb, Ch., Wikström; H. (1982) The use of Cytodex[R] 3 microcarriers and reduced-serum media for the production of nerve growth promoters from chicken heart cells. Devel. Biol. Stand. (in press).

10. Pharmacia Fine Chemicals (1981) Microcarrier cell culture: principles and methods. Technical Book Series, Uppsala, Sweden.

11. Phillips, P.D., Cristofalo, V.J. (1981) Growth regulation of WI-38 cells in a serum-free medium. Exp. Cell Res. 134: 297-302.

12. Sanford, K.K., Earle, W.R., Evans, V.J., Waltz, H.K., Shannon, J.E. (1951) The measurement of cell proliferation in tissue cultures by enumeration of cell nuclei. J. Natl. Cancer Res. Inst. 11: 773-795.

13. Walthall, B.J., Ham, R.G. (1981) Multiplication of human diploid fibroblasts in a synthetic medium supplemented with EGF, insulin and dexamethasone. Exp. Cell Res. 134: 303-311.

14. Weinstein, R., Hoover, G.A., Majure, J., van der Spek, J., Stemerman, M.B., Maciag, T. (1982) Growth of human foreskin fibroblasts in a serum-free, defined medium without platelet-derived growth factor. J. Cell. Physiol. 110: 23-28.

15. van Wezel, A.L., van der Velden-de Groot, C.A.M., van Herwaarden, J. (1980) The production of inactivated polio vaccine on serially cultivated kidney cells from captive-bred monkeys. Devel. Biol. Stand. 46: 151-158.

Growth of Normal Human Cells in Defined Media

Richard G. Ham

Department of Molecular, Cellular and Developmental Biology, Campus Box 347,
University of Colorado, Boulder, CO 80309, USA

INTRODUCTION

Until quite recently, the requirements for growth in culture of normal human cells were poorly understood. Good growth of human diploid fibroblasts had been possible for many years, but only with substantial amounts of serum (Hayflick and Moorhead, 1961). Methods had also been developed for certain types of normal human epithelial cells, such as keratinocytes (Rheinwald and Green, 1975) and mammary epithelial cells (Stampfer et al., 1980), but these typically required feeder layers, conditioned media, or special supplements for satisfactory growth. This report reviews recent progress toward a complete understanding of the growth requirements of several different types of normal human cells.

Defined medium systems will be considered individually for six different types of normal human cells: fibroblasts (Bettger et al., 1981); chondrocytes (Jennings, 1982); keratinocytes (Tsao et al., 1982); bronchial epithelial cells (Lechner et al., 1982); mammary epithelial cells (S. Hammond, M. Stampfer, R. Ham, unpublished); and prostatic epithelial cells (Chaproniere-Rickenberg and Webber, 1982). A separate discussion of each of these systems is made necessary by the differences in growth requirements that exist among the six cell types. These discussions are preceded by a more general description of the methods employed in our laboratory for the development of defined media. In addition, after the requirements of these six cell types are described individually, they are compared and used as a basis for discussion of the best ways to develop defined media for additional types of normal human cells, some of which cannot yet be grown well in any type of medium, defined or otherwise.

METHODS FOR DEVELOPMENT OF DEFINED MEDIA

Although the qualitative and quantitative growth requirements of individual cell types differ substantially from one cell type to another, even within the same species, our experience has shown that a similar approach can be used for the analysis of growth requirements and the development of a defined medium for each new cell type that is studied. That approach has been described in detail in a recent review (pages 28-33 of Ham, 1981), and will only be summarized briefly here.

The obvious first step is to obtain enough growth so that growth-response assays can be performed. Any means that will work is acceptable for this step, including the use of complex undefined supplements, the use of conditioned medium, or the use of feeder layers of irradiated cells. In most cases, our laboratory has bypassed this step by allowing someone else to accomplish it. Many different laboratories are devoting large amounts of energy to obtaining growth in culture of many diverse types of cells from humans and other species. Generally, when we are ready to work with a new cell type, we select one that other investigators have already succeeded in growing reasonably well in a complex undefined culture system.

The next major step is to optimize the basal nutrient medium and other aspects of the culture system so that good clonal growth can be obtained with minimal amounts of dialyzed serum or other supplements. In most cases the first phase of optimization is to survey all available media, including recently developed optimized media for other normal cell types, to determine which one will support clonal growth with the smallest amount of dialyzed supplement. The optimization process is then carried out with that medium.

Optimization is both a qualitative and a quantitative process. One of its major objectives is to include in the medium every nutrient required by the cell type in question. Conventional media are frequently deficient in certain B vitamins such as biotin and vitamin B_{12}, and trace elements such as iron, copper, zinc, and selenium, which must be added for satisfactory serum-free growth. In addition, quantitative requirements have proven to be very important. In the absence of undefined supplements, cells tend to be intolerant of marginal deficiencies or excesses of medium components. Thus, adjustment of every component of the nutrient medium to its experimentally determined optimum concentration is often critically important for satisfactory serum-free growth of normal cells.

Optimization studies are always done with suboptimal concentrations of the dialyzed supplements so that improvements in growth can be detected readily. In addition, because secondary requirements often cannot be detected until the first-limiting requirement has been satisfied, it is necessary each time that growth is improved to reduce the concentration of the dialyzed supplement further and test a second time for possible qualitative and quantitative requirements that were not previously detectable due to the amount of dialyzed supplement that was present (Ham and McKeehan, 1978b).

The goal of optimization is to reduce the requirement for dialyzed supplements as low as possible. For some permanent lines, optimization may completely eliminate the need for macromolecular supplements. This was found to be the case during the development of medium F12 for Chinese hamster lines (Ham, 1965; Hamilton and Ham, 1977), and also during the development of medium MCDB 411 for mouse neuroblastoma C1300 (Agy et al., 1981). However, in the case of normal cells, we have thus far always found that optimization alone will not totally eliminate the requirement for undefined macromolecular supplements.

The final phase in the development of defined media for normal cells consists of replacing the remaining requirement for serum or other undefined additives with appropriate mixtures of hormones, growth factors, carrier proteins, enzyme inhibitors, attachment factors, lipids, supplemental nutrients, or other defined additives as needed. This procedure was pioneered by Dr. Gordon Sato and his colleagues (Sato, 1975; Hayashi and Sato, 1976; Barnes and Sato, 1980) and is reviewed in this volume by Dr. Sato. In theory, it should be possible to replace any amount of serum with a sufficiently complex and concentrated mixture of defined additives. However, in practice, this has generally not worked well for normal cells, which typically require large amounts of serum for growth in conventional media, if they can be grown at all in such media. We have found that for normal cells, it is far more effective to reduce the requirement for undefined additives to a minimal level through optimization of the basal nutrient medium and other aspects of the culture system before attempting the replacement. When the serum requirement for optimal growth has been reduced to two percent or less, it is generally relatively easy to replace the remainder with defined additives, as will be described in the following sections for individual cell types.

DEFINED MEDIUM FOR SPECIFIC TYPES OF NORMAL CELLS

Fibroblasts

The human diploid fibroblast was the first normal human cell type for which we optimized a culture medium, and also the first one to be grown in a defined medium. The starting point for these studies was the system developed by Hayflick and Moorhead (1961), in which good monolayer and clonal growth was obtained with 10% whole calf serum added to Eagle's basal medium. We selected clonal growth as the most sensitive assay for the adequacy and freedom from toxicity of the culture medium (Ham, 1972). We also elected to use only dialyzed supplements whenever possible in order to maintain maximum control over the small molecular composition of the culture medium. An initial survey of media revealed that medium F12 was the best starting point for the optimization process. Adjustment of the concentrations of cysteine and glutamine generated medium MCDB 102, which supported far better clonal growth with dialyzed serum (Ham et al., 1977). Addition of selenium and reduction of the concentration of zinc led to MCDB 103, which substantially reduced the amount of dialyzed serum required for clonal growth (McKeehan et al., 1976). A complete round of optimization of all medium components then yielded MCDB 104, which, when used in conjunction with low temperature trypsinization and polylysine-coated culture dishes, supported optimal clonal growth of human diploid fibroblasts with 2% dialyzed serum (McKeehan et al., 1977). Subsequent modifications led to media designated MCDB 105, 107, 108, and 110, but failed to reduce the serum requirement significantly below that in MCDB 104.

At this point, attempts to replace the remaining serum requirement with defined additives were initiated. Insulin (INS), dexamethasone (DEX), and epidermal growth factor (EGF) each individually stimulated a minor increase in ^{3}H-thymidine incorporation. When tested in combination, these three substances, were found to be highly synergistic, both in thymidine incorporation assays and in clonal growth assays (Walthall and Ham, 1981). However, the best growth that could be obtained was still substantially less than with dialyzed serum.

We next turned our attention to lipid requirements. About one fourth of the dry mass of a typical cultured cell is composed of lipids, and it is well known that cultured cells preferentially utilize lipids from exogenous sources when they are available. However, the defined medium that we were using was virtually devoid of lipids, with only a trace of linoleic acid in its formula. We therefore prepared and tested a lipid supplement, designated liposome B, whose composition is similar to that of intracellular membranes. It consists of soybean lecithin, cholesterol, and sphingomyelin in a weight ratio of 6:3:1, plus small amounts of vitamin E, and vitamin E acetate, all dispersed in a saline solution as liposomes. When added at a total lipid concentration of 10 µg/ml, this supplement caused a major improvement in growth of human diploid fibroblasts under defined conditions (Bettger et al., 1981). An additional supplement containing prostaglandins E_1 and $F_{2\alpha}$, reducing agents, and phosphoenolpyruvate was further beneficial in the presence (but not the absence) of INS, DEX, EGF, and liposome B. Most of the effect appeared to be due to the prostaglandins.

The composition of the defined medium for human diploid fibroblasts that resulted from these studies is given in Table 1. On the basis of total colony area per petri dish, the clonal growth that is obtained in this medium is about 60% of the maximum that can be obtained with dialyzed fetal bovine serum in the same basal medium. The colonies that form in the defined medium are large, but are not as dense in their centers as colonies grown in serum, apparently due to a greater sensitivity to density-dependent inhibition in the defined medium. Preliminary studies have shown that this problem can be overcome at least partially by adding platelet-derived growth factor (PDGF) to the defined medium at day 7 of a 12-14 day clonal growth assay. However, we have not been able to obtain enough PDGF to incorporate it routinely into the defined medium.

Members of our laboratory group have also recently developed defined media for fibroblasts from chicken embryos and sheep. At roughly the same time as Dr. McKeehan optimized the medium for human fibroblasts, he also did parallel

TABLE 1. DEFINED MEDIA FOR NORMAL FIBROBLASTS

Species	Human	Chicken	Sheep
Basal medium	MCDB 110	MCDB 202	MCDB 202
Insulin μg/ml	0.95	20	10
Dexamethasone M	1.4×10^{-6}	--	1.0×10^{-6}
EGF ng/ml	30	20	--
FGF ng/ml	--	--	100
Liposome B μg/ml[a]	10	10	30
Supplement A	+[b]	-	-

[a] Each 10 μg/ml of Liposome B provides 6 μg/ml of soybean lecithin, 3 μg/ml of cholesterol and 1 μg/ml of sphingomyelin, plus 0.06 μg/ml of vitamin E and 0.2 μg/ml of vitamin E acetate.

[b] Supplement A provides 2.5×10^{-8} M prostaglandin E_1, 2.0×10^{-6} M prostaglandin $F_{2\alpha}$, 6.5×10^{-6} M dithiothreitol, 6.5×10^{-7} M reduced glutathione, and 1.0×10^{-5} M phosphoenolpyruvate.

optimization studies with chicken embryo fibroblasts, which resulted in the development of medium MCDB 202 (McKeehan and Ham, 1977). Use of this medium, together with low temperature trypsinization and polylysine-coated culture dishes reduced the amount of dialyzed serum needed for optimal growth of chicken fibroblasts to about 2 percent. Human fibroblasts also grew quite well in this medium, although chicken fibroblasts did not grow well in the medium optimized for human fibroblasts (Ham and McKeehan, 1978a). Recently, we have achieved clonal growth of chicken fibroblasts in a serum-free medium consisting of MCDB 202 supplemented with 20 μg/ml insulin, 20 ng/ml EGF, and 10 μg/ml liposome B (Graves and Ham, 1982). Glucocorticoids do not appear to be important in this system.

MCDB 202 is also a satisfactory basal medium for serum-free growth of sheep fibroblasts. For these cells, however, fibroblast growth factor (FGF) is a far more effective mitogen than EGF. Our current defined medium for sheep fibroblasts consists of MCDB 202 supplemented with 10 μg/ml insulin, 1×10^{-6} M dexamethasone, 100 ng/ml FGF, and 30 μg/ml liposome B. All four of these supplements are needed for satisfactory serum-free growth (Broad and Ham, unpublished).

Chondrocytes

We have reported many years ago that good clonal growth and expression of differentiated properties could be obtained in primary cultures of rabbit ear chondrocytes in medium F12 supplemented with fetal bovine serum and chicken embryo extract (Ham and Sattler, 1968; Ham et al., 1970). Quantitative optimization studies subsequently revealed that these cells exhibit unusually broad plateaus of optimal growth response, and that no significant improvement in growth over that obtained in MCDB 104 could be achieved by further optimization. Serum replacement also proved to be quite easy. Substantial clonal growth, together with a low level of expression of cartilage-like differentiation (detected by staining with acidified alcian green) was obtained by supplementing MCDB 104 with 5.0 μg/ml liposome B, 1.0 μg/ml insulin, and 100 ng/ml FGF (Jennings and Ham, 1981). EGF was much less effective as a mitogen in this system than FGF, which had previously been reported to be beneficial to rabbit chondrocytes, even in the presence of serum (Gospodarowicz and Mescher, 1977).

For our studies with human chondrocytes, we began with the system that had worked well for rabbit chondrocytes. Human chondrocyte suspensions were prepared from rib cartilage removed from young individuals during corrective chest surgery or at autopsy. Excellent clonal growth and expression of cartilage-like differentiation were obtained in medium F12 supplemented with serum plus chicken embryo extract. Although growth was poor in the defined medium that had been developed for rabbit chondrocytes, further supplementation of that medium with 1×10^{-7} M dexamethasone (or hydrocortisone) resulted in rapid multiplication to form large diffuse colonies. Expression of cartilage-like differentiation was not seen in these colonies. However, we were able to verify that the cells growing in the defined medium were actually chondrocytes by first growing the colonies for a few days in the defined medium and then transferring them to medium F12 supplemented with serum and chicken embryo extract. Under these conditions, the centers of the mature colonies accumulated substantial amounts of extracellular matrix, which was stained brightly green by acidified alcian green (Ham and Sattler, 1968).

Although some cartilage-like differentiation was observed with the rabbit chondrocytes in their defined medium, it was also far below the level that could be obtained with undefined supplements. Thus, for chondrocytes from both species, it appears likely that a specific differentiation-promoting factor may be needed for full expression of differentiated properties in the defined growth media. We have not yet been able to obtain enough somatomedin C to determine whether it is the missing factor. However, there is also a distinct possibility that expression of cartilage-like differentiation may be dependent on achieving a high density of cells in the centers of the colonies. If this is the case, the critical requirement may be for a factor that promotes more dense growth, rather than for a true differentiation-promoting factor.

Keratinocytes

Soon after it became evident that growth of fibroblasts could be improved and their requirements for serum could be reduced by optimizing their basal nutrient medium, we decided to try the same general approach on a human epithelial cell. When we surveyed the literature early in 1976, we concluded that the best starting point would be the human epidermal keratinocyte, whose clonal growth and serial subculture had just been achieved by Rheinwald and Green (1975) through use of an irradiated 3T3 feeder layer. A survey of alternative media and supplements revealed that growth could be obtained without the feeder layer through use of medium 199 in conjunction with pituitary extract and high levels of hydrocortisone (Peehl and Ham, 1980a).

A broader medium survey then revealed that medium F12 would support enough clonal growth with dialyzed serum to permit medium optimization studies to be undertaken. This process greatly improved growth and reduced the serum requirement. A totally new medium, designated MCDB 151, was developed, which, in the presence of high levels of hydrocortisone, supported good clonal growth of normal human keratinocytes with 2 percent dialyzed fetal bovine serum as its only undefined supplement (Peehl and Ham, 1980b).

At this point, replacement of the remaining requirement for serum with defined supplements became feasible. Trace elements were added to the medium, and it was supplemented with a mixture of insulin, EGF, transferrin, progesterone, ethanolamine, and phosphoethanolamine, which supported serum-free growth and also allowed the level of hydrocortisone to be reduced (Tsao et al., 1982). Adjustment of the iron and zinc levels has since eliminated the need for transferrin. Progesterone, whose effect was marginal at best, has also been deleted (Boyce and Ham, 1982). The composition of the current defined medium for clonal growth of normal human keratinocytes is given in Table 2.

No undefined supplements are needed for relatively short-term cultures in this medium, including clonal growth experiments and limited subculturing. However, supplementation with whole bovine pituitary extract (wBPE) at a protein concentration of 70 μg/ml is distinctly beneficial for longer term cultures, and makes possible initiation of primary cultures, frozen storage, and serial subculture, all in the absence of serum (Boyce and Ham, 1982).

When combined with defined supplements, wBPE can be a valuable tool in the development of media for epithelial cells. In cases where the defined medium is still somewhat deficient, wBPE greatly improves the growth of epithelial cells without promoting fibroblastic overgrowth. We have observed this both for keratinocytes and for mammary epithelial cells, and anticipate that it will also be true for many other types of epithelial cells.

Several of the results of our studies on the growth requirements of normal human keratinocytes could not have been easily anticipated. The first is that these epithelial cells are surprisingly easy to grow in culture when they are provided with an adequate medium. The second is that their growth requirements are not particularly unusual or complex. With the possible exception of ethanolamine and phosphoethanolamine, which had only recently been shown to be required by other types of cells (Kano-Sueoka et al., 1979; Kano-Sueoka and Errick, 1981), there is

TABLE 2. DEFINED MEDIA FOR NORMAL HUMAN KERATINOCYTES, BRONCHIAL EPITHELIAL CELLS, AND MAMMARY EPITHELIAL CELLS

Cell type	Keratinocyte	Bronchial[a]	Mammary
Basal medium	MCDB 153[b]	MCDB 152[c]	MCDB 170[d]
Insulin µg/ml	5.0	5.0	5.0
Hydrocortisone M	1.4×10^{-6}	5.0×10^{-7}	1.4×10^{-6}
EGF ng/ml	5.0	5.0	25
Ethanolamine M	1.0×10^{-4}	5.0×10^{-7}	1.0×10^{-4}
Phosphoethanolamine M	1.0×10^{-4}	5.0×10^{-7}	1.0×10^{-4}
Transferrin µg/ml	--	10	5.0
Prolactin µg/ml	--	--	5.0
Prostaglandin E_1 M	--	--	2.5×10^{-8}

[a] From Lechner et al. (1982), who refer to the complete defined medium as "LHC-1".

[b] MCDB 153 is MCDB 152 (Tsao et al., 1982) with 5×10^{-6} M $FeSO_4$ and 5×10^{-7} M $ZnSO_4$ (Boyce and Ham, 1982).

[c] The basal medium is described by Lechner et al. as MCDB 151 plus trace elements. Also, it is modified by increasing calcium to 1.1×10^{-4} M and sulfate to 2.5×10^{-5} M.

[d] MCDB 170 is MCDB 202 (McKeehan and Ham, 1977) with 7×10^{-5} M cysteine and 5×10^{-7} M zinc.

nothing qualitatively unusual about the components of the defined medium. Thus, the ability of this medium to support the growth of normal human keratinocytes so much more effectively than other media appears to be primarily due to quantitative changes in the concentrations of its components that were made during the process of optimization.

A third unanticipated result is that the optimized defined media for keratinocytes and fibroblasts are each selective against growth of the opposite cell type. In retrospect, this is almost certainly why keratinocytes (and other types of epithelial cells) had always been so difficult to grow in culture. Virtually all standard culture media were originally developed for fibroblast-like cells (Ham, 1974, 1981). Thus, in addition to promoting fibroblastic overgrowth, they also tended to inhibit growth of the epithelial cells.

We do not yet understand all of the reasons for the selectivity of the keratinocyte and fibroblast media. However, one major aspect of that selectivity is the difference in their calcium ion concentrations. Fibroblasts need a high calcium concentration for multiplication, particularly when grown with limiting amounts of serum or defined mitogens. Keratinocytes, on the other hand, require a low calcium concentration for multiplication, and are diverted to a non-proliferative terminal differentiation pathway when the calcium concentration is increased. Thus, in addition to obtaining selective growth of normal human keratinocytes, we have also been able to control their differentiation in the defined medium, simply by manipulating the calcium ion concentration.

Bronchial epithelial cells

A recently published study by Lechner et al. (1982) has shown that normal human bronchial epithelial cells can be grown and subcultured in a defined medium that is closely related to the keratinocyte defined medium described above. The basal nutrient medium is a slight modification of MCDB 152 (Tsao et al., 1982). It is supplemented with insulin, hydrocortisone, EGF, ethanolamine, phospho-ethanolamine, and transferrin (Table 2), and is used in conjunction with culture surfaces that have been coated with a mixture of fibronectin, collagen, and bovine serum albumin.

The addition of as little as 0.5% serum to the defined medium is distinctly inhibitory to growth of bronchial epithelial cells. That inhibition is partially overcome by the addition of cholera toxin, which has little effect on growth in the defined medium without serum. Prior to introduction of a basal nutrient medium that had been optimized for an epithelial cell type, growth of bronchial epithelial cells in medium 199 had required both serum and a feeder layer of growth-arrested Swiss 3T3 cells.

Mammary epithelial cells

Soon after it became evident that normal human keratinocytes could be grown in a defined medium, we elected to begin studies on a second type of normal human epithelial cell to determine how generally applicable our keratinocyte data would prove to be. We selected as our starting point a complex conditioned medium system that had been developed by Stampfer et al. (1980) for growth of human mammary epithelial cells. This study has been carried out in collaboration with Dr. Stampfer, who routinely prepares organoids or primary cultures from normal reduction mammoplasty tissue and sends them to us frozen for use in our studies of cellular growth requirements.

We began by testing the keratinocyte defined medium for its ability to support growth of normal mammary epithelial cells. When supplemented with wBPE and increased calcium, that medium supported moderate growth of the mammary cells, but did not meet our expectations. We therefore surveyed all available media in our laboratory, and found that MCDB 202, which had originally been developed for chicken embryo fibroblasts (McKeehan and Ham, 1977), was far superior to MCDB 153 as a basal medium for the mammary cells when used with wBPE and the keratinocyte defined supplements (Ham, 1982).

Clonal growth of mammary epithelial cells is far better in MCDB 202 supplemented with insulin, hydrocortisone, EGF, ethanolamine, phosphoethanolamine, and wBPE than in the original conditioned medium, which requires a higher cell density for satisfactory cellular multiplication. In addition, our serum-free medium with wBPE supports serial subculture through far more population doublings than were previously possible. In experiments still in progress in Dr. Stampfer's laboratory, cultures in the BPE supplemented medium are still multiplying actively after 15 subculturings with 1:10 splits, whereas those in the original conditioned medium ceased to multiply after about four such passages. Detailed cellular characterization studies are still in progress. However, chromosome number remains diploid and cellular morphology does not change detectably in the long-term serial subcultures.

Very recently, we have successfully replaced wBPE, which was the only undefined component of the medium for human mammary epithelial cells, with a mixture of prolactin and prostaglandin E_1. Although our results are still preliminary and must be verified by further testing, we can now obtain rapid clonal growth of normal human mammary epithelial cells in the defined medium described in Table 2. The basal nutrient medium, MCDB 170, that we are currently using consists of MCDB 202 (McKeehan and Ham, 1977) with cysteine reduced to 7×10^{-5} M and zinc increased to 5×10^{-7} M. These changes, which were both found to be beneficial for growth of mammary epithelial cells with small amounts of wBPE, represent our first steps toward optimization of the nutrient mixture specifically for growth of normal human mammary epithelial cells.

Most of the clonal growth experiments leading to development of the defined medium for human mammary cells were done with second or third passage cultures. However, our first primary culture experiment in the defined medium, which was completed just before this conference, also yielded excellent growth. Organoids prepared by Dr. Stampfer and shipped to us frozen were thawed, washed free of the freezing medium, and placed into culture flasks containing the defined medium. They quickly attached and formed rapidly spreading dense outgrowths that contained large numbers of mitotic cells. During the first 10 days in culture, many of these outgrowths grew to diameters of 5 mm or more.

As was the case for normal human keratinocytes, normal human mammary epithelial cells have also proven to be far easier to grow in culture and to have far simpler growth requirements than would have been anticipated from the difficulties that have characterized past attempts to culture them.

Prostatic epithelial cells

Chaproniere-Rickenberg and Webber (1982) have been able to obtain substantial multiplication of primary cultures of human prostatic epithelial cells in RPMI 1640 supplemented with 1×10^{-8} M zinc chloride, 0.3 I.U./ml (12.5 μg/ml) zinc free insulin, 1×10^{-8} M dexamethasone, 10 ng/ml EGF, and 1.0 μg/ml transferrin. Optimization of the basal nutrient medium has not yet been undertaken for human prostatic epithelial cells.

FUTURE PROSPECTS

There obviously remain many more types of normal human cells that cannot yet be grown in defined media, including a substantial number that do not grow well in any currently available culture system. On the basis of the results presented above, it appears that growth of most of these cell types in defined media could be accomplished rather quickly if enough investigators were willing to undertake systematic studies of their growth requirements, and if the appropriate granting agencies were willing to finance such studies adequately.

Most of the normal human cell types for which defined media have now been developed were until quite recently considered very difficult to grow in culture, even with undefined supplements. However, a comparison of the defined media that have been developed for these cells (Table 3) suggests that their requirements are all relatively simple. It therefore seems reasonable to predict that the growth requirements of those cell types that are still difficult to grow in culture will also be found to be less complex than previously thought when they are studied systematically.

Another feature that is clearly evident in Table 3 is the individuality of the growth requirements of the six cell types that are included there. Four distinctly different basal media are used (MCDB 104/110, MCDB 152/153, MCDB 170, and RPMI 1640), and each of the six defined media contains a different combination of defined supplements. Some of the components that are currently included in some of the media are probably not essential, and it is likely that most of the cells still need additional components for maximal long-term multiplication. Nevertheless, a number of well-defined differences in growth requirements can already be identified: 1) Chondrocytes and fibroblasts require a lipid supplement, whereas the epithelial cells appear not to; 2) Chondrocytes require FGF, whereas the other five cell types all require EGF; 3) Ethanolamine and/or phosphoethanolamine are clearly needed by keratinocytes and bronchial epithelial cells, but appear to have no effect on fibroblasts or chondrocytes; 4) Prostaglandin E_1 is highly beneficial to mammary epithelial cells, moderately beneficial to human fibroblasts, and probably not needed by the other cell types; 5) Prolactin is highly beneficial to the mammary cells, but not the others.

Individuality of growth requirements will undoubtedly prove to be one of the major keys to understanding the growth requirements of additional types of normal

TABLE 3. DEFINED MEDIA FOR SIX NORMAL HUMAN CELL TYPES

Cell Type	Fibroblast[a]	Chondrocyte	Keratinocyte	Bronchial	Mammary	Prostate
Basal Medium	MCDB 110	MCDB 104	MCDB 153	MCDB 152[b]	MCDB 170	RPMI 1640[c]
Insulin	+	+	+	+	+	+
Glucocorticoid[d]	+	+	+	+	+	+
EGF	+	-	+	+	+	+
FGF	-	+	-	-	-	-
Liposome B	+	+	-	-	-	-
Transferrin	-	-	-	+	+	+
Ethanolamine	-	-	+	+	+	-
Phosphoethano-lamine	-	-	+	+	+	-
Prostaglandin E_1	+	-	-	-	+	-
Prolactin	-	-	-	-	+	-

[a] The fibroblast defined medium also contains prostaglandin $F_{2\alpha}$, reduced glutathione, dithiothreitol, and phosphoenolpyruvate, none of which are present in the other five media.

[b] Calcium and sulfate levels are altered. Cf. Table 2.

[c] Zinc is added to original formula.

[d] Dexamethasone or hydrocortisone.

human cells. For example, we are currently attempting to define the growth requirements of human capillary endothelial cells. The best starting medium for optimization studies with these cells was found to be MCDB 402 (Shipley and Ham, 1981), which has unusually high concentrations of many components. Preliminary optimization studies suggest that human capillary endothelial cells will ultimately prove to have growth requirements that are significantly different from those of any of the cell types we have previously worked with.

Procedures for systematic analysis of growth requirements of cell types that have not previously been studied are outlined briefly at the beginning of this presentation, and in detail on pages 28 to 33 of Ham (1981). Cumulative experience in this and other laboratories has consistently shown that these procedures work well. In each case, the cells in question "know" exactly what they need for multiplication. Our task is to ask them the right experimental questions in a systematic manner, and to listen patiently for their answers without attempting to impose our own biases on them (Ham, 1982). As long as this is done, it is possible, at least in theory, to define the growth requirements of any cell type that can be made to multiply sufficiently in culture to perform growth-response assays.

ACKNOWLEDGMENTS

The research described in this report was supported by Grants CA-15305, CA-30028, and GM-26455 from the National Institutes of Health. I am grateful to the many past and present members of my research group who have contributed to the results presented here and to Karen Brown for preparation of the manuscript.

REFERENCES

Agy, P. C., G. D. Shipley and R. G. Ham. 1981. Protein-free medium for C-1300 mouse neuroblastoma cells. In Vitro 17:671-680.

Barnes, D. and G. Sato. 1980. Methods for growth of cultured cells in serum-free medium. Anal. Biochem. 102:255-270.

Bettger, W. J., S. T. Boyce, B. J. Walthall and R. G. Ham. 1981. Rapid clonal growth and serial passage of human diploid fibroblasts in a lipid-enriched synthetic medium supplemented with EGF, insulin, and dexamethasone. Proc. Natl. Acad. Sci. U.S.A. 78:5588-5592.

Boyce, S. T. and R. G. Ham. 1982. Quantitative and qualitative characterization of control of differentiation of normal human epidermal keratinocytes in chemically defined clonal culture and serum-free subculture. 32nd. Symposium on the Biology of Skin, in press.

Chaproniere-Rickenberg, D. M. and M. M. Webber. 1982. A chemically defined medium for the growth of adult human prostatic epithelium. Cold Spring Harbor Conferences on Cell Proliferation 9:1109-1115.

Gospodarowicz, D. and A. L. Mescher. 1977. A comparison of the responses of cultured myoblasts and chondrocytes to fibroblast and epidermal growth factors. J. Cell. Physiol. 93:117-127.

Graves, D. C. and R. G. Ham. 1982. Serum-free clonal growth of chicken embryo fibroblasts. In Vitro 18:305 (Abstract No. 127).

Ham, R. G. 1965. Clonal growth of mammalian cells in a chemically defined, synthetic medium. Proc. Natl. Acad. Sci. U.S.A. 53:288-293.

Ham, R. G. 1972. Cloning of mammalian cells. Methods Cell Physiol. 5:37-74.

Ham, R. G. 1974. Nutritional requirements of primary cultures. A neglected problem in modern biology. In Vitro 10:119-129.

Ham, R. G. 1981. Survival and growth requirements of nontransformed cells. Hdbk. Exp. Pharmacol. 57:13-88.

Ham, R. G. 1982. Importance of the basal nutrient medium in the design of hormonally defined media. Cold Spring Harbor Conferences on Cell Proliferation 9:39-60.

Ham, R. G. and W. L. McKeehan. 1978a. Development of improved media and culture conditions for clonal growth of normal diploid cells. In Vitro 14:11-22.

Ham, R. G. and W. L. McKeehan. 1978b. Nutritional requirements for clonal growth of nontransformed cells. In: Nutritional Requirements of Cultured Cells. (H. Katsuta, ed.). Japan Scientific Societies Press, Tokyo, pp. 63-115.

Ham, R. G. and G. L. Sattler. 1968. Clonal growth of differentiated rabbit cartilage cells. J. Cell. Physiol. 72:109-114.

Ham, R. G., S. L. Hammond, and L. L. Miller. 1977. Critical adjustment of cysteine and glutamine concentrations for improved clonal growth of WI-38 cells. In Vitro 13:1-10.

Ham, R. G., L. W. Murray, and G. L. Sattler. 1970. Beneficial effects of embryo extract on cultured rabbit cartilage cells. J. Cell. Physiol. 75:353-360.

Hamilton, W. G. and R. G. Ham. 1977. Clonal growth of Chinese hamster cell lines in protein-free media. In Vitro 13:537-547.

Hayashi, I. and G. H. Sato. 1976. Replacement of serum by hormones permits growth of cells in a defined medium. Nature 259:132-134.

Hayflick, L. and P. S. Moorhead. 1961. The serial cultivation of human diploid cell strains. Exp. Cell Res. 25:585-621.

Jennings, S. D. 1982. Clonal growth of human hyaline cartilage in a defined medium. In Vitro 18:305-306 (Abstract No. 129).

Jennings, S. D. and R. G. Ham. 1981. Clonal growth of primary cultures of rabbit chondrocytes in a defined medium. In Vitro 17:238 (Abstract No. 155).

Kano-Sueoka, T. and J. Errick. 1981. Effects of phophoethanolamine and ethanolamine on growth of mammary carcinoma cells in culture. Exp. Cell Res. 136:137-145.

Kano-Sueoka, T., D. M. Cohen, Z. Yamaizumi, S. Nishimura, M. Mori, H. Fujiki. 1979. Phosphoethanolamine as a growth factor of a mammary carcinoma cell line of rat. Proc. Natl. Acad. Sci. U.S.A. 76:5741-5744.

Lechner, J. F., A. Haugen, I. A. McClendon, and E. W. Pettis. 1982. Clonal growth of normal adult human bronchial epithelial cells in a serum-free medium. In Vitro 18:633-642.

McKeehan, W. L. and R. G. Ham. 1977. Methods for reducing the serum requirement for growth in vitro of nontransformed diploid fibroblasts. Develop. Biol. Standard. 37:97-108.

McKeehan, W. L., W. G. Hamilton, and R. G. Ham. 1976. Selenium is an essential trace nutrient for growth of WI-38 diploid human fibroblasts. Proc. Natl. Acad. Sci. U.S.A. 73:2023-2027.

McKeehan, W. L., K. A. McKeehan, S. L. Hammond, and R. G. Ham. 1977. Improved medium for clonal growth of human diploid fibroblasts at low concentrations of serum protein. In Vitro 13:399-416.

Peehl, D. M. and R. G. Ham. 1980a. Growth and differentiation of human keratinocytes without a feeder layer or conditioned medium. In Vitro 16:516-525.

Peehl, D. M. and R. G. Ham. 1980b. Clonal growth of human keratinocytes with small amounts of dialyzed serum. In Vitro 16:526-540.

Rheinwald, J. G. and H. Green. 1975. Serial cultivation of strains of human epidermal keratinocytes: The formation of keratinizing colonies from single cells. Cell 6:331-344.

Sato, G. H. 1975. The role of serum in cell culture. In: Biochemical Actions of Hormones. Litwack, G. (ed.) New York, Academic Press, Vol. III. pp. 391-396.

Shipley, G. D. and R. G. Ham. 1981. Improved medium and culture conditions for clonal growth with minimal serum protein and for enhanced serum-free survival of Swiss 3T3 cells. In Vitro 17:656-670.

Stampfer, M., R. C. Hallowes, and A. J. Hackett. 1980. Growth of normal human mammary cells in culture. In Vitro 16:415-425.

Tsao, M. C., B. J. Walthall, and R. G. Ham. 1982. Clonal growth of normal human epidermal keratinocytes in a defined medium. J. Cell. Physiol. 110:219-229.

Walthall, B. J. and R. G. Ham. 1981. Multiplication of human diploid fibroblasts in a synthetic medium supplemented with EGF, insulin, and dexamethasone. Exp. Cell Res. 134:303-311.

Investigations on the Cultivation of Insect Cell Lines in Serum-Free Media

H. G. Miltenburger

Zoologisches Institut der Technischen Universität, D-6100 Darmstadt, FRG

During the last two decades the sophisticated techniques of cultivating mammalian cells in vitro have been increasingly applied to the culturing of invertebrate cells. Up to now more than 130 cell lines from 56 different species of invertebrates (mostly insects) have been established. In 1962 Grace demonstrated that insect cells can be continuously subcultured as cell lines (6). During the years to follow cell lines, particularly from pest insects belonging to the group lepidoptera (butterflies) were established. At present about 50 lepidopteran cell lines are available. Several cell lines have been derived from other insect groups like diptera, coleoptera and hymenoptera. Particular attention has been paid to lepidopteran cells in culture since in vitro replication of lepidopteran pathogenic viruses has been shown to follow a mechanism similar to that for replication in vivo. These viruses are members of the baculovirus group and are natural pathogens of many lepidopteran pest species. The larvae are killed by the virus infection within a few days. On account of species specificity or very limited host range some of these viruses are used as biological insecticides in integrated pest control. The virus material for such pesticides is produced in green houses in mass populations of the natural hosts. During the past few years there have been several review articles published dealing with baculoviruses as biological pesticides (11, 12, 16, 17). The fact that baculoviruses, and in particular the nuclear polyhedrosis viruses (NPV) replicate well in several lepidopteran cell lines initiated investigations on the possibilities of commercially producing baculoviruses in vitro. This requires the production of large quantities of cells for substrate. Several laboratories have therefore made efforts to develop defined, cheap and qualitatively good nutrient media for insect cell culturing. The composition of insect cell culture media was originally mainly based on insect haemolymph analysis. The majority of them guaranteed the maintenance of primary

cultures for only a few days or weeks. As the cell cultures require
supplementing with a natural protein haemolymph was added. An important step towards the long term maintenance of insect cell cultures
has ben the successful replacement of haemolymph by mammalian serum
(19). In addition it has been shown that biological complexes like
whole egg ultrafiltrate and bovine plasma albumin can replace haemolymph. As in mammalian cell cultures the serum introduces into the
media a variety of unknown and undefined compounds which help in
supporting cell proliferation. Hormones are one example. It has also
been found that proteins are necessary for efficient attachment of
cells to the surface of the culture vessel for monolayer formation.
The development in the late sixties of semi-synthetic nutrient media
suitable for insect cells and containing bovine serum, or foetal
bovine serum (FBS) instead of haemolymph has been the reason for the
establishment of most insect cell lines during the past 15 years.
Today there are more than 40 known media for insect cell culturing.
The general composition is demonstrated by Grace's medium which is
still widely used in insect tissue culture. As mentioned above one
major reason for tissue culture studies with cells from pest butterflies was to learn more about the interaction of insect pathogenic
baculoviruses with cells in vitro. It was hoped that methods would
be developed for the mass production of such viruses in cell cultures. Since our laboratory has contributed to this project over the
past years I shall report on an example of insect cell culturing
with possible practical application for lepidopteran cell culture
and baculovirus replication in media with and without sera.
For our in vitro studies we decided to start with a model system for
the evaluation of the mechanisms of cell-virus interaction. One
important pest butterfly in agriculture is the cabbage moth, Mamestra
brassicae (Mb). The larvae of this species can cause great damage and
economic loss in cabbage cultures. Baculovirus-infected larvae die
within one or two weeks following the uptake of a nuclear polyhedrosis virus with the food. Death is due to the mass replication of the
virus in nearly all organs and cells of the body. The virus which
replicates in Mb hardly replicates at all in other species. However, there is another nuclear polyhedrosis virus which has also been
shown to replicate well in cabbage moth larvae. This is a NPV isolated from the butterfly species Autographa californica (Ac), the
alfalfa looper. As Ac-NPV has been shown to be more virulent in cell
cultures than Mb-NPV we began to study cell-virus interaction with

Ac-NPV. Also since Ac-NPV were used in in vitro experiments in other laboratories we are able to make comparisons.

There were no cell lines from the cabbage moth. Therefore we firstly had to establish cell lines. We were able to derive five permanent cell lines from about 2000 tissue explants of four/five instar larvae. In the beginning we used a slightly modified Grace-medium supplemented with 10 % FBS. After several months of careful treatment the cell lines could be established. The predominantly spindle-like cells firmly adhere to the vessel surface. One of these cell lines, IZD-Mb 0503, (IZD = Institute of Zoology Darmstadt) also proliferates well as a suspension culture (13). Morphology, mass-culture-, and colony-growth curves are used as parameters in the regular checking of the cell-line characteristics. Karyotype analysis is impossible in somatic lepidopteran tissues and cell lines, because the cells are pseudo-polyploid or mixoploid with chromosome numbers of up to several hundred per cell. Quantitative analyses of chromosome preparations from our cell lines showed that the chromosomes are, with few exceptions, very small or dot-like obviously having either no or only diffuse centromeres. The different cabbage moth cell lines also can be characterized by determination of the mean DNA content of cell cycle subpopulations using cytofluorometry techniques. In addition isozyme analysis can be used to characterize our cell lines (7, 12). For nearly all experiments we used cell line IZD-Mb 0503 which showed very stable characteristics over the years. In pilot experiments with monolayer cultures we also found that this cell line is particularly suitable for Ac-NPV replication studies in vitro. When treated with infectious haemolymph from Ac-virosis carrying larvae many cells showed severe cytopathic effects after only 12 hours with nuclear granulation, hypertrophy and rounding up. Two or three days after the infection up to 100 cubic proteinaceous polyhedra of 1-3 µm diameter had developed in the nuclei of the cells. Centrifuged cell- and polyhedra-free supernatants from these cultures were infectious when introduced into monolayer Mb-cultures due to a high titer of infectious free virions not occluded by a polyhedron. Normally, the baculo-like virions are within the polyhedra.

Virus replication is dependent on good if not optimal cellular physiology and metabolism. Therefore the nutrient medium is a highly important factor in this system. Alternatively in the case presented here NPV replication can be taken - at least partially - as a quantitative and qualitative expression of cell and medium quality. This can be measured using methods applied routinely in virology. It is obvious that this system offers advantages with respect to medium development particularly because the viruses are not pathogenic in mammals and man (9, 11). In recent electron microscope studies reported by Adams et al. (1) and by our laboratory (3) it was demonstrated that under appropriate medium conditions baculovirus entry into cells in vitro is performed as it occurs in vivo by attachment of enveloped nucleocapsids to the cell membranes and engulfment.

For in vitro mass production of viruses it is necessary to have suspension cultures of larger volumes. Therefore we isolated subclones of our cabbage moth cell line IZD-Mb 0503 which had lost anchorage dependency and which proliferated when floating free in suspension. During this work a major problem was the supply of oxygen to suspension cultures of volume greater than three litres. This difficulty was overcome by an oxygen diffusion technique. This means that the mass production of cabbage moth cells is now possible in

	mg/l		mg/l
L-Arginine HCl	350	Thiamine HCl	0.01
L-Aspartic acid	175	Riboflavin	0.01
L-Asparagine	175	Ca-Pantothenate	0.01
L-Alanine	110	Pyridoxine HCl	0.01
ß-Alanine	100	p-Aminobenzoic acid	0.01
L-Cystine	10	Folic acid	0.01
L-Glutamic acid	300	i-Inositol	0.01
L-Glutamine	300	Biotin	0.01
Glycine	325	Choline Cl	0.10
L-Histidine HCl	1250	Niacin amide	0.01
L-Isoleucine	25		
L-Leucine	40	NaCl	3250
L-Lysine HCl	310	$NaH_2PO_4 \cdot H_2O$	570
L-Methionine	25	KCl	1370
L-Proline	175	$CaCl_2 \cdot 2H_2O$	550
L-Phenylalanine	75	$MgCl_2 \cdot 6H_2O$	1140
DL-Serine	550	$MgSO_4 \cdot 7H_2O$	1390
L-Tyrosine	25	$NaHCO_3$	225
L-Tryptophan	50	KH_2PO_4	50
L-Threonine	90		
L-Valine	50	Lactalbumin hydrolysate	3250
		Yeast extract	2500
Sucrose	1300		
Fructose	200	Fetal calf serum	5 %
Glucose	2350		
		pH	6.4
Neomycinsulfate	500		

Fig. 1. IZD-LP01 medium for culturing Mamestra brassicae cell line IZD-Mb 0503

continuously running laboratory fermenters at volumes of 10 litres
and more (4, 10). For both the monolayer and suspension cultures we
regularly use the nutrient medium IZD-LP01 (Fig. 1).

This medium was developed in our laboratory on the basis of two
media described earlier by Grace (6) and Varma and Pudney (19).
In most insect tissue culture media used by other laboratories 10 %
or more of FBS have to be added whilst our medium requires only 5%
FCS. However, the use of vertebrate serum may be undesirable for
several reasons: it may be toxic for insect cells; it might be the
source of mycoplasm contamination; it contains or may contain uniden-
tifiable components making experiments for evaluating cell nutrition
requirements in serum supplemented media quite difficult. Therefore,
as in vertebrate cell culturing, there is a need for the development
of serum-free media for insect cell cultures. Only a relatively small
number of laboratories are working with insect cell in vitro, in
particular lepidopteran cells, and thus at present there are only a
limited number of reports on the cultivation of insect cells in
serum-free media or in chemically defined media.
Hink (8) and Goodwin and Adams (5) demonstrated cell proliferation of
insect cell lines in serum-free media. Goodwin and Adams reported on
several serum-free insect cell culture media for cell lines from the
gypsy moth, Lymantria dispar. They analysed the capacity of these
media, which were supplemented with peptones, liver digest, yeasto-
late and lactalbumin hydrolysate, to promote proliferation. Since
these media were supplemented with chemically poorly defined components they have to be regarded as semi-defined. On the basis of such
a composition Goodwin and Adams then tried to improve the quality of
serum-free media by supplementing with lipid complexes, glycerol,
folic acid, glutamin, and other compounds. Besides cell population
growth curves they used nuclear polyhedrosis virus replication as
one of the parameters for the evaluation of the effect of the supplements. They found that most of the compounds added did not support
NPV-replication. These results indicate that the nutritional requirements of the virus-infected cells were not fulfilled. Supplementing
the media with lipid complexes containing per litre 5 mg methyl
oleate, 1.5 mg cholesterol, and 25 mg Tween 80 allowed better replication of gypsy moth NPV. However, although the formation of
enveloped nucleocapsids and polyhedra occured in this case the elec-
tron-microscope analysis revealed that many of the polyhedra were
empty i.e. the virions were not occluded. Goodwin and Adams also
studied the effects of styrols. Since many insects require styrol

nutritionally one would expect a compound like cholesterol to be essential for cell culture growth. Cholesterol or related styrols play a vital role in the synthesis of cell membranes in general. In insects cholesterol is also essential for the synthesis of the growth and development hormone ecdysone. Therefore, some insect media include cholesterol at concentrations of 0.2 µg/ml (dissolved in Tween 80 and 95 % ethanol).

A cell proliferation stimulating modification in Goodwin's media was achieved by altering the lipid supplement to 1.75 mg/lα-tocopherol-acetate and increasing the amount of cholesterol to 4.5 mg/l. It is interesting that the addition of up to 35 units per l of insulin did not improve proliferation of several insect cell lines. Glutamine is essential for insect cells in vitro. When a concentration of 2 g/l was present in the medium polyhedra formation occured although many of the polyhedral bodies did not occlude virions. The addition of 24 mg/l of folic acid together with 2g/l glutamine caused virus challenged insect cell monolayers to remain attached to the growth surface even after polyhedra formation. Normally insect cells detach on day 3/4 post infection when virions and/or polyhedra are formed in the nuclei. In addition the nuclei of the cells were heavily packed with polyhedra as compared to cells from cultures grown in serum-free medium without folic acid and 2g/l glutamine. The addition of 5 g/lα-glycerophosphate (α-GP) also had a marked effect on the formation of polyhedra. Polyhedra were consistently formed 2-3 days sooner than in cells grown only in medium lacking α-GP. The addition of glycerol supported cell proliferation very positively. Consequently supplementing the medium with α-GP and glycerol resulted in relatively stable cell proliferation kinetics and NPV-replication. When the serum-free medium was supplemented with 3.6 mg/l folic acid, 2 g/l fresh glutamine, 1 g/lα-GP, glycerol, and B-vitamins, the gypsy moth cell line had a shortened population doubling time thus producing more cells per unit time.

Studies on amino acid requirements of insect cells in vitro have been reported by Mitsuhashi (14). However, the results are difficult to evaluate as media supplemented with vertebrate serum were used in most experiments. This raises the possibility that free amino acids present in the serum interfere with amino acid measurements as do free amino acids formed by the degradation of serum protein. These difficulties could be avoided if the analyses on essential amino acid requirements in insect tissue culture were performed in serum-free medium. In Mitsuhashi's experiments although the serum content was reduced it still amounted to 5 %. Nevertheless, some results are informative. They indicate that both α-L-alanine and ß-alanine are unnecessary or even detrimental for lepidopteran cell lines. When glutamine is omitted in the medium this results in prolonged cell survival without proliferation. The omission of certain amino acids resulted in reduced cell proliferation although this effect varied according to the particular cell line. Whilst 14 amino acids (arginine, glutamine, histidine, isoleucine, leucine, lysine, methionine, phenylalanine, proline, serine, threonine, tryptophan, tyrosine and valine) were necessary for continuous culturing of many cell lines alanine, asparagine, aspartic acid and glutamic acid could be deleted from the cell culture media without negative effects on cell proliferation.

To obtain media devoid of free amino acids sera lacking free amino acids can be prepared by dialysis or ultrafiltration. However, even then it is impossible to entirely exclude the effects of amino acids because free amino acids may be released from the treated serum, probably due to detoriation of serum protein. It is therefore important to try to use protein free culture media for the determination of non-essential amino acids.

At present there is only one protein free culture medium available which can support growth of insect cell cultures. It has been reported by Wilkie et al. (20) and so far is the only completely chemically defined medium for insect cells. In this medium several insect cell lines from different species could be subcultured for many passages. It was also possible to demonstrate complete NPV-replication indicating that the polyhedra contained virions. Unfortunately, this medium did not support the proliferation of our cabbage moth cell line IZD-Mb 0503 very well, demonstrating the specificity of serum-free media with regard to different cell lines. We therefore modified the composition on the basis of data from the literature and from our own experience. Thus a medium was obtained which sufficiently supported the proliferation of our cell line in monolayer (fig. 2). However, this medium had to be supplemented with serveral bioproducts meaning that it is not chemically defined. The cells

	mg/l		mg/l
L-Arginine·HCl	450	Thiamine HCl	2
L-Aspartic acid	175	Riboflavin	0.05
L-Asparagine	300	Ca-Pantothenate	1
L-Alanine	200	Pyridoxine HCl	1
ß-Alanine	100	p-Aminobenzoic acid	2
L-Cystine	50	Folic acid	1
L-Glutamic acid	300	i-Inositol	2
L-Glutamine	500	Biotin	0.05
Glycine	500	Choline Cl	20
L-Histidine·HCl·H$_2$0	3000	Niacin amide	1.2
L-Isoleucine	50		
L-Leucine	50	NaCl	3250
L-Lysine HCl	500	NaH$_2$PO$_4$·H$_2$0	570
L-Methionine	50	KCl	1370
L-Proline	300	CaCl$_2$·2H$_2$0	550
L-Phenylalanine	150	MgCl$_2$·6H$_2$0	1140
DL-Serine	550	MgSO$_4$·7H$_2$0	1390
L-Tyrosine	50	NaHCO$_3$	225
L-Tryptophan	100	KH$_2$PO$_4$	50
L-Threonine	150		
L-Valine	100	Lactalbumin hydrolysate	3250
		Yeast extract	2500
α-D-Glucose	4000		
		Fe SO$_4$ (NH$_4$)$_2$SO$_4$·6H$_2$0	5
Spermidine	1	ZnSO$_4$·7H$_2$0	0.5
Spermine HCl	1	CuSO$_4$·5H$_2$0	0.4
Putrescine	1	MnCl$_2$·4H$_2$0	0.4
α-Amino-n-butyric acid	1		
o-Phosphoryl ethanolamine	2	Tween 80	20
Taurine	1		
Ascorbic acid	0.2	pH	6.3
Hypoxanthine	10		
Methylcellulose (15 cps)	2		
α-Tocopherol acetate	0.01		
Cholesterol	1		
ß-Sitosterol	1		
Stigmasterol	1		

Fig. 2. Serum-free IZD-LP02 medium for culturing <u>Mamestra</u> <u>brassicae</u> Cell line IZD-Mb 0503

needed several passages for adaptation to the serum-free medium conditions. After 8 weeks they proliferated well and the morphology was unaltered although the population doubling time was longer than that in medium containing serum. Subculturing could be done at 4 day intervals with dilutions of 1:5. A minimum of 100,000 cells per 5 ml in a plastic T-50-flask is necessary to seed for successful proliferation. Anchorage dependency is not markedly changed and the cells adhere quite firmly to the vessel surface. Whereas the cabbage moth cell line formed monolayers, a <u>Spodoptera</u> <u>frugiperda</u> (fall army worm) cell line proliferated more or less as a suspension culture in this medium: the cells attached only to a small extent to the vessel surface. The proliferation of the cell line in three experiments is shown in fig. 3.

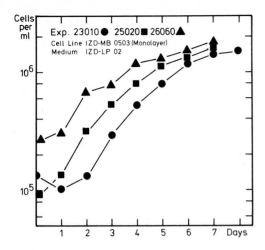

Fig. 3. Growth curves of IZD-Mb 0503 cells in serum-free medium
IZD-LP02. Three independent experiments.

To assess the quality of the medium with regard to metabolic activities infection of cells was performed in monolayer cultures on day 3
or 4 of cultivation with Ac-NPV. The infectious dose was 6.4×10^7-
1.5×10^8 $TCID_{50}$ (Tissue Culture Infective Dose 50 %) per ml in 5 ml
total volume. There were 5×10^5 cells per ml. As is the case with
cells cultured in medium with serum polyhedra had formed in many
cells two days after the infection (figs. 4, 5). 3-4 days after the
infection of the cultures polyhedra with occluded virions could be
found in 36-50 % of the cell nuclei. The mean number of polyhedra
per nucleus was 6.3 and 13.4 in two independent experiments. For
comparison with NPV replication in IZD-LP01 medium see fig. 6. The
infectious supernatants i.g. medium containing newly replicated free
virions (= nonoccluded virions) had 8.2×10^8 $TCID_{50}$/ml in experiment 3 and $7.3 \times 10.^6$ $TCID_{50}$/ml in experiment 4. In the meantime the
IZD-Mb 0503 subclone has been fully adapted to the serum-free
medium. It has been subcultured more than 300 times by now. The
cultivation of the IZD-Mb 0503 cells in serum-free medium in suspension cultures can only be performed in 100 ml spinner vessels, so
far. However during the past two years we have subcultured the
subclone in suspension more than 200 times. The population doubling

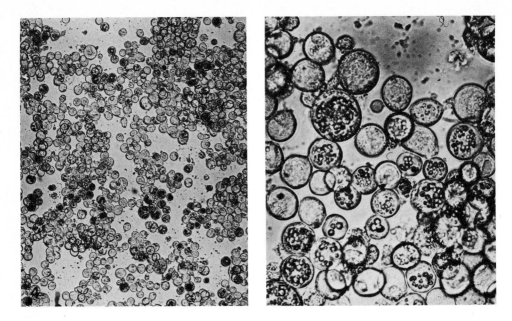

Fig. 4. Monolayer culture of IZD-Mb 0503 cells in serum-free medium
        IZD-LP02 4 days after infection with Ac-NPV. The cytopathic
        effect is seen as rounding up of the cells. In many cells
        polyhedral inclusion bodies have been formed in the nucleus
        (dark particles). Microscopic magnification about 120 times
Fig. 5. Section of fig. 4. The polyhedra are seen in the nuclei.

Replication of Ac-NPV in cell line IZD-Mb 0503

medium IZD-LP 01: with 5% fetal calf serum

medium IZD-LP 02: without serum

Exp.no.	medium	mean number of polyhedra per cell	% cells with polyhedra	culture
1	IZD-LP01	33,0	85	monolayer
2	"	9,5	71	suspension (BIOSTAT)
3	IZD-LP02	6,3	50	monolayer
4	"	13,4	36	monolayer

Fig. 6. Production of Ac-NPV-polyhedra in medium IZD-LP01 and IZD-
        LP02. Experiment 3 was performed in a fermenter BIOSTAT S
        (B. Braun AG, 3508 Melsungen, FRG) at a volume of 10 litres.

time in the serum-free suspension culture is about 44 h. This is considerably longer than in monolayer cultures with serum-free medium (16-20 h) and in serum-supplemented medium (14-16 h). Infection of the IZD-Mb 0503 cells in suspension with Ac-NPV in serum-free medium did not result in polyhedra formation. Also, the determination of the virus titer in the culture supernatant did not indicate the formation of infectious free virions. This means that so far the conditions of the spinner cultures with serum-free medium are not optimal for virus replication.

An interesting formulation of a serum-free insect cell medium was reported recently by Röder (15). He supplemented a basic compound complex of salts, amino acids and vitamins with chicken egg yolk at a concentration of 0.5 % and obtained good cell growth of lepidopteran cells and an unchanged rate of NPV replication. His cell lines have been subcultured more than 200 times so far.

In conclusion

1. Insect cell lines of many species can be propagated in media containing salts, amino acids, vitamins, trace elements and various organic compounds or compound complexes.
2. Generally natural proteins are required by insect cells in vitro for successful and continuous culturing. Bovine serum (fetal, newborn or adult) can be used instead of homologous or heterologous hemolymph.
3. For insect cell culturing only a few serum-free media have been reported which adequately support cell proliferation in monolayer or suspension cultures. So far there is only one chemically-defined medium available for certain lepidopteran cell lines.
4. Mass production of cells from lepidopteran cell lines and mass production of NPV for the in vitro production of viral pesticides may be possible according to the experience and techniques developed during the past years. Most media used for these procedures still have to be supplemented with vertebrate serum. However, it can be expected that these media will be replaced by semi-defined or defined serum-free media in the future.

References

1. Adams J R, Goodwin R H, Wilcox T A (1977) Electron microscope investigations on invasion and replication of insect baculo-viruses in vivo and in vitro, Biol. Cellulaire 28: 261-268
2. Barnes D, Sato G (1980) Methods for growth of cultured cells in serum-free medium, Anal. Biochem. 102: 255-270
3. Bassemir U, Miltenburger H G, David P (1982) Morphogenesis of Autographa californica nuclear polyhedrosis virus in a Mamestra brassicae (cabbage moth) cell line: further aspects on baculo-virus assembly, Cell and Tissue Res. in press
4. Eberhard U (1981) Untersuchungen zur Charakterisierung und Opti-mierung der Produktion von Insektenzellen im Rührkessel Bioreak-tor, Diplomarbeit, Technische Hochschule Darmstadt, Darmstadt, FRG, 59 pp
5. Goodwin R H, Adams J R (1980) Nutrient factors influencing viral replication in serum-free insect cell line culture. In: Kurstak E, 6. Maramorosch K, Dübendorfer A (eds) Invertebrate Systems in vitro, pp 493-509 Elsevier/North-Holland Biomedical Press, Amsterdam Oxford New York
7. Grace T D C (1962) Establishment of four strains of cells from insect tissues grown in vitro, Nature 195: 788-789.
8. Hilwig I, Eipel H E (1980) Flow-cytometric characterization of insect cell lines under the influence of virus infection. In: Miltenburger H G (ed) Safety Aspects of Baculoviruses as Biologi-cal Insecticides, pp 145-158, Bundesministerium für Forschung und Technologie, Bonn, FRG
9. Hink W F (1976) A compilation of invertebrate cell lines and culture media. In: Maramorosch K (ed) Invertebrate Tissue Cul-ture, pp 358-369 Academic Press, New York San Francisco London
10. Miltenburger H G, ed. (1980) Safety Aspects of Baculoviruses as Biological Insecticides, Symposium Proceedings, Bundesministerium für Forschung und Technologie, Bonn, FRG, 301 pp
11. Miltenburger H G, David P (1980) Mass production of insect cells in suspension. In: Griffiths B, Hennessen W, Horodniceanu F, Spier R (eds) Proceedings of the Third General Meeting of the European Society of Animal Cell Technology, pp 183-186, S. Kar-ger, Basel
12. Miltenburger H G (1980) Viral pesticides: hazard evaluation for non-target organisms and safety testing. In: Lundholm B, Stakerud M (eds) Environmental Protection and Biological Forms of Control of Pest Organisms, pp 57-74 Ecol. Bull (Stockholm) 31
13. Miltenburger H G, Wulf H (1978) Zytogenetische und biochemische Untersuchungen zur Charakterisierung von Insekten-Zellinien, Mitt. dtsch. Ges. allg. angew. Ent. 1: 102-106
14. Miltenburger H G, David P, Mahr U, Zipp W (1977) Establishment of lepidopteran cell lines and in vitro replication of insect patho-genic viruses, Z. ang. Ent. 82: 306-323
15. Mitsuhashi J (1980) Requirements of amino acids by insect cell lines. In: Kurstak E, Maramorosch K, Dübendorfer A (eds) Inverte-brate Systems in vitro, pp 47-58 Elsevier/North-Holland Biomedi-cal Press, Amsterdam Oxford New York
16. Röder A (1982) Development of a serum-free medium for cultivation of insect cells, Naturwissensch. 69: 92-93
17. Summers M, Engler R, Falcon L A, Vail P V, eds. (1975) Baculo-viruses for Insect Pest Control: Safety Considerations, American Society for Microbiology US Environmental Protection Agency Washington D.C. 186pp

18. Summers M, Kawanishi C Y, eds. (1978) Viral Pesticides: Present Knowledge and Potential Effects on Public and Environmental Health, Symposium Proceedings, Health Effects Research Laboratory, Office of Health and Ecological Effects US Environmental Protection Agency, Research Triangle Park, North Carolina 312 pp
19. Vago C, Chastang S (1958) Obtention de lignées cellulaires en culture de tissus d'invertébrés, Experientia 14: 110-111
20. Varma M G R, Pudney M (1969) The growth and serial passage of cell lines from Aedes aegypti (L.) larvae in different media, J. Med. Ent. 6: 432-439
21. Wilkie G E I, Stockdale H (1980) Chemically-defined media for production of insect cells and viruses in vitro. In: Griffith B, Hennessen W, Horodniceanu F, Spier R (eds) Proceedings of the Third General Meeting of the European Society of Animal Cell Technology, pp 29-37, S. Karger, Basel

This work was supported by the Federal Ministry for Research and Technology (Bundesministerium für Forschung und Technologie), Bonn, FRG.

Cell Proliferation and Growth Factors

Different Signalling Systems Control the Initiation of DNA Replication in Cultured Animal Cells

Luis Jimenez de Asua and Angela M. Otto

Friedrich Miescher-Institut, P. O. B. 2543, CH-4002 Basel, Switzerland

One of the most fascinating problems of modern biology not yet completely understood is how living organisms replicate their genetic material (DNA) and divide in response to changes in the extracellular environment (1-3). It is generally accepted that in mammalian cells in vivo and in vitro the frequency of cell replication is controlled by the intrinsic requirements of specific organs and by a delicate balance between a variety of mitogens, ions, nutrients and cellular inhibitors present in the intercellular milieu (2,3).

Swiss mouse 3T3 cells, which can be arrested in the Go/G1 phase or Q state of the cell cycle (4,5) provide a useful model system to study under in vitro conditions the interaction of mitogens and hormones on the control of cell proliferation. These cells can be stimulated to divide by epidermal growth factor (6), factor(s) derived from SV28/BHK transformed cells (7,8), fibroblastic growth factor (9,10), platelet-derived growth factor (11), prostaglandin $F_{2\alpha}$ (12) and vasopressin (13). Hydrocortisone, insulin and prostaglandin E_1 or E_2 in these cells can only modulate the effect of these mitogens (3,14).

Most of these mitogens initially interact with receptors at the surface membrane and deliver a repertoire of signals which, interacting with specific intracellular targets, triggers a cascade of events leading to the initiation of DNA replication and cell division (1-3).

A central question as to the mechanisms by which mitogens stimulate DNA replication is whether they act through different signalling systems. Is there a unique cascade or are different cascades of events regulating the initiation of DNA replication? Our objective here is to present some experimental evidence in support of the view that mitogens and hormones may act by eliciting several signalling systems to control the initiation of DNA replication in animal cells. We shall discuss the following points:

Abbreviations: Epidermal growth factor (EGF), prostaglandin $F_{2\alpha}$ ($PGF_{2\alpha}$), prostaglandin E_1 (PGE_1) and prostaglandin E_2 (PGE_2).

1.) Two independent signalling systems mediate the effect of mitogens,

2.) other signalling systems amplify or reduce the effects of mitogens,

3.) the signalling system for the lag phase and rate of entry into S phase can be uncoupled,

4.) different mitogens act through different signals,

5.) some biochemical perspectives.

Experimental system

Swiss mouse 3T3 cells were propagated in Dulbecco's modified Eagle's medium as described before (3). In the assay of the initiation of DNA synthesis and determination
of the rate of entry into S phase cells were plated in 30 mm Petri dishes in Dulbecco's modified Eagle's medium supplemented with low molecular weight nutrients and 6%
fetal calf serum (3). After three to four days the cultures received fresh medium
and were then allowed to become confluent and quiescent (3). The cells were used when
no mitotic figures were observed. The following diagram shows the experimental protocol described above (Fig. 1). In experiments in which colcemid was added to the cultured medium for 8 hours and removed prior to adding a mitogen, cells were washed
twice with serum-free medium prewarmed at 37°C. Conditioned medium retrieved from
parallel quiescent cultures was added to the treated cultures with mitogens as described before (16). The rate constant k was calculated as described in previous
publications (3,16).

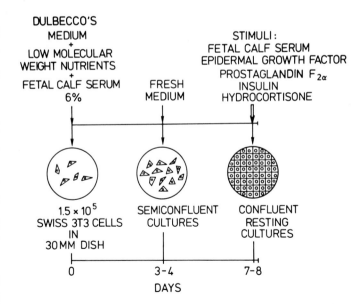

Fig. 1. Diagrammatic scheme for the experimental conditions in which cultures of 3T3
cells become confluent and resting prior stimulation with mitogens and hormones.

RESULTS AND DISCUSSION

1. Two independent signalling systems mediate the effect of mitogens

EGF, FGF, $PGF_{2\alpha}$, or serum stimulate the initiation of DNA replication in confluent resting Swiss 3T3 cells by controlling two different phenomena (3,10,17):

1) Setting in motion a cascade of events necessary for the progression of cells through a relative constant lag phase aof about 12-15 hours.

2) Increasing the rate at which stimulated cells enter into the S phase.

The lag phase, defined as the time between the initial addition of the mitogen and the initiation of DNA replication, requires a very low concentration of any of these mitogens. In contrast, the rate of initiation of DNA replication increases with the mitogen concentration up to a saturating level and can be changed by addition of the same mitogen later during the lag phase. The resulting rate follows apparent first order kinetics which can be quantified by a rate constant k. Table 1 shows the changes in the kinetics for entry into S phase upon addition of different concentrations of EGF and $PGF_{2\alpha}$.

Table 1. Stimulation of DNA replication by two concentrations of EGF, FGF or $PGF_{2\alpha}$ in Swiss 3T3 cells.

Additions	Lag phase hr	Rate constant $\times 10^{-2}$/hr
A None	----	0.04
EGF 4.0 ng/ml	14.5	0.88
EGF 20.0 ng/ml	14.5	1.67
EGF 4.0 ng/ml + EGF 16 ng/ml at 8 hr	14.5	1.66
B None	----	0.06
$PGF_{2\alpha}$ 60 ng/ml	15.0	1.10
$PGF_{2\alpha}$ 240 ng/ml	15.0	1.80
$PGF_{2\alpha}$ 60 ng/ml + $PGF_{2\alpha}$ 240 ng/ml at 8 hr	15.0	1.70
Serum	15.0	29.00

Data from (17) and (3), respectively.

Since both the lag phase and the rate of entry into S phase have different modes of control by these mitogens we suggest that either EGF, FGF or $PGF_{2\alpha}$ operate by delivering and regulating at least two independent signalling systems. Signal(s) 1 stimulates a cascade of events that determines the progression through the lag phase. Signal(s) 2 determines the final rate of initiation of DNA replication.

We have found that in Swiss 3T3 cells $PGF_{2\alpha}$ and EGF are required to be present in the culture medium for at least 8-10 hours to allow some cells to enter into S phase (18; unpublished data). This suggests to us that these mitogens need to trigger and maintain signal 1 for this length of time to allow an event to occur which is required by the cells to proceed through the remainder of the lag phase.

2. Other signalling systems

There is evidence that in confluent resting Swiss 3T3 cells hormones and other compounds, which by themselves do not initiate DNA synthesis, can elicit signals which amplify or reduce the stimulatory effect of mitogens. The length of the lag phase is the same for the different mitogens and is probably intrinsic to the cell. However, it depends on the mitogen whether and when the signal of a hormone has an amplifying, a reducing or no effect.

A. Amplifying effects. Insulin at a physiological concentration of 50 ng/ml amplifies the mitogenic effect of EGF (Fig. 2) as well as of FGF and $PGF_{2\alpha}$ by increasing the rate of entry into S phase (3,10). As shown in Fig. 2, insulin does not start a lag phase by itself nor alters its length induced by the mitogen. Furthermore, its amplifying effect is observed when added at any time of the lag phase.

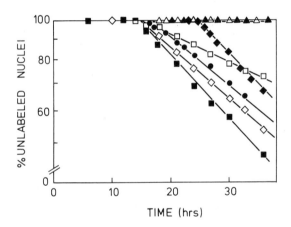

Fig. 2. The effect of non-synchronous additions of EGF (20 ng/ml) and insulin (50 ng/ ml) on the initiation of DNA synthesis in confluent Swiss 3T3 cells. Additions were as follows: (Δ), none; (▲), insulin; (□), EGF; EGF with insulin added at (■), 0 hr; (◇), 8 hr or (●), 15 hr; (◆), insulin with EGF added at 8 hr. Rate constant values were: (Δ), 0.04; (▲), 0.06; (□), 1.52; (■), 3.46; (◇), 2.95; (●), 2.76; (◆), 3.53 x 10^2/hr. Data from (19).

Microtubule-disrupting drugs, such as colchicine, colcemid and nocodazole, also enhance the rate of initiation of DNA synthesis stimulated by either EGF, FGF or $PGF_{2\alpha}$; but in contrast to insulin, these drugs must elicit their signal(s) during the first 8 hours of the lag phase, later additions having no effect (16,20-22). PGE_1 and PGE_2

at a concentration which is not stimulatory in itself (30 ng/ml), enhance or amplify the mitogenic effect of $PGF_{2\alpha}$ at any time of the lag phase; but they have no effect with EGF (14). The effect of hydrocortisone also depends on the mitogen: its signal(s) amplifies only when interacting with signal 2 of FGF (10).

B. Reducing effects. With both $PGF_{2\alpha}$ and EGF, the signal(s) elicited by hydrocortisone reduce the stimulatory effect, but only within the first 5-8 hours of the lag phase (3,17).

3. The signalling systems for the lag phase and the rate of entry into S phase can be uncoupled

Treatment of confluent resting Swiss 3T3 cells with colchicine, colcemid or nocodazole for 8 hours does not initiate DNA synthesis nor change the number of cells in the monolayer (20). Subsequent addition of EGF , FGF or $PGF_{2\alpha}$ stimulates the same rate of entry into S phase as if these drugs had been added together with the mitogens, however, the lag phase was markedly shortened. When colcemid or nocodazole was removed prior to stimulation by a mitogen, the lag phase was likewise shortened, but the enhancement of the rate of entry into S phase was lost in correlation with the reassembly of microtubules. Removal of colchicine from the culture prior to stimulation shortened the lag phase and still allowed enhancement of signal 2, because

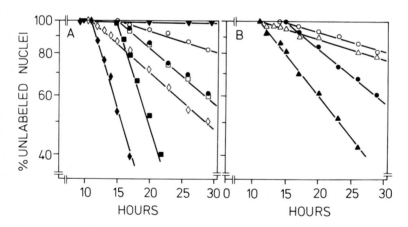

Fig. 3. Dissociation of the length of the lag phase and rate of initiation of DNA replication by preincubation with colcemid. Concentrations used were for EGF 20 ng/ml, insulin 50 ng/ml and colcemid 1 μM. A, Continuous exposure to colcemid: (▼) colcemid alone added 8 hr before other additions, (O) EGF; (●) EGF + insulin, (□) EGF + colcemid, (■) EGF + insulin and colcemid; all at 0 hr. Colcemid added 8 hr before (◇)EGF or (◆) EGF + insulin. B. Removal of colcemid prior stimulation: (O) EGF; (●) EGF + insulin. Colcemid added 8 hr before and removed prior addition of (△) EGF or (▲) EGF + insulin. Values of k (x 10^2/hr and length of lag phase in A and B were: (O) 1.4,15 hr; (●,□) 3.8, 15 hr; (■) 13.8, 15 hr; (◇) 3.8, 11 hr; (◆) 13.8, 11 hr; (△) 1.4, 11 hr; (▲) 5.0, 11 hr. Data from (20).

microtubule reassembly is much slower than upon removal of colcemid or nocodazole
(20-22). Fig. 3 shows how microtubule-disruption long before and during the lag phase
induced by EGF or EGF with insulin affects the kinetics for entry into S phase. These
results indicate that the signals for the length of the lag phase and the rate of
initiation of DNA synthesis can be independently modified and thus can be uncoupled.
Moreover, these results support the concept that mitogens stimulate two different
signalling systems.

4. Different mitogens act through different signals

EGF and $PGF_{2\alpha}$ are two structurally unrelated mitogens (23) and each one displays
similar patterns of interactions with insulin, hydrocortisone and microtubule-disrupting drugs on the initiation of DNA replication (3,16,17,20). The structural difference (EGF is a polypeptide, $PGF_{2\alpha}$ a lipoid), however, indicates that these two mitogens interact with different membrane receptors. On the other hand, hydrocortisone
as well as PGE_1 and PGE_2 exert different effects depending on the mitogen (see above).
This raises the simple question: Do these mitogens trigger a common signalling system
and thus a single cascade of events, or do they elicit different signalling systems,

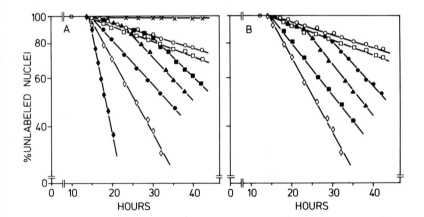

Fig. 4. Fraction of cells that remains unlabelled after synchronous or nonsyn-
chronous addition of EGF (20 ng/ml) and $PGF_{2\alpha}$ (300 ng/ml). A (x), no additions; (O),
EGF; (□), $PGF_{2\alpha}$; (◆), serum. EGF with $PGF_{2\alpha}$ added at: (◊,●,▲,■) 0, 6, 10 or 15 hr.
B (□), $PGF_{2\alpha}$; (O), EGF; $PGF_{2\alpha}$ with EGF added at: (◊), 0 hr; (■), 6 hr; (▲), 10 hr;
(●), 15 hr. Values of k (10^2/hr). In A were (x), 0.06; (O), 1.1; (□), 1.4; (◊), 6.1;
(◆), 25.3; (●,▲,■) average of 3.26. In B were (□), 1.3; (O), 1.1; (◊), 6.1; (■,▲,●),
average of 4.1. The length of the lag phase in A and B was 14.5 hr. Data from (23).

which could activate different cascades of events leading to the initiation of DNA synthesis? One can make the following predictions: If the mitogens trigger a common signalling system, then one could expect additive effects when both mitogens are at subsaturating concentrations and no further enhancement when one mitogen is at a saturating concentration. Alternatively, if different mitogens trigger different signalling systems and as a result different cascades of events, then the stimulation of DNA replication by two or more mitogens could be inhibited or enhanced compared to the effect of one mitogen alone. Other more complicated possibilities are conceivable but for simplicity of the presentation will not be discussed.

EGF and $PGF_{2\alpha}$ added together to resting Swiss 3T3 cells stimulate synergistically the rate of initiation of DNA replication after a constant lag phase of 15 hr (Fig. 4). This result supports the prediction that two different mitogens act through different signalling systems.

Two different signalling systems require coordinate interaction during the lag phase to be able to result in a synergistic effect on the rate of entry into S phase. Adding one mitogen 6 hours after the other results in a synergistic effect which is less than when both mitogens are added together. The length of the lag phase is not changed. This indicates that the signals delivered by EGF and $PGF_{2\alpha}$ interact most effectively during the first few hours. Delaying the addition of the second mitogen for 10 or 15 hours renders a synergistic effect not observed until 15 hours after the addition of the second mitogen. This means that after six hours of the lag phase the second signalling system can no longer be temporally integrated. However, there

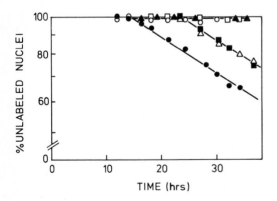

Fig. 5. The effect of non-synchronous addition of EGF (20 ng/ml) and insulin (50 ng/ml) on the initiation of DNA synthesis in clone Swiss 3T3 SL. Additions were as follows: (O), none; (▲), insulin; (□), EGF; (●), EGF with insulin added at 0 hr; or (■), 8 hr; (△), insulin with EGF added after 8 hr. Rate constant values were (O), 0.04; (▲), 0.06; (□), 0.07; (●), 2.15; (■), 2.18; (△), 2.16 x 10^2/hr. Data from ref. (19).

appear to be signals from the first mitogen which persist to interact with the second signalling system. From these results it cannot be concluded whether only signal(s) 2 for regulating the rate of entry into S phase are different or whether also signal(s) 1 for progression through the lag phase are different for these two mitogens.

A variant cell line of Swiss 3T3-K (SL_1) is characterized by its unresponsiveness to EGF alone: however, together with insulin EGF stimulates the initiation of DNA synthesis (Fig. 5). $PGF_{2\alpha}$ alone, or with insulin, stimulates the same kinetics for entry into S phase as in the parent cells (19). As shown in Fig. 5, when insulin and EGF are added one after the other, the progression of the lag phase is induced from the time of the second addition. These results have been interpreted as evidence that the signals(s) 1 of EGF cannot be elicited and that they thus appear to be different from those of $PGF_{2\alpha}$. Furthermore, since insulin contributes with a signal of its own (which alone is not sufficient for stimulating DNA synthesis) to help EGF start the lag phase, it further favors a concept that signal 1 is not comprised of a single, unique signal, but more likely constitutes, together with signal(s) 2, an intricate signalling system.

The scheme in Fig. 6 summarizes the difference in the cascade of events between $PGF_{2\alpha}$ and EGF in stimulating the initiation of DNA replication. To emphasize this concept, the interaction of PGE_1 and PGE_2 with EGF and $PGF_{2\alpha}$ is shown. The interactions of insulin, hydrocortisone and microtubule-disrupting drugs, which are apparently the same for $PGF_{2\alpha}$ and EGF have been omitted for simplicity. However, the similarity in interactions indicates that EGF and $PGF_{2\alpha}$ stimulate some events in common before and after 6 hours of the lag phase. In particular, rate determining events appear to occur at about 10 hours of the lag phase regardless of the stimulating mitogen (3,24,25). The converging lines at 6 hours simply indicate the time up to which EGF and $PGF_{2\alpha}$ interact most efficiently to increase the rate of entry into S phase upon completion of the lag phase.

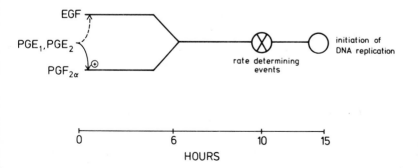

Fig. 6. A diagrammatic presentation of different interactions of PGE_1 and PGE_2 with $PFG_{2\alpha}$ and EGF.

5. Some biochemical perspectives

The kinetics of initiation of DNA synthesis observed upon stimulation by a single mitogen, upon its interaction with hormones, and when two different mitogens interact suggest that different signalling systems regulate the rate of cell proliferation. The major challenge is now to sort out which of the biochemical changes occurring upon mitogenic stimulation in Swiss 3T3 cells are constituents of the signalling system and which are events of the cascade(s) leading to DNA replication.

The binding of mitogens to its specific receptor elicits a series of biochemical changes, some occurring within minutes, others within the first 2 hours. For example, EGF added to quiescent cells triggers changes in surface membrane events such as activating the (Na^+, K^+)-ATPase and increasing influx of Na^+ and nutrients (26). EGF also activates a protein kinase activity associated to the receptor complex (6). After EGF-binding, the receptor complex is aggregated and subsequently internalized and degraded (6). For $PGF_{2\alpha}$ the receptor has not yet been characterized in Swiss 3T3 cells, but it also stimulates the membrane (Na^+, K^+)-ATPase as well as phosphate and glucose uptake (3). Both EGF and $PGF_{2\alpha}$, in contrast to serum, do not change the intracellular levels of cyclic AMP (3,14,27).

There is evidence that continuous protein synthesis is required for progression through the lag phase and for determining the rate of entry into S phase (28). Thomas et al. (29,30) have shown that serum, EGF and $PGF_{2\alpha}$, but also insulin, stimulate the multiple phosphorylation of the S6 ribosomal protein on the 40s subunit and increase polysome formation and the rate of protein synthesis. There is also evidence for synthesis of specific proteins after mitogenic stimulation. Within two hours after serum stimulation in Swiss 3T3 cells many changes in the pattern of cytoplasmic proteins, some being under transcriptional and/or translational control, were observed by Thomas et al. (31). Changes in proteins have also been observed upon stimulation by platelet-derived growth factor in Balb/3T3 cells by Pledger et al. (32). Nilsen-Hamilton et al. (33) have found that EGF and FGF stimulate the synthesis and glycosylation of a protein secreted to the medium. Two nuclear non-histone proteins are stimulated by $PGF_{2\alpha}$ and insulin, one appearing at about 10 hours, which could be related to the initiation of DNA synthesis (3). Recently, it has been found that DNA polymerase α activity stimulated by $PGF_{2\alpha}$ and insulin requires continuous protein synthesis (Otto et al., manuscript in preparation). On the other hand, there is evidence that in Swiss 3T3 cells EGF, FGF and insulin inhibit protein degradation (34). Therefore, it is conceivable that protein synthesis as well as degradation are important in regulating the levels and the activity of proteins involved in DNA replication.

It is not clear how the numerous events occurring at the beginning of the lag phase can ultimately control DNA replication, which is not initiated until about 15 or more hours later and which requires a variety of enzymes probably organized in a replicative complex (35). Furthermore, the question remains which are the essential events stimulated by each mitogen to be able to initiate DNA replication, and which are the optional, modulating events that differ with the mitogen. It is tempting to suggest that certain initial events at the surface membrane may act as signalling system(s), which in turn activate, maintain and/or modulate cytoplasmic and nuclear events organized in one or more cascades. Our approach will be to study biochemical events occurring during DNA replication, which will complement those known to occur in the early part of the lag phase and may help eventually to link the different events to a cascade leading to DNA replication.

Acknowledgements. We thank Drs. Margret Eschenbruch, Ilse Novak-Hofer and Gary Thomas for constructive criticisms to the manuscript. We also thank Mrs. Marie-Odile Ulrich for skilful technical assistance. A.M.O. is a Special Fellow of the Leukemia Society of America.

REFERENCES

1. Holley, R.W. (1975) Nature 258, 487-490.
2. Holley, R.W. (1980) in Control Mechanisms in Animal Cells, eds. Jimenez de Asua,L., Levi-Montalcini, R., Iacobelli, S. and Shields, R. (Raven Press, New York), pp. 15-25.
3. Jimenez de Asua, L., Richmond, K.M.V., Otto, A.M., Kubler, A.-M., O'Farrell, M.K. and Rudland, P.S. (1979) in Hormones and Cell Culture, Cold Spring Harbor Conferences in Cell Proliferation, eds. Sato, G.H. and Ross, R. (Cold Spring Harbor Laboratory, Cold Spring Harbor, New York) Vol. 6, pp. 403-424.
4. Baserga, R. (1976) Multiplication and Division of Animal Cells. Dekker, New York.
5. Brooks, R.F., Bennett, D. and Smith, J.A. (1980) Cell 19, 493-502.
6. Carpenter, G. and Cohen, S. (1979) Ann. Rev. Biochem. 48, 193-216.
7. Bürk, R.R. (1973) Proc. Natl. Acad. Sci. USA 70, 369-372.
8. Bourne, H. and Rozengurt, E. (1976) Proc. Natl. Acad. Sci. USA 73, 4555-4559.
9. Gospodarowicz, D. (1974) Nature 249, 123-127.
10. Richmond, K.M.V., Kubler, A.M., Martin, F. and Jimenez de Asua, L. (1980). J.Cell. Physiol. 103, 77-85.
11. Shier, W.T. and Durkin, J.P. (1982) J. Cell. Physiol. 112, 171-181.
12. Jimenez de Asua, L., Clingan, D. and Rudland, P.S. (1975) Proc. Natl. Acad. Sci. USA 72, 2724-2728,
13. Rozengurt, E., Legg, A. and Pettican, P. (1979) Proc. Natl. Acad. Sci. USA 76, 1284-1287.
14. Otto, A.M., Nilsen-Hamilton, M., Boss, B.D., Ulrich, M.D. and Jimenez de Asua, L. (1982) Proc. Natl. Acad. Sci. USA 79, 4992-4996.
15. Todaro, G. and Green, H. (1963) J. Cell Biol. 17, 299-313.
16. Otto, A.M., Zumbé, A., Gibson, L., Kubler, A.-M. and Jimenez de Asua, L. (1979) Proc. Natl. Acad. Sci. USA 76, 6435-6438.
17. Otto, A.M., Ulrich, M.O. and Jimenez de Asua, L. (1982) J. Cell Physiol. 108, 145-153.
18. Jimenez de Asua, L. (1980) in Control Mechanisms in Animal Cell, eds. Jimenez de Asua, L., Levi-Montalcini, R., Iacobelli, S. and Shields, R. (Raven Press, New York) pp. 173-197.
19. Jimenez de Asua, L., Smith, C. and Otto, A.M. (1981) Cell Biol. Int. Rep. 6, 701-797.
20. Otto, A.M., Ulrich, M.O., Zumbé, A. and Jimenez de Asua, L. (1981) Proc. Natl. Acad. Sci. USA 78, 3063-3067.
21. Otto, A.M. (1982) in Prostaglandins and Cancer: First International Conference (Alan R. Liss, New York) pp. 391-396.

22. Otto, A.M. and Jimenez de Asua, L. (1982) (submitted for publication).
23. Jimenez de Asua, L., Richmond, K.M.V. and Otto, A.M. (1981) Proc. Natl. Acad. sci. USA 78, 1004-1008.
24. Brooks, R.F. (1976) Nature 160, 248-250.
25. Pardee, A.B., Dubrow, R., Hamlin, J.L. and Kletzien, R.F. (1978) Ann. Rev. Biochem. 47, 715-750.
26. Rozengurt, E. (1979) in Hormones and Cell Culture, Cold Spring Harbor Conferences in Cell Proliferation, eds. Sato, G.H. and Ross, R. (Cold Spring Harbor Laboratory, Cold Spring Harbor, New York) Vol. 6, pp. 773-788.
27. Rozengurt, R., Legg, A., Strang, G. and Courtenay-Luck, N. (1981) Proc. Natl. Acad. Sci. USA 78, 4392-4396.
28. Brooks, R.F. (1977) Cell 12, 311-317.
29. Thomas, G., Siegmann, M., Gordon, J., Jimenez de Asua, L., Martin-Pérez, J. and Nielsen, P. (1981) in Protein Phosphorylation, Cold Spring Harbor Conferences in Cell Proliferation, eds. Rosen, O. and Krebs, E. (Cold Spring Harbor Laboratory, Cold Spring Harbor, New York) Vol. 8, pp. 783-799.
30. Thomas, G., Martin-Pérez, J., Siegmann, M. and Otto, A.M. (1982) Cell 30, 235-242.
31. Thomas, G., Thomas, G. and Luther, H. (1981) Proc. Natl. Acad. Sci. USA 78, 5712-5716.
32. Pledger, W.J., Hart, D.A., Locatell, K.L. and Scher, C.D. (1981) Proc. Natl. Acad. Sci. USA 78, 4358-4362.
33. Nilsen-Hamilton, M., Shapiro, J.M., Massoglia, S.L. and Hamilton, R.T. (1980) Cell 20, 19-28.
34. Ballard, F.J., Knowles, S.L., Wong, S.S.C., Bodner, J.B., Wood, C.M. and Gunn, J.M. (1980) FEBS Lett. 114, 209-212.
35. Reddy, G.P.V. and Pardee, A.B. (1980) Proc. Natl. Acad. Sci. USA 77, 3312-3316.

Ectopic Auto-Stimulation of Growth

Robert R. Bürk

Friedrich Miescher-Institut, P. O. Box 2543, CH-4002 Basel, Switzerland*

Abstract. According to dogma nearly every cell in a mammal has the same genes encoded in its DNA and differentiation involves the selective de-repression of a different and small proportion of these genes in the cells of different tissues. The gene for a hormone-like growth factor will be present in all cells but only expressed in a source cell from which the factor will be transported in the circulation to a target cell whose growth it regulates. If, by mutation, translocation, or terato-geny (mis-differentiation) the gene becomes expressed in the target cell, then the target cell will stimulate its own proliferation (auto-stimulation) and escape the normal growth regulation controls. Although the normal factor will be acting on the normal receptor to produce a normal response the cell will behave like a tumour cell. An auto-stimulating cell will also grow in culture independently of added growth factor. It has been possible to demonstrate the production of growth factors by tumour cells in tissue culture and that these factors partially explain the reduced requirement of transformed cells for serum in tissue culture.

The earliest cell lines to be established in culture were derived from tumours. Thus, L-cells came from a mouse sarcoma (1), HeLa from a human cervical carcinoma (2) and H.Ep 2 from a human laryngeal carcinoma (3). This gave rise to the notion that cancer cells are easier to grow in culture than their normal counterparts. The easiness of culture is a rather soft concept. What actually was easy was the discovery of the methodology for culturing these cells. This meeting shows that method-ologies can be developed for the culture of almost all cells.

I think that one of the fundamental problems of culture has been the wish for cell proliferation. In many tissues the proliferation rate is low and if such tissues were maintained in culture we would call them quiescent. However, research requires multiple cultures, therefore it must be possible to increase the amount of a tissue. Thus, growth of the tissue is necessary and so proliferation and differentiation of the cells are necessary. Ideally, one needs two media, embryonic and adult, growth and maintenance. Small numbers of cells could be increased by proliferation in the growth medium and allowed to form a tissue which is then maintained in a maintenance medium. Almost the whole effort of cell culture research has been devoted to the first phase. The second

---

*Present address: Biotechnology Department, Ciba-Geigy Limited, CH-4002 Basel, Switzerland

phase has something to do with organ culture or is called "the problem of differentiation". Since research has required proliferating cells, cancers were an appropriate source of starting cells since they are already proliferating and the problem of initiating proliferation seemed to be thus avoided.

A major difficulty of working with real tumours is that of obtaining the appropriate control of a normal tissue. The result is that it has been difficult to compare the fastidiousness in the medium requirements of cancer cells with their normal counterparts. However, when neoplastic transformation in culture is possible, especially of a cloned cell line, then the comparison is possible. In 1963, Stanners, Till and Siminovitch (4) showed that clones of polyoma-virus-transformed hamster fibroblasts had the ability to grow in a reduced serum concentration compared to the parent. Recently, Lechner and Kaighn (5) using the approach of Ellem et al.(6) have quantitated the serum protein requirement of prostatic carcinoma cells in comparison with that of prostate cells.

The serum requirement of BHK21/13 (7) was early used to establish quiescent cultures in 0.25% calf serum that could be stimulated to proliferate by adding serum to 10% to the cultures (8). In contrast, PyY, a polyoma-virus-transformed clonal derivative of BHK21/13 grew in the 0.25% serum medium. In those days we were not yet able to produce serum-free culture conditions. However, it appeared this was something approaching the in vivo situation in an important aspect, namely the rate of cell proliferation. A culture in 0.25% serum had a very low proliferation rate but could be stimulated to proliferate. There appeared to be an analogy between a normal tissue and its response to a wound. Further, the transformed cells proliferated under the conditions where the normal population was quiescent which also appeared analogous and hopefully homologous to the growth of a tumour in a non-growing tissue. The use of low serum concentrations to produce quiescent cultures became a routine.

A less precise method of producing quiescent cultures has been to allow the cells to proliferate until they exhaust the medium. Thus, 3T3 cells can be left in a medium containing 10% serum and after a few days the culture becomes quiescent. The limiting exhausted component is then replaced by adding serum (9) or defined substances to the depleted medium (10). It has been found that not only platelet-derived growth factor but also epidermal growth factor, prostaglandin $F_{2\alpha}$ with a number of hormones will reinitiate DNA synthesis in such cultures in depleted medium.

An advantage of the depleted medium approach was that scratching a monolayer culture to produce a wound in the layer initiated proliferation
at the edge of the wound (9,11). This scratching seems a closer analogy
to the in vivo situation with respect to the effects of wounding than
the serum addition approach. Incidentally, the scratch experiment showed
that the medium was only globally exhausted and that a local perturba-
tion was sufficient to allow proliferation. These observations can now
be explained by the diffusion boundary layer (12).

An experiment that demonstrates the importance of the topology of the
cultures is to wound them with a razor blade and change the bulk medium
to a limiting one, in the case of 3T3 cells to Dulbecco's plus 2% foetal
calf serum, and then add increasing amounts of a growth factor from SV28
tumour cells (13). It was observed that the cells at the edge of the
wound respond to a ten-fold lower concentration of the growth factor
than the cells 5 mm into the monolayer.

To return to the ease of culturing tumour cells; it was noticed that
various virus-transformed cells have a reduced requirement for serum
for proliferation. Perhaps the tumour cells make their own growth factors (14). The hypothesis is illustrated diagrammatically in Figure 1
(15). Imagine an organism with 26 genes, a-z,and three cell types. There
is differential expression of the genes. F and M are expressed in all
cells. Hexagonal cells are differentiated to express genes G and N.
Further imagine the hexagonal cell requires the growth factors A and B
for its proliferation. These factors are produced in source cells and
pass to the target cell presumably in the blood stream. (For this model,
if a substance is properly produced in the target cell, it is not a
growth factor but a second messenger). In the model the proliferation
of the hexagonal cell is controlled by the substances A and B produced
by the spiky and rounded cells. In reality probably the synthesis,
processing, export, glycosylation, etc., of A and B would be controlled
by more than one gene and further there would be a network of feedback
loops between the various cells regulating the production of A and B.
What then is neoplastic transformation? Suppose gene a which should not
be expressed in its target cell becomes expressed in its target cell.
One can imagine that (i) there is a mutation in the DNA associated with
the regulation of the expression of gene a so that it is no longer recognised by a repressor whose gene could also mutate. Either way there
would be constitutive production of A, the former being dominant, the
latter recessive; (ii) a foreign piece of DNA from a virus could be
introduced near gene a resulting in its inappropriate activation by a
hormone or read through from a strong promoter; (iii) a teratogenic

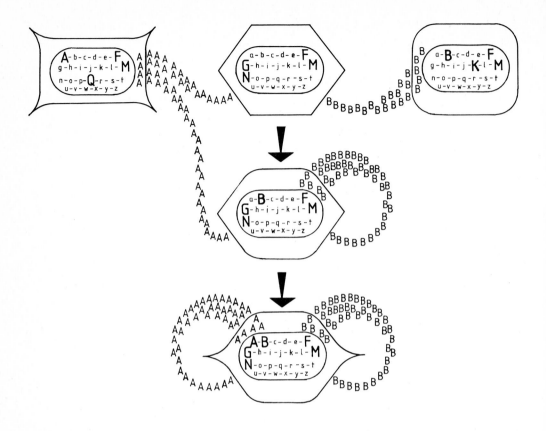

<u>Fig. 1</u>. Ectopic auto-stimulation reproduced from ref. 15 with permis-
sion, Raven Press, New York.

event could result in the loss of e.g. a methylation(s) of the DNA so
that the gene is mis-differentiated and becomes expressed. All these
mechanisms are possible. All result in a hereditable new phenotype. The
teratogenic change in the DNA might be reversible in the whole organism
but the other changes seem unlikely to be reversible at all. The new
phenotype involves the production of a growth factor in its target cell.
If the expression of gene <u>a</u> (which in reality would be a complex of
genes) leads to the production and release of factor A in a manner homologous to that in the proper "spiky" source cell, then the target
cell would be releasing a growth factor which acts on itself to stimulate itself to proliferate. The altered target cell is still dependent
on a source cell for factor B and so its proliferation will still be
regulated by factor B. However, if the cause of the change in the DNA
is still acting or is repeated then the gene <u>b</u> may be expressed so that

factor B is produced ectopically in its target cell. At this point the target cell stimulates its own proliferation independently of the proper controlling sources and, if in fact there are feedback loops, it may well repress the proper sources. It seems to me this cell will now proliferate as long as it receives nutrients and until or unless it produces a novel surface antigen that would make it subject to immune attack by the host. The result would be a benign tumour.

It turns out, however, that growth factors stimulate the migration of cells. There are obvious selective advantages to this combination of activities in wound-healing and in embryogenesis. Experimentally, it is only when there is a great excess of the growth factors that one sees a monolayer culture running wild. On the present hypothesis the cells would be constitutively producing factors and so the concentration would be at a maximum in the tumour causing the cells to migrate out.

Notice that evolutionarily, there is a selective advantage to having multiple, independent parallel but synergistic pathways regulating the rate of proliferation of cells. If one pathway fails, becomes constitutive as described above, then the other pathways still exert some degree of control. Thus, multiple parallel control offers a fail-safe system of regulation. However, the more pathways there are the more genes are involved and the larger the target for carcinogens and the larger the chance of a single failure. This fail-safe mechanism can only be broken by multiple hits which is consistent with the multiple hit nature of many cancer/age curves (16).

Notice also that although the hypothesis described above refers to hormonal or external control, the pathways also involve internal events like the activation of protein kinases. A corollary to the hypothesis is that the internal pathway can be altered by the four mechanisms suggested above resulting in the constitutive activation in the absence of the appropriate hormone of, say, a protein kinase. Thus, one can imagine in the case of cyclic AMP-dependent protein kinase that the regulatory subunit might not be produced so that the catalytic subunit would no longer be regulated (inhibited), the cell would continually behave as though its cyclic AMP had been raised. Conversely, one can imagine an overproduction of the regulatory subunit or a loss of the catalytic subunit which would make the cell behave as though cyclic AMP were continuously low and might expect the transformed phenotype in the case of fibroblasts. It would seem that the tumour viruses produce transformation by altering the internal events of growth regulation and that cellular onc-gene products are the normal proper proteins of growth regulation.

Ectopic production of hormones by tumours is well documented (17). Some of these hormones are involved in growth regulation in some tissues. Clinically, a tumour may be detected by the effect its ectopically produced hormone is having on another tissue (18). Notice ectopic production is not a sufficient condition of the hypothesis, there must also be auto-stimulation. The hormone or growth factor, it would be better to talk of "proliferation hormone", must act on the cell that is inappropriately producing it. The target cell becomes also a source cell. It is clear that one can imagine a corollary whereby a source cell inappropriately acquires receptors and the ability to respond to its own factor. Ectopic auto-stimulation involves a fully normal factor acting in the normal manner on its proper receptor. The prospects of pharmacologically interfering with the process without interfering with the normal process are restricted therefore to inhibiting production in the tumour cell selectively over the proper source.

We have looked for and found growth factors produced by a tumour cell line (19). SV28 is a line of cells derived in a complicated manner from the line BHK21/13 (20). SV28 has hamster chromosomes and SV40 t-antigen. Thirty cells injected subcutaneously in hamsters give rise to tumours in all animals. Further, some 70% of the animals have metastases to diverse sites in the body. The secondary tumours are invasive. SV28 can be said to be a malignant cell line. The parent cell line, BHK21/13 was derived by serial passage and cloning from baby hamster kidney fibroblasts (7). It requires the injection of between 10^4 and 10^5 BHK21/13 cells subcutaneously in hamsters to produce a tumour in 50% of the animals. These tumours do not metastasize or invade. They remain at the site of injection and can be called benign. SV28 cells can be maintained

Table 1. Properties of the Cells	2°,3° Cultures from baby hamster kidney	BHK21/13	SV28
Tumour dose$_{50}$	$> 10^7$	$10^4 - 10^5$	< 30
Metastasis	−	−	+
Agar growth	−	−	+
Agar growth + FGF	−	+	+
Serum requirement	++	+	−
Contact inhibition	+	+	−
Density inhibition	+	±	−
Orientation	+	+	−
Factor A	−	−	+
Factor B	−	+	+

for long periods in culture without serum. Our longest run was some 5
months changing the medium every two hours on the Bellco Autoharvester
Roller machine. The harvest medium is a rich source of growth factors
for 3T3 mouse cells (19). Table 1 summarises the properties of SV28 in
comparison with the cell line BHK21/13 and the secondary and tertiary
cultures of baby hamster kidney fibroblasts.

Using a migration assay (19), originally in the hope of finding a factor
that promotes invasion, we have purified two factors from SV28 conditioned medium (21). Table 2 summarises their properties. Factor A has a
molecular weight in SDS electrophoresis of 23,000 and an isoelectric
point at 10.4. Factor B has an apparent molecular weight of about 46,000
by gel filtration but is inactivated by SDS electrophoresis. Factor B
focusses at pH 9.8. Table 2 summarises the chemical and biological properties of these factors. Both are sensitive to β-mercapto-ethanol,
stable at low pH and insoluble at high pH, i.e. near their iso-electric
point. Both factors stimulate migration of 3T3 cells. However, at saturating doses factor B is more effective than factor A. The fact that
their saturating effects are different suggests they act in different
ways. Further, their saturating effects are additive showing that not
only are they different but that they have been biochemically separated.
Both factors stimulate tritiated thymidine incorporation into resting
cells and raise the labelling index to near 95%. There is some dependence on serum. A concentration of 0.2% serum in the culture medium is
sufficient to allow a full effect of either factor. In comparison, epidermal growth factor and fibroblast growth factor only produce their

Table 2. Properties of SV28-Growth Factors	Factor A	Factor B
Migration	+	++
Thymidine incorporation	+	+
Labelling index	+	+
Serum requirement	+	+
Overgrowth	+	±
Orientation	+	−
Agar growth	?	−
Molecular weight	23,000	46,000
Iso-electric point	pH 10.4	pH 9.8
SDS electrophoresis	resistant	sensitive
β-Mercaptoethanol	sensitive	sensitive

full effect on the labelling index in the presence of ten times more
serum, i.e. 2%. Both factor A and factor B synergise with both epidermal
growth factor and fibroblast growth factor in their effect on ^{3}H-thymi-
dine incorporation. Both factor A and factor B allow the growth of 3T3
cells in the presence of 0.5% foetal calf serum at a rate similar to
that in 10% foetal calf serum and of SV3T3 cells. Thus, 3T3 grow like
SV3T3 in the presence of the factors. Factor A in the presence of 10%
serum gives growth to higher density (overgrowth) while factor B has
little overgrowth capacity. Factor A alters the orientation of the cells
in the culture so that the cells are randomly oriented as if they were
freely crawling over each other. It is as if factor A overcomes contact
inhibition of movement whereas factor B does not overcome contact inhibition of movement. Factor A at high concentration from the Sephadex G75
step may stimulate growth of BHK21/13 cells in semi-solid agar but it
has not been possible to produce enough SDS electrophoresis purified
material to test this. Factor B has been observed not to stimulate growth
in semi-solid agar.

BHK21/13 cells differ from SV28 cells with respect to the production
of the factors. When medium from BHK21/13 cells was tested it was found
to contain one factor which was identified as factor B because it acts

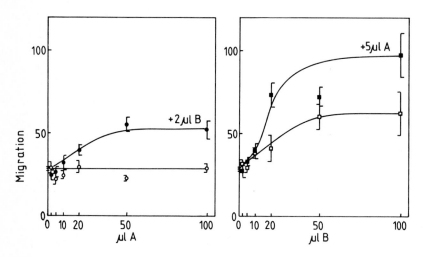

Fig. 2. Synergistic effect of factors A and B on migration of fibroblasts
in secondary cultures from baby hamster kidneys. See ref.15 for assay
conditions.

in the presence of saturating amounts of factor A from SV28 cells but
has no effect in the presence of saturating amounts of factor B from
SV28 cells (15). The factor from BHK21/13 cells could be purified in
the same way that the factor B could be purified from SV28 cells (15).
It is therefore concluded that BHK21/13 cells produce factor B and do
not produce factor A. Secondary or tertiary cultures of baby hamster
kidney fibroblasts did not produce, in a number of independent experiments, any migration stimulating activity (15). Table 1 summarises these
results. It was found that secondary cultures of baby hamster kidney
fibroblasts respond to factor B but not to factor A. However, they do
respond to factor A in the presence of a low dose of factor B (Fig. 2).
There is a clear synergy between factors A and B.

The situation is summarised in Figure 3. The normal baby hamster fibroblasts produce neither factor but respond to factor B which allows them
to respond to factor A. The "benign" BHK21/13 cells produce factor B,

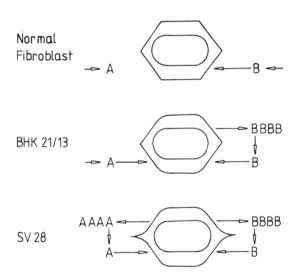

Fig. 3. Increased growth factor production with increased transformation of baby hamster kidney fibroblasts.

presumably respond to it (autostimulation), although there is little effect of added factor B, and respond to factor A. The "malignant" SV28 cells produce factors A and B and presumably respond to them (auto-stimulation), although again addition of the factors has little detectible effect on the already high migration of SV28 cells.

There has apparently been a progression (Fig. 1) from normal to benign to malignant with a progression from no factor to one factor to two factors. It has not yet been possible to identify a proper source of factor A or factor B. It is therefore strictly speaking hypothetical to say the factors are ectopically produced. They could be anachronistically produced. They could be embryonic factors expressed at the wrong time in an adult tissue. They could even be "neo"-transformation factors. Comings long ago proposed that the SV28 factors could be what he named "transforming factors" (22). Since the factors synergise with epidermal growth factor and fibroblast growth factor, they are apparently not epidermal growth factor or fibroblast growth factor. It is also unlikely that they are sarcoma growth factor(s)(23) or transforming growth factor(s) because of the synergy with epidermal growth factor (24). There could be a relationship with epidermal growth factor-dependent transforming growth factor that has been recently reported (25), but factor A and factor B are not dependent on epidermal growth factor. Factor A resembles human platelet-derived growth factor that has molecular weight 28-30,000 and an isoelectric point at pH 9.8 (26, 27,28). Further platelet-derived growth factor has been reported to be produced by a human osteosarcoma (29). That osteosarcoma seems to be an example of ectopic auto-stimulation.

We have shown that a tumour cell line that can be grown without serum produces growth factors that can stimulate growth of a normal cell line that has a high serum requirement. This suggests two things that are important for this meeting. Firstly, that tumour cells, if they are already producing their own growth factors, that is if they are auto-stimulating, can indeed be less fastidious than their normal counterparts in their growth requirements for polypeptide hormones. Secondly. that tumour cells can be a source of growth factors for the growth of normal cells.

REFERENCES

1. Sanford, K.K., Earle, W.R., and Likely, G.D. (1948) J. Nat. Cancer Inst. 9, 229.
2. Gey, G.O., Coffman, W.D., and Kubicek, M.T. (1952) Cancer Res. 12, 264.
3. Moore, A.E., Sabachewsky, L., and Toolan, H.W. (1952) Cancer Res. 15, 598.
4. Stanners, C.P., Till, J.E., and Siminovitch, L. (1963) Virology 21, 448.
5. Lechner, J.F., and Kaighn,M.E. (1979) J. Cell Physiol. 100, 519.
6. Ellem, K.A.O., and Gierthy, J.F. (1977) J. Cell Physiol. 92, 381.
7. Macpherson, I., and Stoker, M. (1962) Virology 16, 147.
8. Bürk, R.R. (1966) Nature 212, 1261.
9. Todaro, G.J., Lazar, G.K., and Green, H. (1965) J. cell. comp. Physiol. 66, 325.
10. Jimenez de Asua, L., Clingan, D., and Rudland, P.S. (1975) Proc. Natl. Acad. Sci. USA 72, 2724.
11. Castor, L. (1969) J. Cell Physiol. 75, 57.
12. Stoker, M.G.P. (1973) Nature 246, 200.
13. Bürk, R.R. (1976) Exp. Cell Res. 101, 293.
14. Bürk, R.R., and Williams, C.A. (1971) in Ciba Foundation Symp.Growth Control in Cell Cultures, eds. G.E.W. Wolstenholme and J. Knight. Churchill Livingstone, London, p. 107.
15. Bürk, R.R. (1980) in Control Mechanisms in Animal Cells, eds. L. Jimenez de Asua et al., Raven Press, New York, p. 245.
16. Doll, R. (1978) Cancer Res. 38, 3573.
17. Rees, L.H. (1975) J. Endocrinol. 67, 143.
18. Bagshawe, K.D. (1974) Brit. Med. Bull. 30, 68.
19. Bürk, R.R. (1973) Proc. Natl. Acad. Sci. USA 70, 369.
20. Wiblin, C.N., and Macpherson, I.A. (1972) Int. J. Cancer 10, 269.
21. Leuthard, P., Steck, G., Bürk, R.R., and Otto, A. (1980) in Control Mechanisms in Animal Cells, eds. L. Jimenez de Asua et al. Raven Press, New York, p. 259.
22. Comings, D.E. (1973) Proc. Natl. Acad. Sci. USA 70, 3324.
23. De Larco, J.E., and Todaro, G.J. (1978) Proc. Natl. Acad. Sci. USA 75, 4001.
24. Todaro, G.J., De Larco, J.E., Fryling, C., Johnson, P.A., and Sporn, M.B. (1981) J. Sup. Struct. Cell. Biochem. 15, 287.
25. Roberts, A.B., Anzano, M.A., Lamb, L.C., Smith, J.M., Frolik, C.A., Marquardt, H., Todaro, G.J., and Sporn, M.B. (1982) Nature 295, 417.
26. Heldin, C.-H., Westermark, B., and Wasteson, A. (1979) Proc. Natl. Acad. Sci. USA 76, 3722.
27. Deuel, T.F., Huang, J.S., Profitt, R.T., Baenziger, J.U., Chang, D., and Kennedy, B.B. (1981) J. Biol. Chem. 256, 8896.
28. Raines, E.W., and Ross, R. (1982) J. Biol. Chem. 257, 5154.
29. Heldin, C.H., Westermark, B., and Wasteson, A. (1980) J. cell. Physiol. 105, 235.

The Growth and Differentiation of Human Endothelial Cells

T. Maciag[1] and R. Weinstein[2]

[1] Department of Pathology and [2] Department of Medicine,
Charles A. Dana Research Institute, Harvard-Thorndike Laboratory, Harvard Medical School, Beth Israel Hospital, Boston, MA 02215, USA

Introduction: The non-thrombogenic nature of veins, arteries and capillaries is maintained in vivo by the presence of the endothelial cell. It has been widely recognized that the identification of factors which influence the growth and differentiation of the endothelial cell will significantly contribute to a better understanding of normal and pathological events in human biology in which the vascular tree has a major impact. These events include tumor growth, atherosclerosis, wound healing, thrombosis and hemostasis. Unfortunately, endothelial cells of human origin have been difficult to study because of their low mitotic index in vivo (1,2). In spite of these difficulties, efficatious methods have been developed for the isolation and propagation of endothelial cells in vitro (3,4,5,6 and 7).

We have concentrated our efforts on the human umbilical vein endothelial cell (HUVEC) because it represents the most accessible source of human endothelium. Furthermore, HUV EC are well characterized in vitro, possessing two unique endothelial cell markers, the Weibel-Palade body (8) and the Factor VIII-related antigen (FVIII:Ag) (9). We initially asked a very simple question: does there exist a growth factor which will stimulate the growth of quiescent populations of HUV EC and permit the serial propagation of HUV EC populations in vitro?

The Identification of Endothelial Cell Growth Factor (ECGF): It has been the experience of most laboratories that the HUV EC undergoes only a limited number of population doublings in vitro. Since low seed density HUV EC populations do not proliferate in Medium 199 and 20% fetal bovine serum (FBS), one can argue that FBS does not contain the requisite growth factors required for HUV EC proliferation. This argument is an extension of the hypothesis, initially proposed by Sato and his colleagues, that serum provides a complex array of growth factors and hormones for cell growth in vitro (10, 11). Unfortunately, the addition of the traditional hormones and growth factors (epidermal growth factor (EGF), platelet-derived growth factor (PDGF), nerve growth factor (NGF), fibroblast growth factor (FGF), insulin-like growth factors (IGF-I, IGF-II), thrombin, insulin and transferrin) individually or in combination with FBS does not extend the proliferative capability of the HUV EC in vitro. However, the addition of a neutral extract prepared from either bovine brain, hypothalamus or pituitary does promote the growth and extend the life span of HUV EC populations in culture (12). This initial observation led to the development of a very sensitive HUV EC growth assay which enabled us to characterize the biochemical nature of endothelial cell growth factor (ECGF) from bovine neural tissue (13).

The Biological Chemistry of Endothelial Cell Growth Factor: Biologically active preparations of crude ECGF can be readily prepared by extraction of bovine neural tissue at pH 7.0 and low ionic strength (12). Characterization of the neutral extract by gel exclusion chromatography and preparative isoelectric focusing indicates that ECGF possesses a high Mr (between 70,000 and 150,000 daltons) and an anionic pI (between pH 4 and 6). Characterization of ECGF prepared by extraction from bovine neural tissue at pH 7.0 and high ionic strength suggests that ECGF possesses a low Mr (between 17,000 and 25,000 daltons) and an anionic pI (between pH 4 and 6). The high Mr form of ECGF and the low Mr form of ECGF are related since it is possible to generate the low Mr form of ECGF from the high Mr form by either acidification to pH 4.5 with a weak acid, increasing the ionic strength or the addition of ethanol (14). The characterization of high Mr and low Mr forms of ECGF is consistent with the identification of high and low Mr forms for other growth factors such as EGF (15,16), the IGF's (17) and NGF (18).

The low Mr form of ECGF has been purified to near homogeneity. ECGF is defined as a single chain protein with a Mr of 22,000 daltons and an isoelectric point between pH 5 and 6. It is biologically active in the HUV EC growth assay in the low nanogram range (14). It is also capable of stimulating the incorporation of (^3H)-thymidine into DNA in Balb/c 3T3 cells in the low nanogram range (14). The biological activity of ECGF is destroyed by heat (60°C, 30 min), strong acids and bases, ionic detergents, trypsin and pronase (12). The biological activity of highly purified preparations of ECGF is quite labile but can be preserved at -80°C in neutral buffers containing 50% glycerol for short periods. Therefore, the use of crude preparations of ECGF for the routine maintenance of HUV EC cultures, is recommended.

The physical properties of ECGF clearly demonstrate its unique biochemical character. Although bovine neural tissue is a rich source of FGF, a potent Balb/c 3T3 cell mitogen, the physical properties of ECGF suggest that these mitogens belong to different families of growth factors. Since bovine brain FGF is a cationic mitogen with a Mr of approximately 13,000 daltons (19), it is physically unrelated to ECGF. Biological activities similar to those described for ECGF have recently been isolated and characterized from bovine retina as eye-derived growth factor (20) and retina-derived growth factor (21) and from bovine pituitary (22) and brain (23) as anionic pI-FGF. Each of these factors possesses a common anionic pI with molecular weights in the range of 22,000 to 12,000 daltons. We have also observed forms of ECGF with molecular weights smaller than 22,000 daltons (23). The lower Mr forms of ECGF may result from proteolytic digestion of the 22,000 dalton form of ECGF during the extraction from bovine tissue at pH 4.5 (14,23).

Biological Attributes of Endothelial Cell Growth Factor: The ability of ECGF to stimulate the growth of quiescent populations of HUV EC in the presence of FBS is the single most important attribute of the growth factor (12,13). The mitogenic activity of ECGF is independent of HUV EC seed density in the presence of a human fibronectin (HFN) matrix (12). Quiescent populations of HUV EC divide in the presence of ECGF with a generation time of approximately 30 to 36 hours.

The second attribute of ECGF is the ability of the mitogen to promote the serial propagation of HUV EC cultures. We have demonstrated (12) that supplementation with FBS, ECGF and HFN matrix can extend the life span of HUV EC to at least 40 cummulative population doublings (CPD). This represents at least 15 passages at a constant split ratio of 1:5. Although the HUV EC population appears to increase size as a function of age in vitro; the extracellular concentration of FVIII:Ag and population doubling time does not significantly change (12). Although we have observed fewer intracellular FVIII:Ag-containing granules in populations of HUV EC beyond 35 CPD, this qualitative decrease in intracellular FVIII:Ag appears to be associated with only the highly senescent cells within the HUV EC population.

The third attribute of ECGF is the ability of the mitogen to reduce the concentration of FBS required for maximum HUV EC growth. We have previously demonstrated that at a constant concentration of FBS, HUV EC growth is proportional to the concentration of ECGF. Titration curves of ECGF biological activity have proved useful during the purification of ECGF as an index of specific activity (14,23). Likewise, HUV EC growth is also proportional to the concentration of FBS at constant concentrations of ECGF (12). Half-maximum growth is routinely achieved at 2.5% (v/v) FBS. These titration curves have proved useful in the evaluation of other growth factors and hormones as potential HUV EC mitogens. We have demonstrated that insulin, transferrin, EGF and thrombin are indeed HUV EC mitogens but only at reduced concentrations of FBS and in the presence of ECGF (24). PDGF, cationic FGF, hydrocortisone, IGF-I and II does not stimulate the growth of low density HUV EC populations under these conditions (24). These observations are consistent with our previous report that hypophysectomized platelet-poor plasma-derived serum can support the growth of HUV EC in the presence of ECGF (12). We anticipate that these results will have value in the formulation of a serum-free, hormone-supplemented medium for the growth of HUV EC populations.

The Differentiation of Human Umbilical Vein Endothelial Cells: The ability of ECGF to support the serially propagation of HUV EC populations naturally led us to study the limitations of the mitogen. Experiments were designed to determine whether HUV EC populations could survive in culture in the absence of ECGF. We observed that HUV EC cultures maintained in the absence of ECGF do not proliferate, but instead, organize into three dimensional, capillary-like structures (25).

The tubular structures were determined to be endothelial cell-derived by a variety of criteria. Transmission electron microscopy revealed that the smallest tubes consisted of a single cell which had wrapped around granular and amorphous debris to form a lumen. These structures contained numerous Weibel-Palade bodies, anatomical structures which are unique to the endothelial cell (25). The cellular junctions which formed the tubular structure consisted of interdigitations of plasma membrane (25). These junctions are quite tight since the tubular structures can withstand the injection of fluorescent dyes into lumen under N_2 pressure. In this instance, the dye can be visualized as being restricted to the luminal area of the tube as it traverses through the tubular structures. These data suggest that the lumin of the tube is continuous for long distances in the culture dish including those areas at which branch points exist. The endothelial cell origin of these capillary-like vessels is further illustrated by immunofluorescent staining of the three dimensional tubular structures for human Factor VIII:Ag (24,25). In addition to containing the Factor VIII:Ag, the tubular structures also contain human urokinase and fibronectin (25).

A second type of tubular structure also appears in the ECGF-free environment. After approximately two months in culture, the HUV EC tubular structures increase in size to form macroscopic tubes (25). Since these larger structures lift off the surface of the dish and float in the culture medium, they can therefore be physically removed from the cell culture environment. Digestion of the macroscopic structure with trypsin readily yields a suspension of viable cells which exclude trypan blue (25). The tube-derived cells are capable of proliferation when introduced into the ECGF-supplemented medium (12,25). The tube-derived cells proliferate to form a confluent monolayer with the morphological characteristics of large vessel endothelial cells. In addition, cells derived in this manner stain positively for human Factor VIII:Ag by immunofluorescence, a further confirmation of their endothelial cell character (25). Together these data strongly suggest that the organized tubular structures are constructed from and contain viable HUVEC. Furthermore, the ability to generate a proliferative population of HUV EC from the organized structures suggest that the tubular, capillary-like structures represent a state of non-terminal HUV EC differentiation (24,25). It should be noted that these experiments can be performed independent of the level of CPD of the HUV EC population.

The Biochemical Mechanism of Human Endothelial Cell Differentiation: The observation that HUV EC organization occures in an environment which minimizes HUV EC proliferation suggests that the endothelial cell itself was capable of providing the information requisite for organization. Other investigators have observed similar endothelial cell behavior with bovine capillary cells in culture (26). Under conditions in which the organizational behavior is enhanced, the presence of sarcoma-conditioned medium and ECGF were demonstrated to be important components of this in vitro angiogenesis system (26). Since (i) sarcoma conditioned medium is widely recognized to contain autocrine growth factor signals and (ii) angiogenesis has historically been postulated to be a growth-oriented phenomena, it was surprising that HUV EC organization should occur under conditions where HUV EC proliferation is minimized (25). We therefore carefully assessed the ability of ECGF to promote HUV EC organizational behavior in vitro.

The organization of HUV EC into viable, tubular structures from a confluent monolayer in vitro, occurs after one to two months in the presence of FBS (25). The addition of either a HFN matrix, ECGF or both to the FBS-supplemented medium does not decrease but indeed increases the time necessary for tube formation (25). Although these data confirmed the reciprocal relationship between HUV-ec growth and differentiation, they did not provide additional insight into the biochemical mechanism of HUV EC organization.

Since HUV EC growth-stimulating signals appeared to delay rather than promote tube development in vitro, we therefore chose to examine the extracellular matrix (ECM) as a source of this information. A simple recycling experiment was designed to evaluate the role of HUV EC-derived ECM in the development of the tubular structures. Confluent dishes of HUV EC were gently treated with trypsin in a manner identical to the general experience of routine subcultivation (12). However, instead of discarding the cell culture dish, the trypsin-treated dish was recycled and the viable HUV EC seeded back into the trypsin-exposed ECM at a cell seed density of 5×10^4 cells per cm^2 in the presence of 10% FBS. The HUV EC population did not proliferate, but instead migrated to form the HUV EC organized structures after one week in vitro (25). Although other interpretations were possible, the data suggested that trypsin was responsible for the proteolytic modification of latent ECM-derived information which stimulated the process of tube development in culture. Confirmation of these suspicions were obtained by the limited digestion of purified HFN with trypsin. A HFN matrix was prepared as previously described (12) and briefly exposed to trypsin. After inhibition of trypsin with soybean trypsin inhibitor, populations of HUV EC were seeded into the culture and supplemented with 10% FBS. HUV EC tube development was observed after only one week in culture (25).

Since endothelial cells are not exposed to trypsin in vivo, other serine proteases were examined as surrogate trypsin candidates. Using an identical assay system, purified HFN matrices were subjected to digestion with purified human alpha thrombin, human plasminogen activator, and human plasmin. We observed that only human plasmin was capable of creatively modifying HFN in a manner which stimulated HUV EC organization (25).

Significance to Tumor Angiogenesis and the Developmental Biology of the Vascular Tree: It has been recognized for almost five decades that fibrinolysis is correlated with tumor growth and metastasis. Furthermore, plasmin generation has been strongly implicated in the vascular physiology of wound healing and angiogenesis (27,28). Similar correlations have been made concerning the relationship of HFN to cell migration, angiogenesis and wound healing (29,30,31). It is therefore not surprising that HUV EC organization in vitro should involve plasminogen activation and fibronectin as key intermediates in the generation of these morphological events. However, what is surprising is the requirement for creative proteolytic modification of latent fibronectin to produce fibronectin-derived information signals. It is the recognition of this proteolytic activation mechanism which leads us to suggest that cells deposit latent biological information in their extracellular matrix as a memory source. When challenged by a pathological event, this latent information is processed by specific hydrolytic enzyme systems which generate biologically active extracellular matrix-derived signals which direct the organizational behavior of the cells at the site of challenge. The interaction between fibronectin and plasmin may be only a single example of perhaps a family of similar senarios which may provide direction for cell migration, proliferation and organization in three dimensions. We envision these biochemical events to involve complicated cascade systems in which hydrolytic enzymes, growth factors, latent matrix information signals and inhibitors interact with high affinity binding sites present on the extracellular matrix to create biochemical effectors which modulate cell behavior.

Additional support for such pathways can be derived from the interaction between growth factors and very specific arginine esteropeptidases. It has been observed that at least two of the traditional growth factors, EGF and NGF, are complexed to specific binding proteins (15,16,18). These binding proteins are serine proteases and play a significant role in the posttranscriptional modification of these respective growth factors (15,18). Since (i) the growth factor binding proteins are complexed to their growth factors as binding protein:growth factor complexes, (ii) the growth factors are stored as enzyme:hormone complexes and (iii) these high Mr growth factor complexes are found to circulate in plasma, the binding proteins may play a more prominent role than was initially anticipated by earlier biosynthetic studies (15). It has been suggested that the binding proteins for EGF and NGF may belong to the plasminogen activator family of proteases (33). Significant kinin-generating activity has also been associated with the growth factor binding proteins (32). Although the ability of these proteases to activate plasminogen has been confirmed (34), these enzymes possess approximately 10 to 20% of the enzymatic activity usually observed with purified urine or tissue-derived fibrinolytic agents (35,36). Nevertheless, it is tempting to speculate that the binding proteins participate in the process of HUV EC organization by their ability to mimic plasminogen activators as fibrinolytic agents.

References

(1) Gimbrone, M.A., Jr., Cotran, R.S. and Folkman, J., J. Cell Biol., 60, 673-684 (1974).

(2) Gimbrone, M.A., Jr., Prog. Hemostasis Thromb., 3, 1-28, (1976).

(3) Jaffe, E.A., Nachman, R.L., Becker, C.G. and Minick, C.R., J. Clin. Invest., 52, 841-850, (1973).

(4) Booyse, F.M., Sedlak, B.J. and Rafelson, M.E., Jr., Thromb. Diath. Haemorrh., 34, 825-839 (1975).

(5) Mueller, S.N., Rosen, E.M. and Levine, E.M., Science, 207, 889-891 (1980).

(6) Schwartz, S.M., In Vitro, 14, 966-980, (1978).

(7) Duthu, G.S. and Smith, J.R., J. Cell Physiol., 103, 385-892 (1980).

(8) Weibel E.R. and Palade G.E., J. Cell Biol., 23:101-112, (1964).

(9) Jaffee E.A., Mosher D.F., J. Exp. Med., 147:1779-1791 (1978).

(10) Hayashi, I. and Sato, G.H., Nature, 259, 132-134 (1976).

(11) Hutchings, S.E. and Sato, G.H., Proc. Natl. Acad. Sci. U.S.A., 75, 901-904 (1978).

(12) Maciag T., Hoover G.A., Stemerman M.B. and Weinstein R., J. Cell Biol, 91:420-426, (1981).

(13) Maciag, T., Cerundolo, J., Ilsley, S., Kelley, P.R. and Forand, R., Proc. Natl. Acad. Sci. U.S.A., 76, 5674-5678 (1979).

(14) Maciag, T., Hoover, G.A. and Weinstein, R., J. Biol. Chem., 257, 5333-5336, (1982).

(15) Frey, P., Forand, R., Maciag, T., and Shooter, E.M., Proc. Natl. Acad. Sci. U.S.A., 76, 6294-6298 (1979).

(16) Taylor, J.M., Cohen, S. and Mitchell, W.M., Proc. Natl. Acad. Sci. U.S.A., 67, 164-171 (1970).

(17) Knauer, D.J. and Smith, G.L., Proc. Natl. Acad. Sci., U.S.A., 77, 7252-7256 (1981).

(18) Berger, E.A. and Shooter, E.M., Proc. Natl. Acad. Sci., U.S.A., 74, 3647-3651, 1977.

(19) Gospodarowicz, D., Bialecki, H. and Greenburg, G., J. Biol. Chem., 253, 3736-3743, (1978).

(20) Barritault, D., Arvuti, C. and Courtois, Y., Differentiation 18, 29-42 (1981).

(21) D'Amore, P., J. Cell Biol., 96, 192a (1982).

(22) Gambarini, A.G. and Armelin, H.A., J. Biol. Chem., 257, 9692-9697, (1982).

(23) Lemmon, S.K., Riley, M.C., Thomas, K.A., Hoover, G.A., Maciag, T. and Bradshaw, R.A., J. Cell Biol., 95, 162-169 (1982).

(24) Maciag T., Hoover G.A., van der Spek J., Stemerman M.B., Weinstein R., Cold Spring Harbor Conferences on Cell Proliferation, Vol. 9, 525-538 (1982).

(25) Maciag T., Kadish J., Wilkins L., Stemerman M.B. and Weinstein R., J. Cell Biol., 94:511-520, (1982).

(26) Folkman, J. and Haudenschild, C.C., Nature, 288, 551-556 (1980).

(27) Hiramoto, R., Bernecky, J., Jurandowski, J. and
      Pressman, D., Cancer Res., 20, 592-593, (1960).

(28) Unkeless, J.C., Tobia, A., Ossowski, L., Quigley,
      J.P., Rifkin, D.B. and Reich, E., J. Exp. Med.,
      137, 85-112 (1973).

(29) Wood, S., Arch. Pathol., 66, 550-568 (1958).

(30) Gordon, S., Unkeless, J.C., and Cohn, Z.A., J. Exp.
      Med., 140, 995-1010, (1974).

(31) Clark, C.R. and Clark, E.L., Am. J. Anat., 64, 251-301,
      1939.

(32) Bothwell, M.A., Wilson, W.H. and Shooter, E.M., J. Biol.
      Chem., 254, 7297-7294, 1979.

(33) Orenstein, N.S., Dvorak, H.F., Blanchard, M.H. and
      Young, M., Proc. Natl. Acad. Sci. U.S.A., 75, 5497-5501
      (1978).

(34) Maciag, T., Frey, P., Weinstein, R., Canalis, E. and
      Shooter, E.M., in "Plasma and Cellular Modulatory Proteins,
      (D. Bing editor) Center for Blood Research, Boston, MA,
      95-108 (1981).

(35) Astedt, B. and Holmberg, L., Nature 261, 595-597 (1976).

(36) Soberano, M.E., Ong, E.B., Johnson, A.J., Levy, M.
      and Shoellmann, G., Biochim. Biophys. Acta., 445, 763-
      773 (1976).

3T3 Cell Growth Initiation and Multiplication in Defined Medium Supplemented with Growth Factors and Hormones That Replace Serum

Dieter Paul

Institut für Toxikologie, Medizinische Fakultät der Universität Hamburg, Grindelallee 117, D-2000 Hamburg 13, FRG

Introduction

Most mammalian cells in culture do not grow in basal tissue culture medium unless serum is added as medium supplement. It is clear that several growth factors present in serum support 3T3 cell proliferation (1,2). Using swiss 3T3 mouse cells cultured in a suboptimal culture medium (DME) this laboratory has been involved for several years in characterizing serum growth factors in attempts to use them to substitute for serum in order to grow 3T3 cells in chemically defined medium (3). Other laboratories have shown that by optimizing the composition of culture media the amount of serum protein required for clonal growth of various cell types can drastically be reduced (4,5). Many cell types, most notably of transformed phenotype, can be cultured successfully in serum-free medium supplemented with hormones and growth factors (9). However, extensive work during the last few years aimed at culturing 3T3 cells in defined medium has suggested that in addition to hormones such as insulin, hydrocortisone and growth factors such as Fibroblast Growth Factor (FGF) (6), Epidermal Growth Factor (EGF) (7) or Platelet-derived Growth Factor (PDGF) (8) additional still unknown activities in serum are necessary to replace serum growth promoting activity (10-12).

We have reported that 3T3 cells require a survival factor present in serum (3,13) and have partially purified the activity (2). In its presence 3T3 or SV40 virus-transformed 3T3 (SV3T3) cells survive for long periods of time in serum-free cultures (3). In addition, we have identified and partially purified an additional activity from serum, Serum Growth Factor II (SGF II) (2), which replaces most of the 3T3 cell growth promoting activity present in 3T3 cell-depleted serum. Here we report that 3T3 cells cultured in serum-free medium supplemented with 2 hormones and 3 pure or highly purified growth factors initiate DNA synthesis and progress through at least two cycles as in the presence of 10% serum.

Materials and Methods

Cell cultures. Swiss 3T3-4a and SV3T3 cells were obtained from Dr. Marguerite Vogt (Salk Institute) and cultured routinely in DME supplemented with 10% calf serum in Falcon or Nunc plastic dishes (maximal density (3T3): 2×10^6 cells per 10 cm dish) and incubated at 37° C in a humidified 10% CO_2/90% air incubator. Cells were transferred after treatment with trypsin (0.05 µg/ml) at room temperature. Autoradiographic analysis after (^{3}H)-thymidine incorporation (2) for 40 hours showed that cells are free of mycoplasma infection and that the labeling index of confluent 3T3 cultures never exceeded 1- 2%. For experiments an enriched medium (MX-76) was utilized containing common components of DME or F12 (minus thymidine) media at whichever concentration is higher. Present, but at concentrations different from those in DME or F12 media are (in mg/l): Ala:18; AsN:50; Gly:100; Hypoxanthine:25; Biotin:0.2; Vitamin B_{12}:0.005; NaCl:6400. Additional components: OH-Proline:20; p-aminobenzoic acid:1; Ascorbic acid:0.025; Glutathion (red):1; Linoleic acid: 0.8.

For purification of SGF II mitogenic activity of fractions was assayed in 3T3 cells in the presence of insulin (1 µg/ml) and dexamethasone (500 ng/ml) by determination of acid-insoluble radioactivity after incubating the cultures with (^{3}H)-thymidine (10 µCi/dish, 6µM) from 16-25 hrs after addition of the fractions to be tested. Survival Factor activity wa assayed in SV3T3 cell cultures in serum-free medium. In the absence of any additions cells attach and start spreading within an hour after plating but they round up and eventually come off the dish in an over night assay. Presence of Survival Factor activity is easily recognized in cultures in which cells are still attached and spread up to a week after plating.

Assays for DNA synthesis initiation and cell multiplication in serum-free medium were usually conducted starting 24 hrs after plating trypsin-treated cells in medium containing Survival Factor (1 µg/ml). Materials to be tested were added at 24 hrs after plating the cells and cultures were incubated for additional 24 hrs. (^{3}H)-thymidine was present in such cultures from 30-48 hrs after plating. For determination of cell number per culture, cells were trypsinized at different times after start of the assay and counted in a Coulter Counter.

Serum fractionation. The preparation of SGF II and Survival Factor from calf serum will be described in detail in a forthcoming paper (D.Paul, manuscript in preparation). Briefly, for preparation of SGF II calf serum was extracted with chloroform/methanol as described (14). Fraction B was dried, dissolved in water and subjected to gel fil-

tration on G200-Sephadex (pH 2). Active fractions eluting at a position equivalent to <3000 daltons were pooled, lyophilized and run on
a G25-Sephadex column (pH 7). Fractions containing activity were pooled and adsorbed to a DEAE-cellulose column. After washing the column
the activity was eluted at low pH (pH 2) and the material concentrated
by ultrafiltration using a UMO-5 filter (Amicon).The material does
not show appreciable adsorption at 280 nm and does not stain with ninhydrin unless subjected to acid hydrolysis (6 M HCl, 130° C for 24 hrs).

For preparation of Survival Factor, calf serum was subjected to
gel filtration at pH 2 (G100-Sephadex). After neutralization of pooled
active fractions the supernatant was extracted with chloroform/metha-
nol (14).The resulting fraction A was acidified and the activity recovered by precipitation at pH 4.7. Active material was adsorbed to Con-
A-Sepharose (1 M NaCl, 0.02 M phosphate buffer pH 7) and eluted with
methyl-α-D-mannopyranoside (100 mM). After dialysis the material was
further fractionated by isoelectric focussing in a sucrose gradient
using ampholytes (Pharmacia) pH 3.5-10. Dialyzed material (pI 4.3-4.8)
was purified by re-isoelectric focusing using ampholytes pH 4.0 - 6.0.
Active fractions (pI 4.4-4.7) were pooled, dialyzed and stored at
-20° C.

Results and Discussion

Previous results have indicated that growth factors in serum
which support growth of 3T3 cells can be replaced by FGF, insulin and
dexamethasone in the presence of low serum (12,15).However, when the
depleted medium is removed and then replaced by fresh, serum-free medium, the response to FGF,insulin and dexamethasone is much reduced,
presumably because additional distinct growth factors present in depleted serum are required for DNA synthesis initiation (Table I).When
cultures are washed before fresh serum-free medium is added back, the
response to serum is unchanged, showing that the responsiveness of
cells is not altered by the manipulations (Table I). It is concluded,
that FGF,insulin and dexamethasone do not replace serum completely and
that additional activities are required to initiate DNA synthesis in
serum-free cultures. Similar conclusions have been drawn with EGF(10)
or PDGF (D.Paul, unpublished observations) as replacements for FGF in
such systems.

The composition of the culture medium very much affects the response of the cells to serum. For example, it has been shown that the
serum requirement for clonal growth of various cell types is reduced
by improving the medium and the general culture conditions (4,5).We
have developed an improved medium (MX-76) which has been used for the

TABLE I. Cells (10^5 per 3 cm dish) were cultured in 0.3% serum.At
day 3 additions were made as indicated into untreated cultures in depleted medium or into cultures where the medium
was removed and replaced with fresh serum-free medium with
or without washes with serum-free medium as indicated(FGF:
10 ng/ml; insulin:1 µg/ml; Dexamethasone: 500 ng/ml).Cul-
tures were pulsed with(^{3}H)-thymidine and prepared for auto-
radiography.Results are presented as percent labeled nuclei
(average of 3 cultures).The error did not exceed ± 3%.

Initiation of DNA synthesis in 3T3 cells in depleted and serum-free medium

Addition	Depleted medium (0.3 % serum)	Fresh serum-free medium		
		no wash	1 wash	2 washes
	(percent labeled nuclei)			
No	4	3	2	2
Serum (10%)	96	97	97	100
Insulin + dexamethasone	30	16	12	8
FGF	33	18	12	8
Insulin + dexamethasone + FGF	88	65	45	30

experiments shown here and the composition of which is outlined in Materials and Methods. Although similar to the formulation that was
found useful for clonal growth of 3T3 cells in the presence of low serum levels (4), it is far from optimal and much work is required to im-
rove its composition in order to increase the mitogenic response of
the cells to growth factors in the absence of serum.

The initiation of DNA synthesis in 3T3 cells in response to insulin and dexamethasone with or without FGF proceeds more efficently in
the presence of SGF II which we have isolated from calf serum (2).Its
activity is low when assayed alone in cultures in which depleted medium has been washed out, but it increases the response of the cells to
insulin and dexamethasone (Table II). Using this assay, SGF II has
been highly purified by procedures which are briefly outlined in Materials and Methods.Its moelcular weight is approximately 500 daltons as
judged by ultrafiltration and by gel filtration on G25-Sephadex.The activity is heat stable (3 min 100° C). Quantitative determination of
SGF II is achieved by staining with ninhydrin after hydrolysis with
HCl (the active material does not stain with ninhydrin). Preliminary
data indicate that when ∿50 ng/ml of the highly purified material are

TABLE II. Cells (10^5/3 cm dish) were cultured in the presence of 0.3% calf serum.Some cultures were used at day 2 without medium change.In parallel cultures the medium was removed at day 2, the cultures washed with serum-free medium and fresh serum-free medium was added back to the cultures with the additions as indicated.Cultures were pulsed with (^{3}H)thymidine, prepared for autoradiography and the fraction of labeled nuclei was scored.See legend of Table I for further details.

Initiation of DNA synthesis in 3T3 cells by SGF II and hormones

Additions	Mitogenic Response (percent labeled nuclei)	
	fresh,serum-free medium	depleted medium (0.3% serum)
Serum (10 %)	96	98
No additions	2	3
SGF II (50 ng/ml)	5	8
Insulin (1 ug/ml)	5	22
Dexamethasone (500 ng/ml)	3	4
Insulin + Dexamethasone	20	39
Insulin + Dexamethasone + SGF II	42	38

added to the cultures in the presence of insulin and dexamethasone, maximal response is obtained.As can be seen in Table II most of the growth promoting activity present in depleted medium which is required for optimal DNA synthesis initiation in response to FGF,insulin and dexamethasone (Table I) can be replaced by SGF II in cultures essentially free of serum (Table II).

In order to assay DNA synthsis initiation in 3T3 cells in the complete absence of serum, it is necessary to plate cells in serum-free medium since it cannot be excluded that traces of serum remain in the cultures after washing cells that have been plated in serum (Table II). We have found previously that 3T3 cells attach in the absence of serum but that they require Survival Factor to survive for more that 1-2 days (2,3,13).SV3T3 cells, which require identical survival activity in serum die within 12-24 hrs after plating them in serum-free medium (3).Therefore, we have used SV3T3 cells to assay for Survival Factor for reasons of convenience (over night assay).Using the procedure oulined in.Materials and Methods we have highly purified Survival Factor from calf serum. The molecular weight of Survival Factor is

150-158,000 daltons as judged from gel filtration on calibrated G200-Sephadex columns and from SDS-polyacrylamide gels and has an isoelectric point of $4.5^{\pm}$ 0.2. The activity is heat labile and is lost after incubation with trypsin. The data suggest that it is a glycoprotein. The activity of Survival Factor cannot be replaced by coating the dishes with poly-L-lysine, poly-DL-ornithine or poly-L-histidine (c.f.ref.4).

When 3T3 cells plated in serum-free medium were incubated in serum-free medium, 10-20% of the cells detached within 24 hrs (Table IV). Remaining cells did not show significant mitogenic rseponse in the presence of the mixture FGF, insulin and dexamethasone although cells were intact as shown by their responsiveness to serum (Table III). When cells were plated into medium containing 1 µg/ml ($\sim$10 nM) Survival Factor only or in combination with SGF II did not stimulate cells to initiate DNA synthesis. However, addition of FGF, insulin and dexamethasone 24 hr after plating cells in the presence of Survival Factor and SGF II leads to initiation of DNA synthesis as effectively as in response to serum as shown by (^{3}H)-thymidine incorporation data and by autoradiographic analysis (Table III). Cells plated in Survival Factor only (data not shown) or in SGF II only were less responsive that in the presence of SGF II plus Survival Factor (Table III). Taken together, the results indicate that for optimal growth induction two serum factors (SGF II and Survival Factor) and FGF, insulin and dexamethasone are required to replace serum activity in DNA synthesis initiation assays (Table III).

When cells plated out in the presence of Survival Factor and SGF-II were subsequently stimulated by FGF, insulin and dexamethasone, they divide about twice and few cells proceed through further divisions (Table IV). Cells which were plated in SGF II only and then stimulated with FGF, insulin and dexamethasone, 80% of the cells enter S (Table III) but they double only once within 96 hrs (Table IV). It thus appears Survival Factor is required to keep cells attached and responsive for longer periods. Presumably, additional hormones, growth factors or carrier proteins for lipids and ions, nutrients (lipids) or trace metals become limiting after cells have proceeded through a few cycles in chemically defined medium described here. Alternatively, growth factors and hormones can be depleted within the time of the assay resulting in limited cell proliferation (Table IV). Addition of pure human transferrin (1 µg/ml) obtained from Behringwerke and further purified on DEAE-Sephadex A-50 (P. Aisen, personal communication) did not substantially improve the responsiveness of the cells. Similar results as shown in Tables III and IV have been obtained using EGF (20 ng/ml) or

TABLE III

Initiation of DNA synthesis in 3T3 cells in serum-free medium by growth factors and hormones

Additions		Mitogenic Response	
0 hrs	24 hrs	cpm per culture	percent labeled nuclei
No	No	159	4
No	Ins	180	4
No	Ins + Dx	328	4
No	Ins + Dx + FGF	568	7
No	Serum (10 %)	8395	86
SF + SGF II	No	257	4
SF + SGF II	Ins	3197	37
SF + SGF II	Ins + Dx	6427	45
SF + SGF II	Ins + Dx + FGF	11388	95
SF + SGF II	Serum (10 %)	11130	95
SGF II	No	227	4
SGF II	Ins	2370	-
SGF II	Ins + Dx	5455	30
SGF II	Ins + Dx + FGF	7622	80
SGF II	Serum (10 %)	7818	92
Serum (0.3%)	No	--	4
Serum (0.3%)	Ins	--	25
Serum (0.3%)	Ins + Dx + FGF	--	88
Serum (0.3%)	Serum (10 %)	--	95

Cells in stock dishes were thoroughly rinsed, trypsinized washed with serum-free medium (three times) and plated at 10^5 cells per 5 cm dish in MX-76 medium without serum in the presence of the additions as indicated in the left column (0-time). Twenty four hours later additions were made as indicated in the second column. Cultures were then pulsed with (3H)thymidine from 42-48 hours and TCA precipitable radioactivity determined. The results are shown in cpm per culture (the error did not exceed $\pm$ 8%). Parallel cultures were incubated from 24-52 hours with (3H)-thymidine from 24-52 hours and prepared for autoradiography. The results are expressed in percent labeled nuclei. Additions of growth factors and hormones as in Table II. SF, Survival Factor: 1 μg/ml; FGF: 10 ng/ml.

TABLE IV

Induction of cell division in serum-free medium
by growth factors and hormones

| Additions | | C e l l   n u m b e r   p e r   d i s h   x 10^{-4} | | | |
O hrs	24 hrs	24 hrs	54 hrs	80 hrs	96 hrs
No	No	13 ± 2	4 ± 1	O	--
No	Ins+dx+FGF		8 ± 1	2	--
No	serum		23 ± 1	66 ± 4	--
SF + SGF II	No	17 ± 2	15 ± 3	15 ± 3	14 ± 3
SF + SGF II	Ins+dx		- -	22 ± 4	22 ± 4
SF + SGF II	Ins+dx+FGF		29 ± 4	52 ± 5	58 ± 3
SF + SGF II	serum		31 ± 2	80 ± 7	--
SGF II	No	15 ± 1	11 ± 3	8 ± 4	--
SGF II	Ins+dx		- -	12 ± 2	--
SGF II	Ins+dx+FGF		23 ± 4	30 ± 3	28 ± 2
SGF II	serum		29 ± 4	56 ± 8	--

Cells (10^5/ 5 cm dish) were plated as described in the legend to Table
III in serum free medium in the presence of the additions as indicated
in the left column.Twenty-four hrs later additions were made to triplicate cultures as described in Table III.Cells were trypsinized at the
time of the additions (24 hrs), at 54, 80 or 96 hrs and counted in a
Coulter Counter.Results are expressed as average cell number per dish
± error.(SF,Survival Factor;dx,dexamethasone;ins, insulin).

PDGF (0.5 U/ml) instead of FGF (D.Paul, unpublished observations).Thus, in 3T3 cells
FGF or EGF or PDGF show similar mitogenic properties. The results presented in Table III and additional data not shown (D.Paul, unpublished observations) indicate
that the effects of growth factors and hormones contributing to the mitogenic stimulus are synergistic and not additive. Insulin or dexamethasone or FGF induce DNA
synthesis in a small fraction of the cell population, whereas the mixture of FGF,
insulin,dexamethasone, SGF II and Survival Factor lead to an effective mitogenic
stimulus in the bulk of the cells which then proceed to divide (Table IV).

Different cell types appear to require a different composition of a growth
factor mixture for DNA synthesis initiation (2,9). For example, rat embryo fibroblasts in secondary cultures are not responsive to dexamethasone or Survival Fac-
tor(D.Paul, unpublished observations).Primary fetal rat liver cells (16) do not require Survival Factor cr FGF or EGF although cells display EGF-receptors(17).Tri-
iodothyronine (T_3) stimulates proliferation in these cells (18) wheras T_3 is inactive in 3T3 cells or in rat embryo fibroblasts. Prostaglandin E_1 but not $F_{2\alpha}$ stimulates DNA synthesis in primary fetal rat liver cells (19) wheras the converse

response is observed in 3T3 cells (20). Thus, it is becoming increasingly clear from studies in cell culture that locally active tissue factors such as prostaglandins (20), which are characteristic for specific micro-environments, and cell attachment to substrata (21) (basal membrane) are as important elements as systemic factors in affecting the responsiveness of cells to mitogenic stimuli. In addition, the situation is further complicated by the observation that endogenous growth inhibitors of mammalian cell proliferation (e. g. interferon (22), corticotropin (23), kidney epthelial cell growth inhibitors (24) presumably are also involved in regulating cell proliferation.

Acknowledgments

I thank Ms. A. Piasecki for excellent technical assistance, Drs. D. Gospodarowitz (UC San Francisco) and K. Brown (Cambridge University) for gifts of FGF and EGF, respectively. The support of Fr. H. Marquardt is gratefully appreciated. This work was supported by a grant of the Deutsche Forschungsgemeinschaft (Bonn).

References

1. Holley, R.W., Nature 258: 487 (1975)
2. Paul, D., Ristow, H.J., Rupniak, H.T. and Messmer, T.O. in : Molecular Control of Proliferation and Differentiation, (W. Rutter, ed), Acad. Press, N.Y. 8, 65 (1977)
3. Paul, D., Lipton, A., Klinger, I. Proc. Natl. Acad. Sci. USA 68: 645 (1971)
4. Shipley, G.D. and Ham, R.G. In Vitro 17: 656-670 (1981)
5. McKeehan, W.L., McKeehan, K.A. and Calkins, D. J. Biol. Chem. 256: 2973 (1981)
6. Gospodarowicz, D. J. Biol Chem. 250: 2515-2520 (1975)
7. Savage, C.R., and Cohen, S. J. Biol. Chem. 247: 7609-7611 (1972)
8. Heldin, C.H., Westermask, B. and Wastesen, C. Proc. Nat. Acad. Sci. USA 76: 3722-3725 (1979)
9. Bottenstein, J., Hayashi, I., Hutchings, S., Masui, H., Mather, J., McClure, D.G., Ohasa, S., Rizzino, A., Sato, G., Serrero, G. and Wofe, R. Methods Enzymol. 58: 94-109 (1979)
10. Mierzejewski, K. and Rozengurt, E., Biochem. Biophys. Communic. 83: 874-880 (1978)
11. Serrero, G.R., McClure, D.B. and Sato, G. in Hormones and Cell Culture (Ross, R. and Sato, G. eds). Cold Spring Harb, N.Y.: Cold Spring Harbor Laboratory pp. 523-530 (1979).
12. Gospodarowicz, D. and Moran,J.S. Proc.Nat.Acad. Sci.USA 71: 4584-4588 (1974)
13. Lipton, A., Paul,D., Henahan,M. and Holley, R.W. Expt.Cell Res. 74: 466-470 (1972)
14. Kaplan,A.E. and Bartholomew,J.C.Expt. Cell Res. 73: 262-266 (1972)
15. Holley,R.W., and Kiernan, J.A. Proc.Nat.Acad.Sci.USA. 71:2942-2946 (1974)
16. Leffert,H.L. and Paul, D. J.Cell Biol. 52: 559-568(1972)
17. Paul,D., Brown,K., Rupniak,H.T. and Ristow,H.J. In Vitro 14: 76-84 (1974)
18. Leffert,H.L. J.Cell Biol. 62: 792-801 (1974)
19. Leffert,H.L. In: Workshop on Rat Liver Pathology (Newberne,J. and Butler,W.eds) Elsevier Amsterdam pp 276 (1978)
20 Jimenez de Asua,L., O'Farrell,M.K.,Clingau,D. and Rudland,P.S, Proc.Nat.Acad. Sci.USA 74: 3845-3849 (1977).
21. Moscona,F. and Folkman, J. Nature 272: 345-347 (1978)
22. Balkwill,F. and Taylor-Papadimitron,J. Nature 274: 798-800 (1978)
23. Hornsby,P.J. and Gill,G.N. Endocrinology 100:926-936 (1978)
24. Holley,R.W.,Böhlen,P.,Fava,R.,Baldwin,J.H., Kleeman,G. and Armour,R. Proc.Nat. Acad.Sci.USA 77:5989-5992 (1980)

Growth-Promoting Activity of Thrombin in Fibroblasts: Temporal Action and Early Biochemical Events in the G0 → G1 Transition

J. Pouysségur, J. C. Chambard, A. Franchi, G. L'Allemain, S. Paris, and E. Van Obberghen-Schilling

Centre de Biochemie, CNRS, Université de Nice, Parc Valrose, F-06034 Nice, France

INTRODUCTION

Polypeptide growth factors and hormones have been shown to play an essential role in the regulation of cell proliferation and cell differentiation. However, the molecular mechanisms by which these extracellular signals act on quiescent cells to induce the G0→G1 transition, DNA replication and subsequent cell division or differentiation are unknown. The introduction by Sato and coworkers of cell culture in serum-free hormone-supplemented medium (1) has greatly facilitated the experimental analysis of the mechanisms of growth factor action. The addition of purified growth-promoting polypeptides to G0-arrested fibroblasts induces a multiple array of biochemical events leading to activation of protein synthesis and subsequent DNA synthesis. Changes in ionic membrane permeability and in protein phosphorylation occur rapidly after stimulation (2-8). These changes, which appear to be ubiquitous, raise the central question of how distinct growth factor receptors translate the variety of external signals into a common activation of cellular metabolism and cell proliferation. The purpose of this paper is to present the growth-promoting activity of α-thrombin in serum-free conditions. We will analyze the temporal action of thrombin during the G0 → G1 transition of the cell cycle and the post-receptor, early-stimulated biochemical events : activation of a Na^+/H^+ exchange and stimulation of protein phosphorylation. This approach to the mode of action of growth factors was performed using a cell line of Chinese hamster lung fibroblasts (CCl39) which posesses the following interesting features : it is non-tumoral (9), it can reversibly enter a non-proliferative G0/G1 state (10), it grows in a chemically defined medium (11) and it is amenable to genetic analysis (12-13).

MATERIAL AND METHODS

Human α-thrombin (3,000 NIH units/mg) and bovine pancreas crystalline insulin (23.6 IU/mg) are from Sigma. For the sources of other materials, see our previous reports (4,8,9).

Cell Culture and Growth Arrest Conditions. The Chinese hamster lung fibroblast line CCl39 (ATCC) was maintained in Dulbecco's Modified Eagle's Medium supplemented with 5% Fetal Calf Serum (FCS). Cells were arrested in G0/G1 essentially as described (10): confluent monolayers were washed twice with serum-free medium and incubated for 30 hours in a serum-free mixture (1:1) of DMEM and Ham's medium (F12).

Measurements of Na^+, Rb^+ and H^+ Fluxes. Na^+ and Rb^+ influxes were measured as described in (4). Briefly, G0-arrested cells in 35mm-dishes were incubated, unless otherwise specified, in 1 ml of DMEM buffered with 20 mM Hepes, at 37°C. Activators: serum, purified growth factors, and the inhibitor, amiloride, were added 1 min before initiating the uptake. Uptakes were initiated by the addition of either $^{22}Na^+$ (2 μCi/ml) or $^{86}Rb^+$ (0.5 μCi/ml). For Na^+ uptake, ouabain was present at 5 mM.

Proton efflux was measured on cell suspensions essentially as described (14,15).

Protein Phosphorylation and SDS-PAGE. In standard experiments, G0-arrested cells were ^{32}P-labeled by incubation for 45 min in P_i-free DMEM containing 1 μM $^{32}P_i$ (100 μCi/ml) and buffered, at pH 7.40, with 20 mM Hepes. Cells were then incubated for an additional 15 min in the presence of serum and, where indicated, inhibitors. Cell monolayers were solubilized in SDS and proteins were reduced and separated on SDS-polyacrylamide slab gel electrophoresis (SDS-PAGE) as described (8).

[^3H]Thymidine Incorporation. For measurements of DNA synthesis, G0-arrested cells were incubated for 24 hours with 1 μCi/ml of [methyl-^3H] thymidine, 3 μM, in the presence of different concentrations of serum or growth factors. Thymidine incorporation into DNA or autoradiography were performed as reported (9).

pH Determination. Intracellular pH of quiescent CCl39 cells was determined using [^{14}C]5,5-dimethyl-2,4-oxazolidinedione, (^{14}C-DMO). Cells were incubated for 20 min at 37°C with 0.5 μCi/ml DMO (55 mCi/mmole) in the presence or absence of growth factors. Monolayers were then rapidly washed four times with cold PBS (washing took 7±1 sec). Extracellular and intracellular water space were determined respectively with [^{14}C]mannitol and [^3H]3-0-methylglucose. pH_i was calcultated from the DMO distribution taking 6.13 for the pK_a of DMO (16,17).

<u>RESULTS</u>

1. <u>Thrombin, a Potent Mitogen for Growth of Chinese Hamster Lung Fibro-</u>
   <u>blasts in a Chemically Defined Medium</u>

   CC139 cells are highly serum dependent for growth and can be arrested
in the G0/G1 phase of the cell cycle by serum deprivation (10). These
arrested cells reinitiate DNA synthesis in response to a variety of growth
factors including α-thrombin, PDGF, EDGF (18), EGF, insulin. When the
cells are "deeply" arrested in the G0 state (30 hours of serum starvation
individual growth factors : PDGF, EDGF, EGF are not, or poorly, effective
in the reinitiation of DNA synthesis with the exception of highly purified α-thrombin (Table 1). Insulin at high concentrations (10 μg/ml) also
fails to reinitiate DNA synthesis ; however, as in many cell systems, it
strongly potentiates thrombin- or PDGF-induced DNA synthesis (Table 1).
It is interesting to note that two purified growth factors : α-trhombin
(1 U/ml, 10 nM) and insulin are as efficient as 10% fetal calf serum (FCS
in the reinitiation of DNA synthesis (Table 1). IGF-I or Multiplication-
Stimulating Activity (MSA) can replace insulin at much lower concentration, their action being mediated through distinct IGF-I and MSA receptors present at the surface of CC139 cells (19).

   When the cells are plated in the serum-free mixture DMEM/F12 (1:1)
containing transferrin, they start to degenerate after 2 days. The addition of insulin (10 μg/ml) maintains the cell population in a quiescent
state for more than 6 days whereas human α-thrombin alone supports expo-

<u>TABLE 1.</u>   REINITIATION OF DNA SYNTHESIS OF GO-ARRESTED CC139 CELLS

Addition(s)	% labeled nuclei	
		+ insulin (10 μg/ml)
None	0.2	0.3
FCS 0.1%	5.5	
" 1 %	19	
" 10 %	44	
α-thrombin 1 U/ml	19	43.5
α-thrombin 10 U/ml	29.5	46.3
α-thrombin 1 U/ml + Hirudin	-	0.9
PDGF (platelet extract 5 μg/ml)	0.2	7.3
PDGF (" " 50 μg/ml)	1.5	16

Cells were arrested in G0/G1 by serum starvation for 30 hours (Material
and Methods). For determination of labeling index, cells were exposed
to growth factors and [methyl-^{3}H]thymidine for 24 hours before they were
processed for autoradiography.

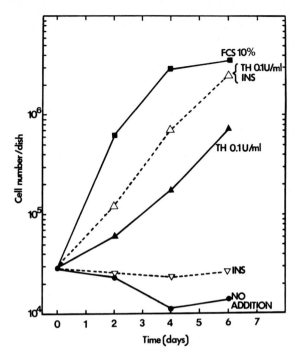

Fig.1. Growth-promoting activity of thrombin. The ability
of highly pure α-human thrombin at 0.1 U/ml (▲), thrombin
(0.1 U/ml) plus insulin (10 µg/
ml) (△), 10% FCS (■), insulin
alone (10 µg/ml) (▽), or no
addition (●) to promote continued proliferation of CC139
is compared. Time "0 days"
corresponds to the time at
which cultures were changed
to serum-free DMEM/F12 medium.
Cells from duplicate 35-mm
dishes representing each condition were trypsinized at 48h
intervals to determine cell
number per dish.

nential growth without any lag. Addition of insulin potentiates the
growth-promoting activity of thrombin (Fig.1). These results confirm
and extend those obtained on the reinitiation of DNA synthesis (Table 1).
The mean doubling time of CC139 cells in the defined medium : 5 µg/ml
transferrin, 10 µg/ml insulin and 0.1 U/ml α-thrombin is 19 hours, a
growth rate close to the 15 hours obtained with 10% FCS. Continuous subculturing and clonal growth can be obtained by passaging the cells in fibronectin-coated dishes (11).

From this serum-free medium we have selected stable variants capable
of growing in medium containing insulin and transferrin (unpublished data) or variants autonomous for growth that are able to grow in the absence of exogenous growth factors (20). We have demonstrated that this selection towards relaxation for growth factor dependence is a prerequisite
for tumoral growth of CC139 cells in nude mice (9,20).

2. Temporal Action of Thrombin

The synergistic action of thrombin and insulin observed with CC139
cells closely resembles that observed in Balb/c-3T3 cells with PDGF and
Insulin-like growth factors. Since it has been proposed that a class of
growth factors called "competence factors" (PDGF, FGF, ...) deliver a stable mitogenic signal after only a brief exposure (2-3 hours) to G0-arres-
ted cells (21), we were prompted to analyze whether thrombin behaves like

a "competence" factor. Therefore, we asked the following questions :
1) Is a short exposure of G0-arrested cells to thrombin sufficient to
induce mitogenicity? 2) If yes, could we ascertain that cell-associated
thrombin has been totally removed? And finally 3) what is the minimal
time of thrombin-receptor occupancy required to observe a maximal mitogenic response?

G0-arrested CC139 cells exposed for various periods of time to α-
thrombin, revealed that a 3-hour exposure of the cells to thrombin is
enough to obtain the maximal mitogenic response either in the absence or
in the presence of insulin (22). To answer the second question, we compared the dissociation of cell-associated [^{125}I]thrombin after extensive
washing (5 rinces) followed by incubation in the absence or presence of
hirudin, a specific thrombin inhibitor (23) that forms highly stable
thrombin-hirudin complexes. Fig.2 shows that dissociation of [^{125}I]throm-
bin is slow and incomplete using the normal washing procedure (5 times)

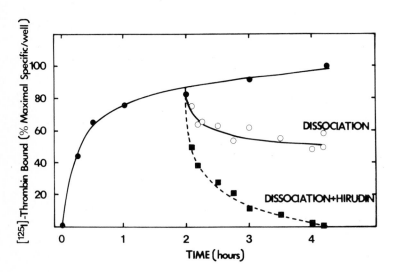

Fig.2. Effect of hirudin on dissociation of [^{125}I]thrombin. Cells were
incubated with .01 U/ml of tracer at 15°C for the indicated periods of
time. Following incubation, cultures were harvested as described in "Methods" and cell-associated radioactivity was determined. Percentage of
maximal specific [^{125}I]thrombin bound per tissue culture well is plotted
as a function of incubation time. Non-specific binding was determined in
the presence of a large excess of thrombin (10 U/ml). After 2 hours of
association parallel cultures were washed 5 times and the dissociation
of [^{125}I]thrombin followed by measuring the residual specifically bound
tracer in the absence (○) or presence (■) of a 100-fold excess of hirudin (1 thrombin-neutralizing unit/ml). Total [^{125}I]thrombin bound at
equilibrium (4 hours) amounted to 11.9% of tracer added ; 80% of the total binding was specific.

whereas in presence of hirudin, dissociation is accelerated and goes to completion in 2 hours at 15°C. Given these results, we reexamined the temporal action of thrombin on DNA synthesis reinitiation. We found that if hirudin was added to cells after a 3-hour thrombin pulse, the thrombin-induced response was abolished as well as the synergistic effect with insulin (22). As far as the third question is concerned, we found that hirudin, added as late as 8 hours after thrombin exposure to the cells, blocked the mitogenic response (data not shown). Hirudin had no inhibitory effect on the stimulation of DNA synthesis induced by growth factors structurally unrelated to thrombin such as FGF or PDGF (22).

The so-called "competence" factors (PDGF, FGF, ...) share in common with thrombin : a synergistic effect with insulin-like growth factors, an activation of the amiloride-sensitive Na^+/H^+ exchanger (see below) and the stimulation of the phosphorylation of a common set of proteins (8). Because of this similarity of action and on the basis of the present study. we would like to propose that thrombin and the so-called "competence" factors must occupy their receptors for the entire G0→G1 period (more than 8 hours) to trigger the mitogenic response of G0-arrested cells. The mitogenicity obtained after only brief exposure of the cells to thrombin, and perhaps to PDGF and FGF as well, could be explained by incomplete removal of the growth factor polypeptides from the cells. A similar conclusion was reached for the mode of action of phorbol esters (24).

3. Growth Factor-stimulated Protein Phosphorylation, an Early Event in the Activation of G0-arrested Cells

Exposure of ^{32}P-labeled, G0-arrested cells to FCS for 15 min resulted in marked alterations in the degree of phosphorylation of several polypeptides. The major changes consistently observed throughout all the experiments concern the stimulation of phosphorylation of a nuclear protein of Mr 62,000, the ribosomal protein S6 of Mr 33,000 and a cytosoluble polypeptide of Mr 27,000 (Fig.3, ref.8). These changes do not appear to be mediated through cAMP or Ca^{++}-dependent phosphorylating systems since 8-BrcAMP or Ca^{++} ionophore A23187 at different concentrations failed to mimic early growth factor-induced phosphorylation. Further, we found that all individual growth factors, α-thrombin (Fig.3), PDGF, FGF, EDGF, capable of reinitiating DNA synthesis of CCl39 cells, also stimulate in common the phosphorylation of the three polypeptides (8). In contrast, and suggesting a different mechanism of action, the insulin-like growth factors, insulin or MSA, do not stimulate the phosphorylation of the protein of Mr 27,000 (Fig.3). However, insulin or MSA which potentiate

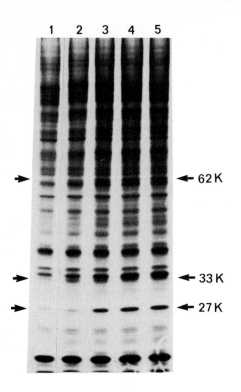

← 62 K

← 33 K

← 27 K

FIG.3. Growth factor-stimulated protein phosphorylation in G0-arrested CC139 cells. Cells were ^{32}P-labeled as described in "Methods" and stimulated for 15 min with the following growth factors :

Lane 1: no addition (control)
Lane 2: insulin 10 µg/ml
Lane 3: human α-thrombin 1 U/ml
Lane 4: α-thrombin 1 U/ml +
        insulin 10 µg/ml
Lane 5: 10% FCS.

The figure is an autoradiogram of SDS-PAGE of whole cell extracts.

the mitogenic action of α-thrombin, PDGF, and EDGF (19, unpublished results) were also found to potentiate phosphorylation of the ribosomal protein S6 (8). These results support the existence of two classes of growth factors and suggest that protein phosphorylation is an early event involved in the control of the cellular G0→G1 transition. Indeed, variants selected for autonomous growth (20) display "constitutive" levels of growth factor-sensitive phosphoproteins (unpublished results).

4. Thrombin Stimulates an Amiloride-sensitive Na^+/H^+ Exchanger and DNA
   Synthesis in a Similar Dose-dependent Manner

Fig.4 shows that : 1) α-thrombin alone added to quiescent CC139 cells stimulates the very early events : Na^+ influx (Fig.4A), Rb^+ influx (Fig. 4B) in a dose-dependent manner strikingly similar to that observed for thrombin stimulation of DNA synthesis (Fig.4C) and 2) interestingly, insulin potentiates both the thrombin-induced monovalent ionic fluxes and thrombin-induced DNA synthesis. This result indicates that potentiation between the two types of growth factors for DNA synthesis takes place very early since it is expressed at the level of membrane ionic permeability one minute, or less, after growth factor addition. Stimulation of Rb^+

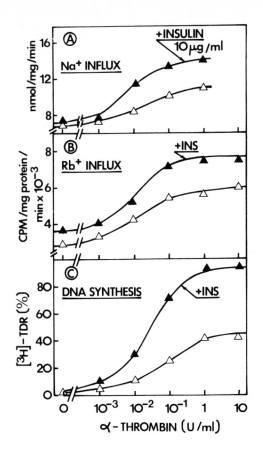

Fig.4 A,B,C. Potentiating effect of insulin on α-thrombin stimulation of Na^+ influx, Rb^+ influx and DNA synthesis in G0-arrested CC139 cells. $^{22}Na^+$ and $^{86}Rb^+$ uptake rates, and [^{3}H]thymidine incorporation were measured following stimulation by increasing concentrations of α-thrombin alone (△) or α-thrombin + 10 μg/ml insulin (▲). Rates of $^{22}Na^+$ influx (A) and $^{86}Rb^+$ influx (B) were measured over an incubation period of 5 min in presence of growth factors. [^{3}H]thymidine incorporation (C) was measured over an incubation period of 24 hours in presence of growth factors (100% corresponds to 55±10% labeled nuclei, a value close to the 60±5% obtained with 10% FCS).

influx parallels that of Na^+, this result being consistent with the well documented activation of the Na^+,K^+ ATPase secondary to an increase in intracellular [Na^+] (2). Previously we have characterized silent fast Na^+ channels in the plasma membrane of CC139 cells (25). These channels can be activated by a combination of neurotoxins and specifically inhibited, as those of excitable cells, by tetrodotoxin (25). Growth factor-stimulated Na^+ influx in quiescent CC139 cells is not affected by tetrodotoxin (25) but is blocked by amiloride (Fig.5A). Half-maximal inhibition is obtained with 5 μM amiloride. This sensitivity to amiloride, and the fact that this drug was reported to block a Na^+/H^+ exchange in various differentiated cell types (14,26,27), prompted us to analyze the movement of protons in CC139 cells. When incubated in Na^+-free medium these cells accumulate intracellular H^+. The addition of external Na^+, or Li^+ to the cell suspension immediately stimulates H^+ release. This Na^+-dependent proton release is saturable with an apparent K_m for Na^+ around 13 mM at a physiological pH and is completely

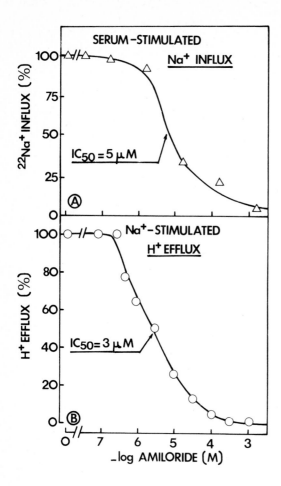

Fig.5 A,B. Amiloride effect on serum-stimulated Na^+ influx and Na^+-stimulated proton efflux in CC139 cells. $^{22}Na^+$ influx rates (A) were measured as described in "Methods" on G0-arrested cells, with an external $[Na^+]$ of 14 mM. 0% corresponds to the basal Na^+ influx rate, 100% to the Na^+ influx stimulated by 10% Fetal Calf Serum (1.5-fold). H^+ efflux rates (B) were measured as in (15) on confluent cultures of CC139 cells preincubated 60 min in a Na^+-free medium. Initial rates of H^+ efflux were measured at pH 7.40 after addition of 20 mM NaCl to the external medium. Amiloride, at various concentrations, was added 2 min before NaCl addition.

inhibited by amiloride (Fig.5B)(15). The parallel amiloride dose-response curves suggest a tight coupling between growth factor-stimulated Na^+ influx and H^+ release in CC139 cells. Further characterization of this Na^+/H^+ exchange system has shown that: 1) it is reversible, 2) it has two distinct sites for Na^+ and H^+, 3) amiloride competes for the Na^+ site with a K_i of 1 μM, pH 7.4) and the stoichiometry of the Na^+/H^+ exchange is 1:1 (15).

5. <u>Regulation of Intracellular pH is Linked to Growth Factor-stimulated Ribosomal Protein S6 Phosphorylation</u>

If the stimulation of the Na^+/H^+ exchanger is one of the initial signals of growth factor action and, if this signal is required for the growth factor-induced biochemical cascade of events, we would expect a pleiotypic inhibitory effect of amiloride.

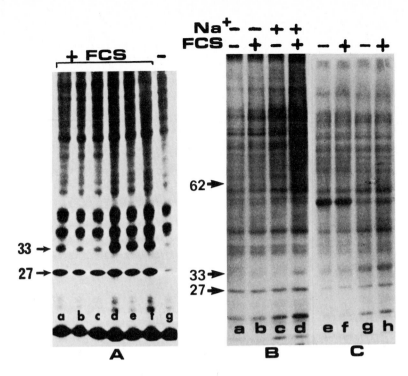

FIG.6 A,B,C. Effect of intracellular pH on serum-stimulated ribosomal protein S6 phosphorylation. A: Before stimulation by 10% FCS, ^{32}P-labelled, arrested cells were preincubated 5 min with the following inhibitors: carbonyl-cyanide, m-chlorophenyl hydrazone (cccP), lane a, 0.025 mM, lane b, 0.25 mM ; 2 mM dinitrophenol, lane c ; 1 and 10 μg/ml oligomycin lane d and e respectively ; no inhibitor, lane f. The inhibitors were maintained during the 15 min of stimulation by 10% FCS ; lane g, unstimulated. B: ^{32}P-labeled cells were preincubated 60 min in Na^+-free medium pH 7.40 and stimulated 20 min with 10% dialyzed FCS (+) either in absence of Na^+ (lane b) or with 20 mM $NaCl_3$ (lane d). Lanes a (no Na^+) and c (20 mM Na^+) were unstimulated. C: ^{32}P-labeled cells were preincubated in medium containing 130 mM Li^+ and then shifted for 20 min to Na^+,Li^+-free medium pH 6.7 in the absence or in the presence of 10% FCS (lane f). Lanes g and h are identical to e and f except that 0.5 mM amiloride was added when the cells were shifted to the Na^+,Li^+-free medium.

We recently reported that, indeed, phosphorylation of the ribosomal protein S6 is inhibited by amiloride at a concentration which abolishes growth factor-stimulated Na^+ influx (4,5). Because movements of Na^+ induced by toxins which activate fast Na^+ channels had no effect on phosphorylation (5), we hypothesized that H^+ efflux is required for growth factor-stimulated S6 phosphorylation. Therefore, we predicted that any condition which would prevent growth factor-induced proton release should prevent S6 phosphorylation. Addition of amiloride is one way to prevent H^+ efflux, however secondary effects have been reported for this drug

(28). For this reason, we investigated three ways of increasing intra-cellular [H^+] independent of amiloride : 1) cells were incubated with weak acids (dinitrophenol and carbonylcyanide m-chlorophenyl hydrazone, cccP), 2) cells were incubated in Na^+-free medium ; these conditions block the H^+ extrusion by the Na^+/H^+ exchanger leading to intracellular H^+ accumulation (14,15), 3) we reversed the Na^+/H^+ exchanger by rever-sing the inwardly-directed Na^+ gradient ; the cells were loaded with 130 mM Li^+ and when shifted to a Na^+,Li^+-free medium, pH 6.7, they ra-pidly took up H^+ from the medium (15). These three conditions which lead to acidification of the cell interior, as incubation with amiloride, pre-vent growth factor-stimulated protein S6 phosphorylation (Fig.6). Addi-tion of 20 mM Na^+ to cells incubated in Na^+-free medium (second condi-tion) restores S6 phosphorylation (Fig.6B). Addition of amiloride in the third condition prevents H^+ uptake through the Na^+/H^+ exchanger and restores S6 phosphorylation (Fig.6C).

Altogether, these results, showing a link between protein phospho-rylation and the functionning of the Na^+/H^+ exchange, support the idea that the regulation of intracellular pH is a key event in the control of cell division.

DISCUSSION AND CONCLUSIONS

A very striking observation is the ubiquity of rapid increases in Na^+ influx, H^+ efflux of many differentiated cell systems in response to a variety of external stimuli. It has been observed in sea urchin eggs after fertilization (29), in hepatocytes (30), lymphocytes (31), frog muscle cells (32), neuroblastoma cells (31), platelets (33)... . Therefore, it is not surprising that a variety of growth factors (e.g. thrombin, FGF, PDGF...) which bind to their own receptor sites in a gi-ven cell, elicit a common early ionic response. Two models outlined in Fig.7 could account for this convergent phenomenon. According to model I, activation of Na^+ influx and H^+ release are secondary to the activa-tion of the intermediate metabolism. Alternatively, in model II, the Na^+/H^+ exchange system serves as an initial transmembrane signaling de-vice upon activation by external agents. In model I, the interaction of growth factors with their receptors deliver (a) signal(s) that activate protein kinases and/or phosphatases and therefore metabolism. Increase in intracellular H^+ production as a consequence of metabolism activation activates the Na^+/H^+ exchange system and initiates the cascade of catio-nic movement across the membrane : H^+ efflux activates Na^+ influx via the Na^+/H^+ antiport ; the Na^+ influx in turn activates the Na^+/K^+ ATPase leading to increased K^+ influx. Therefore, activation of these

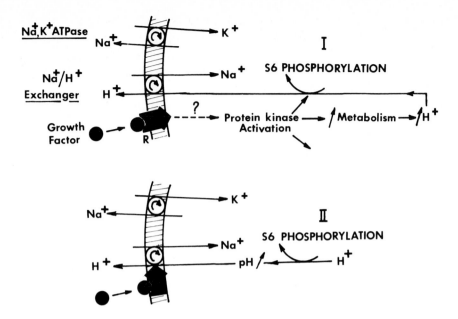

FIG.7. Schematic representation of the growth factor-stimulated S6 phosphorylation and its coupling to the Na$^+$/H$^+$ exchange system. The large black arrow (R) represents a membrane growth factor receptor.

ionic movements are common to all cell systems as is common activation of glycolysis or other metabolic pathways linked to the onset of protein and nucleic acid synthesis. In contrast, in the second model, the interaction of growth factors with their specific membrane receptors directly activates the Na$^+$/H$^+$ exchange system leading to an increase in intracellular pH as one of the first signals.

In this respect, preliminary results have shown that FCS or thrombin + insulin, when added to quiescent CC139 cells, stimulates a rapid alkalinization of the cell interior sensitive to amiloride (Δ pH = + 0.15-0.20 units). A similar increase in intracellular pH was also reported for mouse fibroblasts (34) and human fibroblasts (35) upon growth factor action.

These results would tend to favor model II. However, the permanent activation of the Na$^+$/H$^+$ exchanger in the presence of growth factors could result from the increase in proton production due to metabolism activation (model I). Therefore, a combination of both models could account for : 1) the increase in intracellular pH and 2) the permanent stimulation of the Na$^+$/H$^+$ exchanger in growth factor-stimulated cells. Among the major unanswered questions are first, how does the growth factor-receptor interaction modify the Na^+/H^+ antiport or its energetic coupling to account for the increase in pH and secondly, does the increase in intracellular pH serve as an intracellular signal for mitogen action ?

From the work presented here and discussed in more detail in specific reports (4,8,11,15,22) we can draw the following conclusions and summarize :

1) The non-tumoral Chinese hamster lung fibroblast cell line CCl39 grows in a completely defined medium (transferrin, insulin and α-thrombin).

2) α-thrombin, alone, at high concentrations (1 U/ml, 10 nM) can support continued growth in serum-free medium. Therefore, insulin or IGF-I are not essential for growth of CCl39 cells.

3) Short exposure of G0-arrested cells to thrombin apparently triggers the mitogenic response. In fact, complete removal of cell-associated thrombin with hirudin, prevents the mitogenic response. Therefore, we propose that thrombin and the so-called "competence factors" (FGF, PDGF,...) must occupy their receptors for the entire G0→G1 period (> 8 hours) in order to induce DNA synthesis.

4) Two classes of growth factors are distinguished on the basis of early biochemical events :
- Class I, including PDGF, FGF, EDGF, thrombin, ... which individually are able to induce DNA synthesis of G0-arrested cells, stimulates :
   i) an amiloride-sensitive Na^+/H^+ exchanger in the membrane.
  ii) the phosphorylation of a common set of proteins : ribosomal protein S6 and the cytosoluble 27K protein.

- Class II, growth factors of the insulin-like growth factor family (insulin, MSA, IGF-I) which are not mitogenic per se for CCl39 cells : do not induce the phosphorylation of the 27K protein, nor do they activate the Na^+/H^+ exchanger. This class of growth factors potentiates the mitogenic response of the first class by potentiating the early biochemical events : activation of the Na^+/H^+ exchanger, stimulation of protein phosphorylation.

5) These growth factor-stimulated protein phosphorylations and the Na^+/H^+ exchanger activation are tightly associated with growth control since both events are "constitutively" expressed in tumoral clones selected for autonomous growth (data not shown).

6) Finally, we have found that ribosomal protein S6 phosphorylation is coupled to growth factor-stimulated H^+ efflux since :

i) amiloride, at a concentration which blocks H^+ efflux, blocks S6 phosphorylation.

ii) conditions which acidify the cell interior (protonophores, reversal of the Na^+/H^+ exchanger) also prevent growth factor-induced S6 phosphorylation.

Therefore, we conclude that regulation of the internal pH through the common activation of the Na^+/H^+ exchanger is an essential step of growth factor action.

ACKNOWLEDGMENTS

We gratefully acknowledge Mrs. Geneviève Oillaux for very efficient secretarial assistance. This research was supported by grants from the "Centre National de Recherche Scientifique" (LP 7300 and ATP n°136), the "Institut National de la Santé et de la Recherche Médicale" (CRL n°80-2016), the "Délégation Générale à la Recherche Scientifique et Technique" (n° 81-L0733) and the "Fondation pour la Recherche Médicale".

REFERENCES

1. Bottenstein, J., Hayashi, I., Hutchings, S., Masui, H., McClure, D., Ohasa, S., Rizzino, A., Sato, G., Serrero, G., Wolfe, R., and Wu, R. Methods in Enzymology (Jakoby, W. and Pastan, I. eds). Acad. Press N.Y., 58, 94-109 (1979)
2. Rozengurt, E. Adv.Enzyme Regul. 19, 61-85 (1981)
3. Moolenaar, W.H., Mummery, C.L., Van der Saag, P.T. and de Laat, S. Cell 23, 789-798 (1981)
4. Pouysségur, J., Chambard, J.C., Franchi, A., S. Paris and Van Obberghen-Schilling, E. Proc.Natl.Acad.Sci.USA 79, 3935-3939 (1982).
5. Pouysségur, J., Paris, S. and Chambard J.C. in: Ions, Cell Proliferation and Cancer (A. Boynton and W. McKeehan eds) Acad. Press N.Y. (1982) in press.
6. Nilsen-Hamilton, M. and Hamilton, R. Nature 279, 444-446 (1979)
7. Haselbacher, G., Humber, R. and Thomas, G. Febs Letters 100, 185-190 (1979).
8. Chambard, J.C., Franchi, A., Le Cam, A. and Pouysségur, J. J.Biol. Chem. (1982) in press.
9. Pérez-Rodriguez, R., Chambard, J.C., Van Obberghen-Schilling, E. and Pouysségur, J. J.Cell Physiol. 109, 387-396 (1981).
10. Pouysségur, J., Franchi, A. and Silvestre, P. Nature 287,445-447(1980).
11. Pérez-Rodriguez, R., Franchi, A. and Pouysségur, J. Cell Biol.Int.Rep. 5, 347-357 (1981).
12. Pouysségur, J., Franchi, A., Salomon, J.C. and Silvestre, P. Proc. Natl.Acad.Sci.USA 77, 2698-2701 (1980).
13. Franchi, A., Silvestre, P. and Pouysségur, J. Int.J.Cancer 27, 819-827 (1981).
14. Moolenaar, W., Boonstra, J., Van der Saag, P. and de Laat, S. J.Biol. Chem. 256, 12883-12887 (1981).
15. Paris, S. and Pouysségur, J. J.Biol.Chem. (1983) in press.
16. Boron, W.F. and Roos, A. Am.J.Physiol. 231, 799-809 (1976).
17. Johnson, C.H. and Epel, D. J.Cell Biology 89, 284-291 (1981).
18. Barritault, D., Plouet, J., Courty, J. and Courtois, Y. J.Neurosci. (1982) in press.
19. Van Obberghen-Schilling, E. and Pouysségur, J. Exp.Cell Res. submitted.

20. Pérez-Rodriguez, R., Franchi, A., Deys, B. and Pouysségur, J. Int. J.Cancer 29, 309-314 (1982).
21. Stiles, C.D., Capone, G.T., Scher, C.D., Antoniades, H.N., Van Wyle, J.J. and Pledger, W.J. Proc.Natl.Acad.Sci.USA 76, 1279-1283 (1979).
22. Van Obberghen-Schilling, E., Pérez-Rodriguez, R. and Pouysségur, J. Biochem.Biophys.Res.Commun. 106, 79-86 (1982).
23. Markwardt, F. in: Methods in Enzymology, Acad. Press N.Y. 19, 924-932 (1970).
24. Dicker, P. and Rozengurt, E. J. Cell Physiol. 109, 99-110 (1981).
25. Pouysségur, J., Jacques, Y. and Lazdunski, M. Nature 286, 162-164 (1980).
26. Aickin, C. and Thomas, R.C. J.Physiol.(Lond.) 273, 295-316 (1977).
27. Rindler, M.J. and Saier, M.H. Jr. J.Biol.Chem. 256, 10820-10825(1981)
28. Lubin, M. in: Ions, Cell Proliferation and Cancer (A Boynton and W. McKeehan eds). Acad. Press N.Y. (1982) in press.
29. Johnson, J.D., Epel, D. and Paul, M. Nature 262, 661-664 (1976).
30. Koch, K. and Leffert, H. Cell 18, 153-163 (1979).
31. Kaplan, J.G. Ann.Rev.Physiol. 40, 19-41 (1978).
32. Moore, R.D., Fidelman, M.L., Hansen, J.C. and Otis, J.N. in: Intra-cellular pH : Its Measurment, Regulation, and Utilization in Cellu-lar Functions (Liss, A.R. ed.) New York pp. 385-416 (1982).
33. Horne, W., Norman, N., Schwartz, D. and Simons, E. Eur.J.Biochem. 120, 295-302 (1981).
34. Rozengurt, E. in: Ions, Cell Proliferation and Cancer (A. Boynton and W. McKeehan eds) Acad. Press N.Y. (1982) in press.
35. Moolenaar, W.H. in: Ions, Cell Proliferation and Cancer (A. Boynton and W. McKeehan eds) Acad. Press N.Y. (1982) in press.

Pure Platelet-Derived Growth Factor Stimulates Human Fibroblasts to Proliferate in Plasma-Free Culture

C. Betsholtz[1], C.-H. Heldin[2], Å. Wasteson[2], and B. Westermark[1]

[1] Institute of Pathology, University of Uppsala, Sweden
[2] Institute of Medical and Physiological Chemistry, University of Uppsala, Sweden

INTRODUCTION

Platelet-derived growth factor (PDGF) is released from platelets when they aggregate (1). It stimulates connective tissue cells to proliferate in vitro (2-5) and has been ascribed a role in wound healing (6) and in the pathogenesis of atherosclerosis (7). Data concerning the role of PDGF in the cell cycle are conflicting. For 3T3 cell cultures PDGF alone is not capable of inducing DNA synthesis but induces a state of "competence" to respond to other hormones which stimulates "progression" through G_1 (8-10). Others have found that PDGF alone is sufficient for stimulation of proliferation of normal human glial cells (2). In this study, we have investigated the role of PDGF in the cell cycle of human skin fibroblasts, a cell type which expresses a high number of PDGF receptors (11). We have found that human fetal or neonatal fibroblasts are able to initiate DNA synthesis and divide in serum-free culture in the absence of added growth factors. When this spontaneous proliferation is inhibited by increased cellular density, reduced cell spreading or subphysiologic extracellular Ca^{2+} concentrations, PDGF becomes mitogenic. In addition, proliferation in the absence of PDGF, EGF or other hormones which usually are added to serum-free culture systems seems to be a feature specific for fetal or neonatal fibroblasts; their adult counterparts have an obligatory requirement for exogenous growth factors.

RESULTS AND DISCUSSION

Fig 1 shows the result from an experiment where human skin fibroblasts of different age, plated sparsely in serum-free MCDB 105, were stimulated with PDGF or EGF. In the fetal (GM 10, 12 fetal weeks) or the neonatal (AG 1523, 3 days) cultures, we had to lower the extracellular Ca^{2+} concentration below regular and physiologic levels (1.0 mM) to obtain growth factor induced DNA synthesis. The adult cultures, however, (GM 3440, 21 years; GM 24, 30 years) incorporated ^{3}H-thymidine to a significantly higher degree in the presence of PDGF or EGF. In order to examine if the neonatal fibroblasts plated at 1.0 mM Ca^{2+} were able to traverse a complete cell cycle in the absence of added growth factors, we used a miniclone technique where cells were seeded in petri dishes containing adhesive palladium islands surrounded by nonadhesive agarose. The procedure for preparing these islands has been described (12,13). Briefly, plastic petri dishes were covered with an agarose film. A titanium grid with 4x100 round holes was placed in the agarose-coated dish which was placed in a vacuum chamber where palladium was evaporated. By this method, round palladium

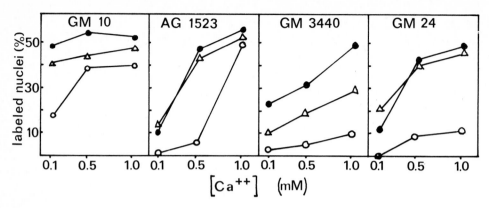

Figure 1. Human skin fibroblasts of different age, regularly grown in Eagle's medium plus 10% (vol/vol) newborn calf serum, were trypsinized, washed and plated serum-free at 5000 cells/cm^2 in MCDB 105 supplemented with the Ca^{++} concentrations indicated in the figure. 48 hrs later, 0.7 mM PDGF or 1.7 nM EGF was added together with ^{3}H-thymidine. Another 48 hrs later, cultures were fixed and processed for autoradiography (16). o———o , control; ●———● , PDGF; △———△ , EGF.

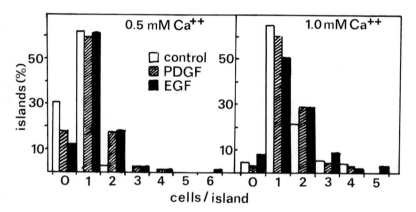

Figure 2. Human neonatal foreskin fibroblasts (AG 1523) were plated serum-free in petri dishes containing palladium islands. 24 hrs later attached cells were scored on the individual islands and unattached cells were removed by washing the dishes once. 0.7 nM PDGF or 1.7 nM EGF was added. 48 hrs later, cells on individual islands were once again scored. The figure shows the percentage distribution of cell number on islands initially containing a single cell.

islands, 121 um in diameter, were created onto which cells could attach, spread and multiply. Because agarose is efficiently cell repellent, the cells were entirely confined to the palladium surfaces. The results from an experiment in which islands initially contained exclusively single cells are shown in fig 2. It is obvious that PDGF or EGF stimulates proliferation in 0.5 mM Ca^{2+}, but not in 1.0 mM Ca^{2+} where background proliferation is high. Apparently a single pure growth factor, or just providing a physiologic Ca^{2+} concentration, can stimulate these cells not only to initiate DNA synthesis, but also to divide in serum-free MCDB 105.

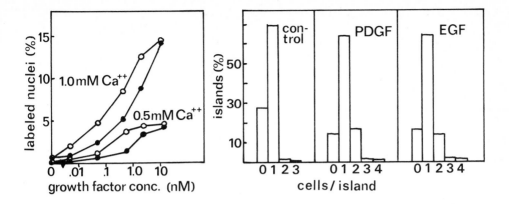

Figure 3. (left) AG 1523 cells were grown to confluency in serum-supplemented Eagle's medium, washed 5 times with phosphate buffered saline and preincubated for 48 hrs in MCDB 105 (0.5 or 1.0 mM Ca^{++}). The cells were then exposed to PDGF or EGF at concentrations indicated in the figure, and ^{3}H-thymidine for 48 hrs followed by fixation and processing for autoradiography (16).●——●, PDGF; ○——○ , EGF.

Figure 4. (right) AG 1523 cells were seeded in petri dishes containing small size palladium islands (72 um in diameter). The experiment was performed as in fig 2.

The intrinsic proliferation activity of neonatal fibroblasts in 1.0 mM Ca^{2+} present in sparse cultures is strongly inhibited in confluent cell cultures. Under these conditions addition of PDGF or EGF increases the fraction ^{3}H-thymidine labeled nuclei from 0.5% to 15% (fig 3). The mechanisms underlying density-dependent inhibition of growth is still poorly understood, but it has been proposed that reduced cell spreading might be an important parameter (14,15). The relation between cell surface area and proliferation rate can be studied by seeding cells on palladium islands which are to small to permit adequate spreading of single cells (13). When neonatal skin fibroblasts are plated on islands, 72 um in diameter, a result analogous to that on confluent cultures is obtained (fig 4); spontaneous proliferation in 1.0 mM Ca^{2+} is suppressed and a PDGF- or EGF-induced proliferative response is revealed.

Our experimental system, in which human fibroblasts in plasma-free culture are stimulated to proliferate in the presence of pure growth factors, or in a medium free from exogenous proteins (fibroblasts of fetal or neonatal origin) should provide an useful model for studying density-dependent inhibition of growth.

REFERENCES

1. C. Busch, Å. Wasteson & B. Westermark, (1976) Thromb. Res. 8,493
2. C.-H. Heldin, Å. Wasteson & B. Westermark, (1980) Proc. Natl. Acad. Sci. USA 77,6611
3. R. Ross & A. Vogel, (1978) Cell 14,203
4. H.N. Antoniades, C.D. Scher & C.D. Stiles, (1979) Proc. Natl. Acad. Sci. USA 76,1809

5. D.R. Clemmons & J.J. Van Wyk (1981) J. Cell. Physiol. 106,361

6. S.D. Balk, (1973) Proc. Natl. Acad. Sci. USA 70,675

7. L.A. Harker & R. Ross, (1979) In Seminars in Thrombosis & Hemostasis, Vol 5, p. 274

8. W.J. Pledger, C.D. Stiles, H.N. Antoniades & C.D. Scher, (1977) Proc. Natl. Acad. Sci. USA 74,4481

9. E.B. Leof, W. Wharton, J.J. Van Wyk & W.J. Pledger (1982) Exp. Cell Res. 141,107

10. R.B. Rutherford & R. Ross (1976) J. Cell Biol. 69,196

11. C.-H. Heldin, Å. Wasteson & B. Westermark (1981) Proc. Natl. Acad. Sci. USA 78, 3664

12. B. Westermark, (1978) Exp Cell Res. 111,295

13. J. Pontén & L. Stolt, (1980) Exp. Cell Res. 129,367

14. A. Zetterberg & G. Auer, (1970) Exp. Cell Res. 62,262

15. J. Folkman & A. Moscana, (1978) Nature 273,345

16. J. Pontén, B. Westermark & R. Hugosson (1969) Exp. Cell Res. 58,393

Synergistic Effect of Retinoic Acid on DNA Synthesis of Prostaglandin $F_{2\alpha}$ Stimulated Swiss 3T3 Cells

M. Eschenbruch, A. M. Otto, and L. Jimenez de Asua

Friedrich Miescher-Institut, P. O. Box 2543, CH-4002 Basel, Switzerland

Introduction

In confluent resting Swiss mouse 3T3 cells, prostaglandin $F_{2\alpha}$ ($PGF_{2\alpha}$) stimulates the initiation of DNA synthesis and cell division. This effect is enhanced by insulin and reflected by an increase in the rate into S phase (1). Recently it has been demonstrated that PGE_1 and PGE_2 (at concentrations that do not stimulate DNA synthesis) have a synergistic effect on $PGF_{2\alpha}$ alone, or with insulin (2). In this communication we report that retinoic acid, as well as analogues of retinoic acid, enhanced the effect of $PGF_{2\alpha}$ and insulin. This synergy was not further increased by PGE_1 or PGE_2. Indomethacin, an inhibitor of prostaglandin synthesis, did not affect the synergy of retinoic acid with $PGF_{2\alpha}$, indicating that retinoic acid did not extert its effect by increasing prostaglandin synthesis.

Materials and Methods

Swiss mouse 3T3-K cells (3) were propagated as described before (1). Initiation of DNA synthesis was assayed by radioactive labelling of cells with $1\mu M$ [methyl-^{3}H] thymidine ($3\mu Ci/ml$) for 28 hr followed by autoradiography, or determining the amount of radioactivity in the acid-insoluble material (1).

Insulin, retinoic acid and retinyl acetate were obtained from Sigma Chemical Co. (St.Louis, MO). Other retinoids were gifts from Dr. W. Bollag, Hoffmann-La Roche, Basel. Stock solutions of retinoids were made in DMSO so that when added to cultures, the concentration of DMSO was not above 0.5%. Prostaglandins were a gift from Dr.J.Pike, Upjohn Company. [Methyl-^{3}H] thymidine (18 Ci/mmol) was obtained from Radiochemical Centre, Amersham.

Results

The effects of retinoic acid on $PGF_{2\alpha}$-stimulation of DNA synthesis is shown in Fig.1. Retinoic acid alone at concentrations from $10^{-8}M$ to $10^{-5}M$ had no effect. However, at a concentration of $10^{-6}M$ it increased by 25% the labelling index obtained by $PGF_{2\alpha}$ alone or $PGF_{2\alpha}$ plus insulin (Fig.1A). Similarly, retinoic acid decreased the level of $PGF_{2\alpha}$ required to give a maximal effect by a factor of 10 (Fig.1B). Retinoic

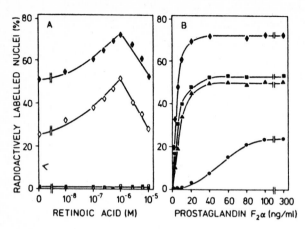

Fig.1. Synergistic effect of retinoic acid on the initiation of DNA synthesis of $PGF_{2\alpha}$-stimulated Swiss 3T3 cells.
A: - Dose-response curve of retinoic acid: □ alone, ◇ with $PGF_{2\alpha}$, ◆ with $\overline{PGF_{2\alpha}}$ and insulin, ■ insulin alone.
B: - Dose-response curve of $PGF_{2\alpha}$; ● alone, ■ with insulin. ▲ with retinoic acid, ◆ with insulin and retinoic acid.

Concentrations: $PGF_{2\alpha}$; 300 ng/ml (A)
            Insulin; 60 μg/ml (A, B)
            Retinoic acid; 1 μM (B)

acid at a concentration of 10^{-5}M had no effect, and higher concentrations were toxic. (The toxicity of retinoic acid varied with the amount of serum present in the medium; results not shown).

Some analogues of retinoic acid were also tested for their synergistic effect on $PGF_{2\alpha}$-stimulation of DNA synthesis. The results obtained with 13-cis retinoic acid, retinyl acetate, trimethylmethoxyphenyl acid as well as the arotinoid ethylamide and an arotinoid keto derivative [for structures see (4)] are shown in Fig.2.

The retinoids at a concentration of 1μM, alone or in combination with insulin (not shown), had no stimulatory effect. All of them, however, enhanced the effect of $PGF_{2\alpha}$ alone, or with insulin, to reach a level of up to two-thirds of the stimulation obtained with serum. Dose response curves of these analogues were similar to that obtained with retinoic acid.

When PGE_1 or PGE_2 were added together with $PGF_{2\alpha}$ they synergistically enhanced the stimulation of DNA synthesis which is reflected in an increase in the labelling index by 30% as shown by (2). When retinoic acid and either PGE_1 or PGE_2 were added together with $PGF_{2\alpha}$ no further increase in DNA synthesis was observed. Indomethacin, which inhibits PGE_2 synthesis in Swiss 3T3 cells (5) had no effect on the synergy of

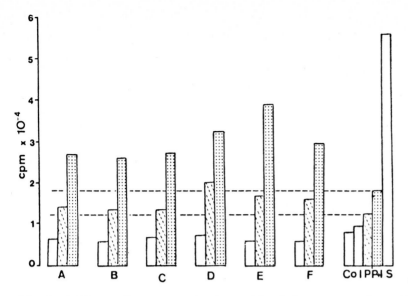

Fig.2. Effect of some retinoic acid analogues on the stimulation of DNA synthesis by $PGF_{2\alpha}$ and insulin.

open bars:	retinoid alone (1 μM)
hatched bars:	retinoid + $PGF_{2\alpha}$ (300 ng/ml)
dotted bars:	retinoid + $PGF_{2\alpha}$ + insulin (60 ng/ml)

Co: control
I: Insulin
P: $PGF_{2\alpha}$
S: Serum, 10%

A: 13-cis retinoic acid
B: TMMP acid
C: retinoic acid
D: retinyl acetate
E: arotinoid ethylamide
F: arotinoid, keto derivative

PGE_1 and PGE_2 added alone or together with retinoic acid to confluent Swiss 3T3 cells did not have any stimulatory effect on DNA synthesis.

retinoic acid with $PGF_{2\alpha}$, indicating that retinoic acid does not act through an increase in prostaglandin production.

Discussion

Retinoic acid has been shown to have a variety of effects on mammalian cells (6). With regard to cell growth, initiation of the rate of proliferation has been reported for several normal and transformed cells (7-11). Furthermore, retinoic acid can inhibit the effect of mitogens such as sarcoma growth factor (12) and the comitogenic effect of TPA on lymphocyte proliferation (13). In contrast there is an enhancing effect of retinoic acid on the stimulation of 3T3 cells by mitogens such as EGF, vasopressin, fibroblast -derived growth factor and insulin (14). These results are in agreement with those presented in this communication where it was shown that retinoic acid enhanced the mitogenic effect of $PGF_{2\alpha}$ alone or with insulin. It did not, however, enhance the synergistic interaction of PGE_1 or PGE_2 with $PGF_{2\alpha}$, which suggests that the mechanism of action of retinoic acid is not via the prostaglandin synthesis pathway.

From results obtained in other cellular systems the synergistic effect of retinoic acid could be explained by one of the following possibilities: i) Retinoic acid may increase the number of binding sites for $PGF_{2\alpha}$, as has been reported for EGF (15). This could be the result of activation of a putative receptor by glycosylation (16). ii) Retinoic acid, after binding to a specific protein and translocation to the nucleus, could regulate the transcription of specific proteins involved in the initiation of protein synthesis.

Experiments to test these hypotheses are underway.

References

1. Jimenez de Asua, L., O'Farrell, M.K., Clingan, D. and Rudland, P. Proc.Natl.Acad.Sci.USA,74 (1977), 3845.
2. Otto, A.M., Nilsen-Hamilton, M., Boss, B.D., Ulrich, M.-O. and Jimenez de Asua, L. Proc.Natl.Acad.Sci.USA,79 (1982), 4992.
3. Todaro, G.J. and Green, H. J.Cell Biol. 17 (1967), 299.
4. Bollag, W. and Matter, A. Ann.N.Y.Acad.Sci. 359 (1981), 9.
5. Shier, W.T. and Durkin, J.P. J.Cell.Physiol. 112 (1982), 171.
6. De Luca, L.M. and Shapiro, S.S., eds."Modulation of cellular Interactions by Vitamin A and Derivatives (Retinoids)". Ann.N.Y.Acad. Sci., Vol. 359, 1981.
7. Lacroix, A., Anderson, G.D.L. and Lippman, M.E., Exp.Cell Res.130 (1980), 339.
8. Jetten, A.M., Jetten, M.E.R., Shapiro, S.S. and Poon, J.P., Exp. Cell Res. 119 (1979), 289.
9. Dion, L.D., Blalock, J.E. and Grifford, G.E. J.Natl.Cancer Inst. 58 (1977), 795.
10. Lotan, R., Neumann, G. and Lotan, D. Ann.N.Y.Acad.Sci.359 (1981), 150.
11. Patt, L.M., Itaya, K. and Hakomori, S.-I. Nature 273 (1978), 379.
12. Todaro,G.J., DeLarco,J.E.and Sporn, M.B. Nature 276 (1978), 272.
13. Kensler, T.W. and Mueller, G.C. Cancer Res. 38 (1978), 771.
14. Dicker, P. and Rozengurt, E. Biochem.Biophys.Res.Com. 91 (1979),1203.
15. Jetten, A.M. Nature 284 (1980), 626.
16. DeLuca, L.M. Vitamines and Hormones 35 (1977), 1.

A.M.O. is a special fellow of the Leukemia Society of America, Inc.

The Secretion of Growth Regulatory Molecules by PC13 Embryonal Carcinoma Cells

John K. Heath and Clare M. Isacke

Department of Zoology, University of Oxford, South Parks Road, Oxford OX1 3PS, U. K.

INTRODUCTION

PC13 embryonal carcinoma (EC) is a malignant teratocarcinoma cell line derived
from the early postimplantation mouse embryo. PC13 EC cells may be induced, by treatment with retinoic acid (RA), to undergo differentiation in vitro into a benign cell
type, PC13 END, which phenotypically resembles the visceral endoderm of the early
postimplantation mouse embryo (1,2). There is a pronounced change in growth regulatory properties associated with this differentiation step. Serum free culture conditions have been developed which will support the multiplication of PC13 EC cells
in vitro. The medium, termed ECM, comprises transferrin (5 µg.ml.), human low density
lipoprotein (LDL, 50 µg.ml.) and human high density lipoprotein (HDL, 50 µg.ml.) in a
basal medium of MCDB104:DME (1:1). The medium does not contain deliberately added
growth factors. PC13 END cells will survive in this medium, but their proliferation
is dependent upon exogenous growth factors, such as epidermal growth factor (EGF) or
insulin (3,4). The susceptibility of PC13 END cells to the action of these hormones
is partially due to the appearance of specific cell surface receptors upon differentiation (3,4). It is thus clear that PC13 EC cell proliferation is regulated in a
different fashion to PC13 END. There would appear to be some developmentally regulated factor (or factors) which control PC13 EC cell proliferation, and which may be
related to their malignant phenotype. Here we examine the possibility that such
molecules may be growth regulatory polypeptides secreted by PC13 EC cells. The
identification of such molecules would be useful in understanding the control of cell
proliferation in the mouse embryo, and if these factors were active upon PC13 EC cells
themselves, could account for their growth factor independent phenotype.

RESULTS

As a preliminary step to investigating the secretion of growth regulatory molecules by PC13 EC cells, PC13 END cells were co-cultured with PC13 EC cells in ECM
serum-free medium. Whilst the labelling index of PC13 END cells alone in ECM is low,
a marked stimulation of PC13 END cell labelling is observed upon introduction of PC13
EC cells into the culture (Table 1). Similar results were obtained when PC13 EC cells
were co-cultured with NRK rat fibroblast cells in medium containing 0.25% foetal calf
serum (Table 1). These observations suggest that PC13 EC cells do indeed have the
capacity to regulate the proliferation of heterologous cell types. To establish

whether this effect was due to cell-cell contact, or the secretion of soluble factors into the medium, and to allow precise definition of the biological activity of these factors, serum free culture conditions for mouse C3H/10T½ fibroblast cells were developed. This medium, termed ECM/F comprises ECM supplemented with Insulin (1 μg.ml.) and dexamethasone (5x10-7M). The proliferation of C3H/10T½ cells in this medium is dependent upon the addition of an exogenous mitogen, such as EGF (Table 1). C3H/10T½ cells were plated in ECM/F which had been conditioned by PC13 EC cells for 48 hours. A marked stimulation of labelling index (Table 1) was observed. Thus PC13 EC cells secrete molecules which can substitute for EGF in controlling the proliferation of mouse fibroblasts.

TABLE 1

Effect of PC13 EC cells on the multiplication of PC13 END cells and fibroblasts.

CELLS	TREATMENT	% LABELLED CELLS
PC13 END	ECM	5
PC13 END	ECM + PC13 EC[1]	20
NRK	0.25% FCS	10
NRK	0.25% FCS + PC13 EC[1]	33
C3H/10T½	ECM/F	2
C3H/10T½	ECM/F + EGF (20 ng.ml.)	46
C3H/10T½	ECM/F conditioned by PC13 EC[2]	67

10^5 cells were plated into 35 mm diameter wells in 2 mls of experimental media or 5 cm dishes with 5 mls of experimental media. ^{3}H-thymidine was added 24 hours later at 1 μCi/ml. and the cells were cultured for a further we hours and processed for auto-radiography. 1) 345 x 10^3 EC cells were added. 2) ECM/F was conditioned by PC13 EC cells for 48 hours, filtered (0.2 μm filter) and used immediately.

Many types of malignant cells have been found to secrete factors which induce the proliferation of anchorage dependent fibroblast cells in semi-solid media (5). ECM conditioned by PC13 EC cells was tested for the ability to induce multiplication of NRK cells in medium containing 0.3% agarose. Colony size was measured after 13 days incubation. It was found that ECM, conditioned by EC cells could induce significant anchorage independent growth of NRK cells in these conditions (Table 2). The action of PC13 EC cell conditioned ECM was significantly enhanced in the presence of EGF (1 ng.ml.) (Table 2). Although this activity is significant it is important to note that the size of anchorage independent NRK colonies induced by PC13 EC cell conditioned medium is not as great as that observed with factors secreted by some other malignant cell types (data not shown). The activity of this EC cell secreted factor would therefore appear to be relatively weak, or be dependent upon some as yet undefined co-factor.

TABLE 2

Multiplication of NRK cells in 0.3% agarose. Effect of PC13 EC cell conditioned media.

ADDITIVES	% COLONIES 50 μ DIAMETER
None	0
PC13 EC cell conditioned ECM	16
1 ng.ml. EGF	6
PC13 EC cell conditioned ECM + 1 ng.ml. EGF	80
PC13 END cell conditioned ECM	8

5×10^3 NRK cells were plated into 1.5 mls. of F12:DME (1:1), 5% FCS, 0.3% agarose + 50% supplement where indicated. Colony size was measured in 100 randomly chosen colonies with a micrometer eye-piece at 400X magnification after 13 days culture.

In order to determine whether these various activities are due to single or multiple molecular species, PC13 EC cell conditioned ECM was lyophilised, solubilised in 1M acetic acid, and subjected to Biogel P-60 gel filtration in 1M acetic acid. Each fraction was tested for the ability to induce DNA synthesis in PC13 END, and NRK cells, and the ability to stimulate anchorage independent multiplication of NRK cells in 0.3% agarose in the presence of 1 ng.ml. EGF. Multiple peaks of activity were observed. Fractions active on PC13 END cells were observed with apparent molecular weights 30K, 10K and 8K daltons. Fractions active on NRK cells were found with apparent molecular weights 30K, 15K and 8K daltons. Fractions that could induce anchorage independent multiplication of NRK cells were observed with apparent molecular weights 15K and 8K daltons. There would consequently appear to be a complex mixture of growth regulatory molecules secreted by PC13 EC cells. Whether these are structurally related remains to be determined by biochemical purification.

Acknowledgements:

This work was financially supported by the Cancer Research Campaign.

REFERENCES

1) Adamson, E.D. et al. Cell 17:469-476
2) Rayner, M. and Graham, C.F. J. Cell Sci. in the press.
3) Rees, A. et al. Nature 281: 309-311
4) Heath, J. et al. J. Cell Biol. 91: 293-297
5) DeLarco, J. and Todaro, G. P.N.A.S. 75: 4001-4005.

Growth Regulation of L-929 Mouse Fibroblasts by Steroid Hormones and Anti-Hormones in Serum Containing and Serum Free Media

I. Jung-Testas and E. E. Baulieu

Université Paris XI, INSERM U 33, Laboratoire de Hormones, F-94270 Bicêtre, France

ABSTRACT

Mouse L-929 fibroblasts contain 3 distinct steroid hormone receptors, RG for glucocorticosteroids, RA for androgens and RE for estrogens. There is no progesterone receptor. Sedimentation coefficient of receptors in low salt medium is $\sim$ 7-8 S and affinity for their respective hormones is very high (K_{Deq} $\sim$ 1 nM). RA binds androgens, anti-androgens (e.g. cyproteron acetate) and progesterone, and somewhat estradiol (but not DES, a synthetic estrogen). RE binds exclusively estrogens and anti-estrogens (e.g. tamoxifen), including DES. RA and RE do not bind glucocorticosteroids. RG binds glucocorticosteroids and progesterone, but neither androgens nor estrogens. At physiological concentrations, androgens or estrogens increase the rate of cell multiplication, and specific anti-hormones inhibit the related growth effect. In the presence of dexamethasone, cell multiplication is strongly decreased, and this effect can be abolished by addition of a new antiglucocorticosteroid, RU 486, of high affinity for RG. Moreover, plasma membrane seems affected by steroid hormones since cell adhesiveness is increased in the presence of androgens or estrogens but decreased in the presence of glucocorticosteroids, effects which are also abolished by the corresponding anti-hormones. These observations were made using culture medium supplemented with charcoal extracted calf serum, and were confirmed in serum free culture medium (SF). The doubling time in SF medium is longer, 24 h instead of 18 h. However, after long term cultures in SF medium (4 months) no change in receptor concentrations was observed and the 18 h doubling time was immediately restored in serum containing culture medium.

1. Introduction

Steroid hormones bind to specific receptor proteins inside the target cell. After binding, the hormone receptor complex undergoes an "activation" step which permits it to accumulate in the cell nucleus. This latter interaction mediate the specific cellular steroid hormone response (reviewed in Baulieu et al. 1975).

In previous reports (Jung-Testas et al. 1976) we described the presence of two distinct sex steroid receptors in L-929 mouse fibroblasts, an androgen-(RA) and an estrogen (RE) receptor which exhibit all the characteristics of the corresponding sex steroid receptors demonstrated in mammalian target organs (Jensen and DeSombre 1972; Baulieu et al 1975). As these cells contain also a glucocorticosteroid receptor (RG)

(Hackney et al. 1970), but no progesterone receptor, they are of particular interest in studying effects of steroid hormones and anti-hormones at the cellular level. In order to distinguish between the effects of non-specific nutritional factors in serum and those of steroid hormones, we used both serum containing and serum-free culture medium to test hormone effects in vitro.

2. Results

Effects of hormones and anti-hormones on cell growth

a. In serum containing medium (DMEcx). After 10 days of suspension culture in DME medium complemented with 10 % charcoal extracted steroid-free calf serum, growth stimulation of L-929 cells has been observed up to + 100 % when either androgen or estrogen at 10 nM concentration have been added to the culture medium. This growth effect was completely inhibited by the addition of the corresponding anti-hormone at 100 nM concentration. However, anti-androgen did not inhibit estrogen-induced cell proliferation and visa versa (Jung-Testas and Baulieu 1979).

b. In serum-free medium (SF). We developed a completely serum-free culture medium which contains no other growth factors, hormones or proteins, but insulin. The composition of SF medium is listed in Table 1. Contineous growth of L-929 fibroblasts has been obtained without pronounced morphological alterations (Fig. 1).

Table 1. (a) Amounts correct for use with 5 % CO_2 ; (b) Hepes was first diluted in 50 ml distilled water, the pH adjusted to 7.3 and then added to the medium ; (c) Insulin is added just before use.

Components added to Ephrussi modified F 12 powder	mg per 1	Components added to Ephrussi modified F 12 powder	mg per 1
L-glutamic acid	250.0	Thymidine	7.2
L-glutamine	584.0	Sodium bicarbonate (a)	800.0
L-leucine	2.5	Hepes (b)	6,600.0
L-tyrosine	11.0	Streptomycin	100.0
Folic acid	5.0		
D-glucose	1,810.0	Penicillin	100 IU/ml
Hypoxanthine	40.0	Insulin (c)	0.12 IU/ml

The doubling time in SF medium is 24 h instead of 18 h, but replacement of SF medium by usual DME medium results in an immediate recovery of the 18 h doubling time (Fig. 2). There was no change in receptor concentration after 4 months of culture in SF medium.

Again, in SF culture conditions, the presence of dihydrotestosterone (DHT) or estradiol (E_2) increased cell proliferation as well as thymidine incorporation into DNA compared to control cultures (Table 2).

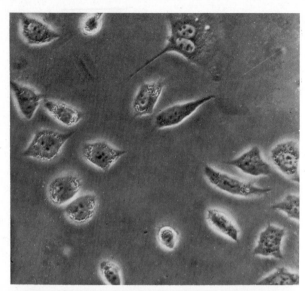

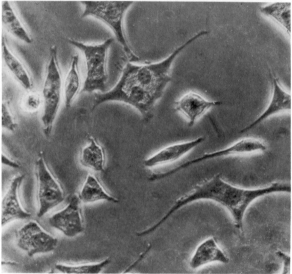

Fig. 1. L-929 cells growing at low density in DME-medium (left), or in SF medium (right). Phase contrast X 450.

Table 2. Effect of DHT or estradiol upon rate of cell number and thymidine incorporation into DNA. 8.10^4 cells were plated in SF medium, and 18 h later, hormone containing medium was given. Three days later, plates were pulsed for 18 h with ^{3}H-methyl-thymidine. Cell counts and measurement of radioactivity were done in triplicates.

Steroid (nM)	cells/dish	^{3}H-methyl-thymidine dpm/dish	^{3}H-methyl-thymidine dpm/10^5 cells
Control	102.000	9.950	9.760
DHT (30)	135.000	16.460	12.190
E_2 (30)	127.000	18.070	14.230

SF medium

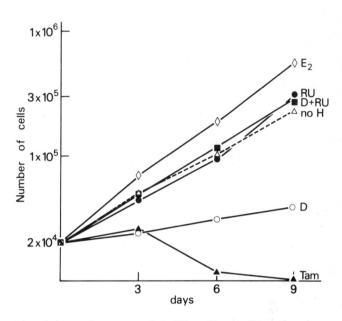

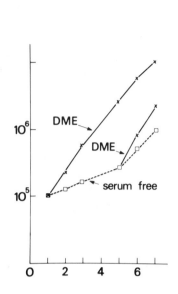

Fig. 2. Growth of L-929
cells in serum containing
(DME) x——x and serum-free
medium □---□ . Abscissa:
days of culture. Ordinate:
cell n°/Petri dish.

Fig. 3. Growth curves of L-929 cells in SF medium in
the absence (noH), or in the presence of steroids:
E_2 = estradiol 40 nM, RU = RU 486 100 nM, D = dexamethasone 100 nM, Tam = tamoxifen 100 nM, D + RU = dex
100 nM + RU 486 100 nM. Medium was changed every two
days.

The addition of glucocorticosteroid to the culture medium results in a decrease
of the growth rate of mouse fibroblasts. At 500 nM concentration cell growth is inhibited to about 50 % in serum containing culture medium (Pratt and Aronow 1966). This
effect is more dramatic in SF medium, since cell growth is almost arrested at 100 nM
concentration (Fig. 3). Growth inhibition can be completely reversed when RU 486, a
new steroid antagonist synthesized by Roussel Uclaf, is added together with dexamethasone to the culture medium. RU 486 is a new anti-fertility steroid which displays
high affinity for both glucocorticosteroid and progesterone receptors (Philibert et
al 1981 ; Herrmann et al 1982). RU 486 alone has no effect on cell proliferation.
Estradiol (40 nM) incrèases cell growth, and tamoxifen (100 nM) inhibits cell growth
leading even to cell death after several days of culture (Fig. 3). Lower tamoxifen
concentration (50 nM) does not influence cell growth, but growth stimulation induced
by 40 nM estradiol is inhibited by 50 nM tamoxifen. In contrary, the presence of
RU 486 together with estradiol does not inhibit the estradiol effect on growth.

Hormone and anti-hormone effects on cell adhesiveness (Table 3)
    It was found earlier that androgens and estrogens increase cell adhesiveness in
SF medium and that dexamethasone has an opposite effect (Jung-Testas and Baulieu

Table 3. Effects of hormones and anti-hormones on L-929 cell adhesiveness in serum-free medium. Plated cells = 4.12 x 10^5/6 cm petri dish. *100 = 5.25 x 10^5 cells counted 30 h later.

Compounds added	Attached cells (Index*)
No Hormone	100*
Dexamethasone 100 nM	54
RU 486 100 nM	93
Dexamethasone 100 nM + RU 486 100 nM	93
Estradiol 40 nM	120
Tamoxifen 100 nM	55
Estradiol 40 nM + tamoxifen 100 nM	67

1979). Therefore cells were plated either in hormone free SF medium, or in the same medium containing hormones, anti-hormones or both together. Again, dexamethasone decreased cell adhesiveness to 50 % of the value obtained in hormone-free medium, and when RU 486 is added together with dexamethasone, 100 nM of each, cell adhesiveness is as efficient as in control cultures. The presence of RU 486 alone in the plating medium does not influence cell adhesiveness. Estradiol increased the plating efficiency and tamoxifen had negative effect on cell plating. The positive effect of estradiol is completely abolished when tamoxifen is present at the same time in the culture medium.

3.   Discussion

The development of chemically defined, protein-free media in which animal cells can be indefinitely cultivated received much attention since long. Evans et al (1956) already succeded in growing fibroblasts in chemically defined culture medium. Hormonal effects on cell growth at low concentrations are indeed difficult to interprete in the presence of unknown factors which occur in serum since the question, if the observed effects are direct or mediated by serum factors, cannot be answered. In our SF-medium, growth stimulation and increase in plating efficiency by androgens and estrogens in L-929 cells is observed and growth inhibition and decrease in plating efficiency by glucocorticosteroids. In the presence of specific anti-hormones these effects are abolished. As L-929 cells contain androgen, estrogen and glucocorticosteroid receptors they might be considered as target cells for steroid hormones. Our results obtained in serum-free medium suggest that the hormonal effects are direct effects mediated by the corresponding receptor. L-929 cells have no progesterone receptor and are therefore of particular interest to study specific anti-glucocorticosteroid action of RU 486.

4. References

Baulieu EE, Atger M, Best-Belpomme M, Corvol P, Courvalin JC, Mester J, Milgrom E,
     Robel P, Rochefort H, DeCatalogne D (1975) Vit Horm 33:649-731
Evans VJ, Bryant JC, Fioramonti MC, McQuilkin WT, Sanford KK, Earle WR (1956)
     Cancer Res 16:77-86
Herrmann W, Wyss R, Riondel A, Philibert D, Teutsch G, Sakiz E, Baulieu EE (1982)
     CR Acad Sci Paris 294:933-938
Jensen EV, DeSombre ER (1972) Ann Rev Biochem 41:203
Jung-Testas I, Bayard F, Baulieu EE (1976) Nature 259:136-138
Jung-Testas I, Baulieu EE (1979) Exp Cell Res 119:75-85
Philibert D, Deraedt R, Teutsch G (1981) 8th Congress on Pharmacology, Tokyo, abstract.
Pratt WB, Aronow L (1966) J Biol Chem 241:5244-5250

Synergistic Interactions of Specific Prostaglandins in Regulating the Rate of Initiation of DNA Synthesis in Swiss 3T3 Cells

Angela M. Otto[1], Marit Nilsen-Hamilton[2], Barbara Boss[2], and Luis Jimenez de Asua[1]

[1] Friedrich Miescher-Institut, CH-4002 Basel, Switzerland
[2] The Salk Institute, San Diego, CA 92138, USA

Prostaglandins (PG) constitute a family of structurally related molecules with diverse functions. They are produced by various animal cells in response to physiological and pathological changes, as e.g. inflammation or cancer. The function of a prostaglandin depends on the target cell and the local presence of other prostaglandins and hormones (1, 2).

In particular, $PGF_{2\alpha}$ has been shown to have mitogenic activity in cultured mouse fibroblastic cells (3). The mitogenic effect of $PGF_{2\alpha}$ is synergistically enhanced by insulin and inhibited by simultaneous addition of hydrocortisone (4). Other prostaglandins, e.g. PGA, B, D, E, have no mitogenic effect or have only a marginal effect compared to that of $PGF_{2\alpha}$ (3). The question is: can other prostaglandins interact with $PGF_{2\alpha}$ to alter its stimulatory effect on cell proliferation?

MATERIAL AND METHODS

Confluent resting Swiss mouse 3T3 cultures were used as a model system for determining stimulation of DNA replication. They were plated in Dulbecco-Vogt's modified Eagle's medium supplemented with 6% fetal calf serum and low molecular nutrients (4, 5). Additions of prostaglandins and hormones were made to the conditioned medium. Determinations of the labelling index, of intracellular levels of cAMP and of 2-deoxyglucose uptake were as previously described (4, 6).

Prostaglandins used were a generous gift of John Pike, Upjohn Company, Kalamazoo, USA.

RESULTS AND DISCUSSION

$PGF_{2\alpha}$ at concentrations as low as 6 ng/ml can alone stimulate the initiation of DNA synthesis in confluent resting Swiss 3T3 cells (6). The resulting labelling index is very low, but can be synergistically enhanced by physiological concentrations of insulin (6). Even though PGD_2, E_1, E_2 and $F_{1\alpha}$ are structurally very similar to $PGF_{2\alpha}$, neither one of them, at a concentration of 100 ng/ml, can stimulate the initiation of DNA synthesis. Only in the presence of insulin can a marginal effect of these prostaglandins on the labelling index be observed (Table 1). When added together with a saturating concentration of $PGF_{2\alpha}$, neither PGD_2 nor $PGF_{1\alpha}$ affected the labelling index observed with $PGF_{2\alpha}$ alone, but PGE_1 and PGE_2 each had a synergistic effect to an extent similar to that of insulin. However, insulin further enhanced the synergy of $PGF_{2\alpha}$ and PGE_1 or PGE_2. On the other hand, PGE_1 and PGE_2 together were no more

TABLE 1. Interactions of $PGF_{2\alpha}$ with other prostaglandins, hydrocortisone and insulin: Effect on labelling index.

Additions	% labelled nuclei at 28 hr	
	without insulin	with insulin
none	0.5	0.7
PGD_2	0.8	5.0
PGE_1	0.6	1.0
PGE_2	0.7	1.8
$PGE_1 + PGE_2$	1.8	3.5
$PGF_{1\alpha}$	1.0	7.5
$PGF_{2\alpha}$	22.0	51.8
$PGF_{2\alpha} + PGD_2$	21.6	52.8
$+ PGE_1$	52.0	77.5
$+ PGE_2$	49.7	78.0
$+ PGE_1 + PGE_2$	53.9	79.0
$+ PGF_{1\alpha}$	23.4	52.0
$PGF_{2\alpha}$ + hydrocortisone	3.3	28.1
$+ PGE_1$ + hydrocortisone	14.4	46.0
$+ PGE_2$ + hydrocortisone	5.5	48.0

Concentrations used were for: PGD_2, PGE_1, PGE_2 and $PGF_{1\alpha}$ 100 ng/ml, $PGF_{2\alpha}$ 300 ng/ml, hydrocortisone 40 ng/ml, and insulin 50 ng/ml.

effective than each one separately. This indicates that PGE_1 and PGE_2 most likely act through a common mechanism to enhance the stimulatory effect of $PGF_{2\alpha}$.

The synergistic effects of $PGF_{2\alpha}$ with PGE_1, PGE_2, and insulin were expressed on the rate of initiation of DNA synthesis and were reflected in proportional increases in cell number at 48 hr (6).

Glucocorticoids such as hydrocortisone inhibit the mitogenic effect of $PGF_{2\alpha}$ (4; Table 1). Likewise, the synergistic effects of PGE_1 and PGE_2 with $PGF_{2\alpha}$ or $PGF_{2\alpha}$ plus insulin were markedly reduced. The effect of hydrocortisone cannot be attributed to its inhibition of prostaglandin synthesis, however, since indomethacin, which also inhibits prostaglandin synthesis, had no effect on DNA synthesis stimulated by $PGF_{2\alpha}$ (not shown; 7).

PGE_1 (100 ng/ml) increases transiently intracellular cAMP levels. This effect was also observed when PGE_1 is added with $PGF_{2\alpha}$. In contrast, PGE_2, alone or with $PGF_{2\alpha}$, did not increase intracellular levels of cAMP (Table 2). This result indicates that the synergistic effects of PGE_1 and PGE_2 with $PGF_{2\alpha}$ is not mediated through this early, transient event.

PGD_2, PGE_1, PGE_2 and $PGF_{1\alpha}$ did not stimulate 2-deoxyglucose uptake within 5 hr after their additions to the culture (Table 2). Only $PGF_{2\alpha}$ was able to stimulate alone. Insulin alone stimulates the early, protein synthesis independent phase of 2-deoxyglucose uptake (4), and it is synergistic with $PGF_{2\alpha}$. Likewise, synergy in 2-deoxyglucose uptake was observed with $PGF_{2\alpha}$ and PGE_1 or PGE_2, but not with PGD_2 or $PGF_{1\alpha}$. Thus, the stimulation of 2-deoxyglucose uptake correlated well with the syner-

TABLE 2. Effects of prostaglandins on intracellular levels of cAMP and
2-deoxyglucose uptake

Additions	cAMP pmol/mg protein at 30 min	at 60 min	2-deoxyglucose uptake pmol/min/mg protein − insulin	+ insulin
none	18.5	19.5	8.8	21.8
PGD_2	−	−	11.7	23.7
PGE_1	91.7	30.4	12.6	26.5
PGE_2	23.2	16.4	10.5	28.2
$PGF_{1\alpha}$	−	−	12.7	44.3
$PGF_{2\alpha}$	17.9	12.1	39.6	106.2
$PGF_{2\alpha}$ + PGD_2	−	−	45.6	111.0
+ PGE_1	95.5	50.8	95.8	169.6
+ PGE_2	9.4	17.5	85.0	158.7
+ PGE_1 + PGE_2	−	−	96.0	−
+ $PGF_{1\alpha}$	−	−	45.9	102.1
Fetal calf serum 10%	5.3	13.6	312.0	−

Concentrations used were as in Table 1. The rate of 2-deoxyglucose uptake was determined in a 10 min-pulse 5 hr after stimulation.

gistic effects observed on the labelling index. No such synergy was observed in the
presence of actinomycin or cycloheximide (not shown). Thus, the expression of the
synergistic interaction of $PGF_{2\alpha}$ with PGE_1 and PGE_2, observed in stimulation of 2-
deoxyglucose uptake as well as in stimulation of DNA synthesis, is most probably under transcriptional and translational control.

ACKNOWLEDGEMENT

A.M.O is a Special Fellow of the Leukemia Society of America, Inc. This work was
supported by National Cancer Institute Grant CA 24395 (to M.N.H.).

REFERENCES

1. Samuelson, B. and Paoletti, R. (eds.) Advances in Prostaglandin and Thromboxane
   Research (1976) Raven Press, New York.
2. Powles, T.J., Bockman, R.S., Honn, K. and Ramwell, P. (eds.) Prostaglandins and
   Cancer: First International Conference (1982) Alan R. Liss, Inc.., New York.
3. Jimenez de Asua, L., Otto, A.M., Ulrich, M.-O., Martin-Perez, J. and Thomas, G.
   (1982) in Prostaglandins and Cancer: First International Conference, eds. Powles,
   T.J., Bockman, R.S., Honn, K. and Ramwell, P. (Alan R. Liss, New York) pp.309-331.
4. Jimenez de Asua, L. Richmond, K.M.V., Otto, A.M., Kubler, A.M., O'Farrell, M.K.
   and Rudland, P.S. (1979) in: Hormones and Cell Culture, Cold Spring Harbor Conferences on Cell Proliferation, eds. Sato, G.H. and Ross, R. (Cold Spring Harbor
   Laboratory, Cold Spring Harbor, New York) Vol. 6, pp. 403-424.
5. O'Farrell, M.K., Clingan, D., Rudland, P.S. and Jimenez de Asua, L. (1979) Exp.
   Cell Res. 118, 311-321.
6. Otto, A.M., Nilsen-Hamilton, M., Boss, B., Ulrich, M-O. and Jimenez de Asua, L.
   (1982) Proc. Natl. Acad. Sci. USA 79, 4992-4996.
7. Hammarstrom, S. (1977) Eur. J. Biochem. 74, 7-12.

Use of Eye Derived Growth Factor from Retina (EDGF) in a Defined Medium for the Culture of Bovine Epithelial Lens Cells

J. Plouët, M. Olivié, J. Courty, Y. Courtois, and D. Barritault[1]

INSERM U.118, CNRS ERA 842, Paris, France

[1] Also from University of Paris XII

Summary

We have previously described that retina and other ocular tissues (iris, choroid, vitreous body) contain a growth factor named Eye Derived Growth Factor or EDGF different from Epidermal Growth Factor (EGF) and Fibroblast Growth Factor (FGF). Since proliferation of bovine epithelial lens cells (BEL cells) is stimulated by addition of EDGF or FGF but not of EGF when cultured in presence of optimal fetal calf serum concentration (6%) in MEM medium, we looked at the effect of these growth factors on proliferation of subcultured BEL cells in a serum free medium. MEM 199 - HAM F12 (1 : 1) supplemented with insulin and transferrin (5 μg x ml^{-1}), of EDGF or 10 ng x ml^{-1} of EGF provided an increase of 70%. No synergistic effect on proliferation was observed with any combination of these growth factors. Hydrocortisone (10^{-8}M) in combination with EDGF provided an increase in proliferation up to 80% of the serum supplemented control, however the cells elongate and looked so different from normal cells that this combination was not used. In the presence of EDGF the following hormones were inefficient : T3 (10^{-12} to 10^{-9}M), PGE$_1$ (1 to 100 ng x ml^{-1}), LHRF (1 to 100 ng x ml^{-1}), testosterone or progesterone (0,1 to 10 ng x ml^{-1}).

Introduction

Bovine Lens Epithelial cells (BEL) can be cultured easily in presence of serum (1) and our laboratory has investigated the growth and synthetic properties of these cells in the presence of 6% fetal calf serum (2, 3). We have purified growth factor (EDGF) from bovine retina which has a Mr of 17.500 and pI at pH 4.5 and can stimulate replicative DNA synthesis in BEL cells at concentration of 14 ng per ml of culture medium (3-6). EDGF is different from Fibroblast Growth Factor (FGF) (5) and Epidermal Growth Factor (EGF (7). In order to obtain more informations as well as on the biological meaning of a growth factor in the retina we attempted to culture BEL cells in a serum free medium where EDGF was compared to EGF and to brain FGF.

Experimental procedure

1. Culture of BEL cells

After 20 to 30 generations, cells were trypsinized and seeded in 35 mm dishes in a M199/F12 (1 : 1) medium supplemented with soybean trypsin inhibitor (199-F 12) or with 6% fetal calf serum (199-F12-FCS). Medium was changed every other day. Cells were counted using a coulter counter and each experiment and measure were done in triplicate.

2. Hormones and growth factors

Insuline, transferrin, PGE_1, T_3, testosterone, progesterone, LHRF were from Collaborative Research. EGF (Korr Laboratories) brain FGF (given by D. Gospodarowicz) or EDGF (6) were tested for mitogenic activity using bioassay (6) based on the ability of growth factors to promote a dose dependent ^3H Thymidine incorporation in DNA of target cells stimulated to pass through Go or G_1 phases. Target cells were BEL cells with FGF or EDGF and Rat 3T3 for EGF, FGF or EDGF. Stimulation Unit (S.U.) was defined as the amount of proteic growth factor which could induce a half of the maximum ^3H Tdr incorporation in DNA of stimulated cells (6). In the experiments described here, EDGF, brain FGF and EGF exhibit a S.U. respectively at $14\ ng \times ml^{-1}$, $20\ ng \times ml^{-1}$ and $1\ ng \times ml^{-1}$ and were used at concentrations of $10\ S.U. \times ml^{-1}$ of culture medium (these doses correspond to maximal stimulation as defined in the bioassay) and added with new medium.

Results and Discussion

1. Effects of growth factors on BEL cells in the presence of serum

Cells seeded at 1.5×10^4 per dish were counted after 8 days of culture (top of Fig.) EDGF or FGF enhanced BEL cell growth by a factor of 3. EGF, even at higher doses (up to 100 S.U., results not shown) had no stimulatory effect on BEL cells under these conditions although these cells have specific receptors (8). Moreover there was no synergetic effect between any of these growth factors. Only shown here for EGF and EDGF.

2. Effects of growth factors and various hormones on BEL cells in the absence of serum (bottom of Fig.).

After 8 days of culture, cells grown only in presence of insulin and transferrin represented 30% of the population versus serum (in 199-F12, cell population reached 20%, results not shown). In presence of insulin and transferrin, EDGF, FGF, EGF alone or any combination of all three factors increased this population up to 70% of the FCS activity. Further more T3, PGE_1, LHRF had no effect on BEL cell proliferation in the range of doses used in presence or absence of any of the three growth factors used. Only hydrocortisone $(10^{-8}M)$ in combination with EDGF showed a slight mitogenic effect (80% of the FCS). However, under these conditions, cells elongate dramatically (as already described by other authors (9)), form clusters and look so different from the in vivo morphology that hydrocortisone was not used for further studies. Testosterone or progesterone were also ineffective (not shown).

Several other investigators have succeeded in growing mammal epithelial lens cells in absence of serum on Petri dishes recovered either by laminin and in presence of EGF or FGF and insulin (10) or recovered biomatrix produced by corneal endothelial cells and in presence of HDL (11).

The results presented here indicate that a growth factor, purified from retina can in vitro stimulate BEL cell proliferation. This may provide us with a model for an in vitro study of the role of retina in lens growth and differentiation.

125

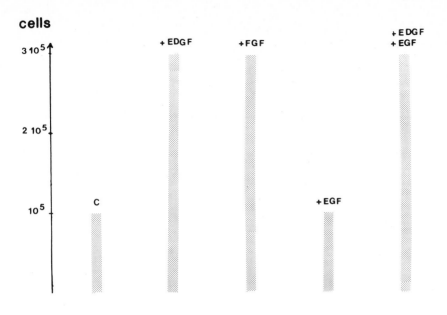

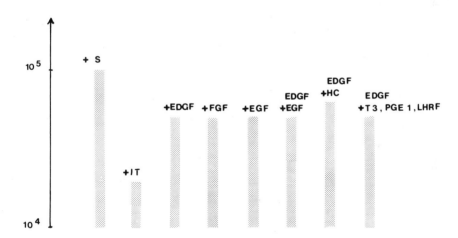

Growth of BEL cells in presence (top) or absence of serum (bottom) after 8 days.
For details, see text.

References
1. Reddan J.R. Cell Biology of the Eye. 1982, 299-375.
2. Courtois Y., Simonneau L., Tassin J., Laurent M. and Malaise E. Differentiation. 1978, 10, 23-30.
3. Courtois Y., Arruti C., Barritault D., Tassin J.,Olivié M. and Hughes R.C. Differentiation, 1981, 18, 11-27.
4. Arruti C., Courtois Y. Exp. Cell Res., 1978, 117, 283-291.
5. Barritault D., Arruti C. and Courtois Y. Differentiation, 1981, 18, 29-42.
6. Barritault D., Plouët J., Courty J. and Courtois Y. Journal of Neurosc. Res., 1982, in press.
7. Plouët J., Barritault D., Courtois Y. and Ladda R. FEBS Letters, 1982, 144, 85-88.
8. Gospodarowicz D., Mescher A., Brown K. and Birdwell R. Exp. Eye Res., 1977, 25, 631-649.
9. Van Venrooij W.J., Groeneveld A.A., Bloemendal H. and Benedetti E.L. Exp. Eye Res., 1974, 18, 527-536.
10. Reddan J.R., De Hart D.J. and Sackman J.E. J. Cell Biol., 1981, 91, 148.
11. Gospodarowicz D. and Massoglia S. Exp. Eye Res., 1982, 35, 259-270.

Effect of Partially Purified Preparation of Human Somatomedin A in the Three Cultured Cell Systems

J. Straczek, M. H. Heulin, F. Sarem, A. Lasbennes, M. Artur, C. Geschier, J. F. Stoltz, F. Belleville, and P. Nabet[1]
F. X. Maquart, P. Gillery, and J. Borel[2]
A. Herman, M. D. Lebeurre, and E. De Lavergne[3]
N. Genetet[4]

[1] Biochemistry Laboratory, Faculty of Medicine, B. P. 184, F-54500 Vandoeuvre, France
[2] Laboratory of Biochemistry, Reims, France
[3] Laboratory of Virology, Nancy, France
[4] Blood Center, Rennes, France

ABSTRACT

Somatomedin and factors of MW < 1000 can be used in cell culture replacing fetal calf serum (FCS) or human plasma. The optimal effects were obtained with the simultaneous use of these two preparations. However when somatomedins are used, the optimal conditions must be determined because at high concentrations they inhibit cell cultures.

1. Introduction

The need to add serum (FCS or human plasma AB, etc...) to cell culture medium is not entirely explainable. These additions while permitting cell culture, present certain inconveniences, in particular it is difficult to study substances released in the medium by the cell (1). Studies have been undertaken to find completely defined serum free media with hormones or growth factors (2). In using three different types of cells we tested synthetic media which were supplemented with partially purified somatomedin A of high ($\sim$ 60 000) or low (<10 000) MW. As we have shown (3) the maximal effect of somatomedin activity needed the presence of a low–MW (< 1000) "cofactor", the latter was tested alone or together with these somatomedins.

2. Material and method

Cell cultures : – Cells from BALB/c derived myeloma line NS,0 (gift of Dr C. Milstein)
– Normal human lung fibroblasts from a 14th week old embryo (Biomerieux 84003) between generations 37 and 39
– Normal infant skin fibroblasts between generations 3 and 10
– Fibroblasts from foreskin of a normal children between generations 5 and 10
– PHA Activated human lymphocytes obtained from normal donors.

Somatomedins (SM) : Low–MW SM (SM–PP$_3$, SM–PP$_4$) was purified from Cohn fraction IV by ultrafiltration cut off 10000 followed by 1000 (SM–PP$_3$ specific activity 2600 mU/mg) and HPLC (SM–PP$_4$ 6000 mU/mg) (4). High–MW somatomedins were purified by fractionated precipitation of human plasma (SM–HP$_1$ 20 mU/mg) followed by ion exchange (SM–HP$_5$ 111 mU/mg) and affinity chromatography (SM–HP$_2$ 1300 mU/mg). Biological activity was determined by sulfation bioassay (^{35}S incorporation in embryonic chick cartilage (5)).

UF$_{1000}$: Human serum ultrafiltrate containing low–MW substances (< 1000) (3).

3. Results

SM and UF$_{1000}$ stimulated the incorporation of ^{3}H Thymidine (^{3}HT) in the cells, but their action when studied separately was significantly lower than that of 5 % FCS (figure 1).

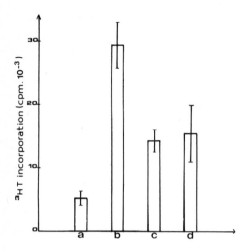

Figure 1 . Effect of growth factor on DNA synthesis : mice myeloma cells (line NS,0) incubated for five days at 37° C. ^{3}HT was added during the final 24 hours – a) medium alone (modified DMEM) ; b) medium + 5 % FCS ; c) medium + 10 % UF$_{1000}$; d) medium + SM–HP$_5$ 15 mU/well.
The bar graphs represent the means of 8 determinations $\pm$ S.D.

<u>Human fibroblasts</u> : The action of 10 % UF$_{1000}$ was shown to be well lower than that of 5 % FCS on the lung and skin fibroblasts in the conditions under which the cultures were studied. However, the effect observed depended on the phase of cell growth (Table I).

Table I . ^{3}HT incorporation in lung or skin fibroblasts – a) medium alone (modified MEM) ; b) medium + 10 % UF$_{1000}$; c) medium + 5% FCS.
A : Trypsination of stock culture followed by immediate incubation in the culture medium to be studied – B) 48 hours preincubation of the trypsinized cells in medium alone followed by incubation in the culture medium to be studied. The results are the means of 7 determinations $\pm$ S.D.

	Lung fibroblasts		Skin fibroblasts	
	(A) Without preincubation	(B) With preincubation	(A) Without preincubation	(B) With preincubation
Incorporation ^{3}HT (cpm)	a 84 $\pm$ 13 b 139 $\pm$ 15 c 8804 $\pm$ 1394	181 $\pm$ 64 675 $\pm$ 189 2196 $\pm$ 373	611 $\pm$ 168 977 $\pm$ 86 4271 $\pm$ 492	207 $\pm$ 39 356 $\pm$ 59 11625 $\pm$ 1395
$R = \dfrac{b-a}{c-a} \times 100$	0,5 %	24 %	10 %	1,3 %

There was a weak effect on protein synthetis and no mitogenic activity when UF$_{1000}$ or SM were used separately in foreskin fibroblasts culture. On the other hand, when used together they were shown to have a synergistic effect on protein synthesis and a mitogenic activity which was measured by DNA synthesis and number of cells (figure 2).

<u>Human lymphocytes</u> : Table II shows the ^{3}HT incorporation in PHA activated lymphocytes in presence of UF$_{1000}$, the latter having an activity which varies from 24 % to 150 % of that of 20 % AB plasma. Figure 3 shows the SM alone excercises a weak effect compared to human

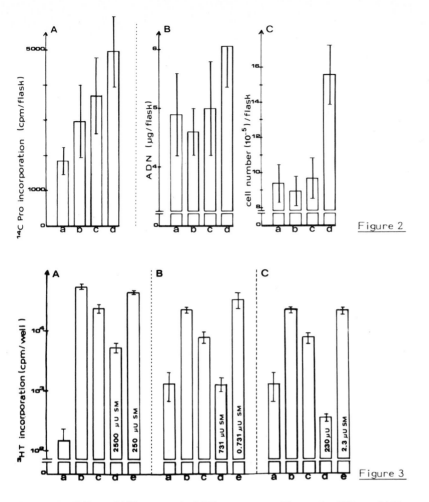

Figure 2 . Effect of UF_{1000} and of SM on protein synthesis (A) ; DNA synthesis (B) and on cell replication (C) measured in confluent cultures of foreskin fibroblasts – a) medium alone ; b) medium + 2 % UF_{1000} ; c) medium $SM-PP_4$ 260 mU/flask ; d) medium + 2% UF_{1000} + $SM-PP_4$ 260 mU/flask. Incubation for 24 hours in the presence of ^{14}C-proline. The results are the mean of 4 determinations $\pm$ S.D.

Figure 3 . Effect of UF_{1000} and SM on PHA activated human lymphocyte cultures.
a) Incubation medium alone (modified 199) ; b) medium + 2,5 % human serum ; c) medium + 10 % UF_{1000} ; d) medium + SM at the indicated concentration ; e) medium + SM + 10 % UF_{1000} (the concentration indicated is that which gives the maximum response).
A : Somatomedin $SM-HP_1$; B) $SM-HP_2$; C : $SM-PP_3$.

serum ; while SM and UF_{1000} when added simultaneously showed an activity similar to that of 2.5 % human serum. However it must be stated that SM must be used at an optimal dose. Concentrations which are to high can be inhibiting (figure 4).

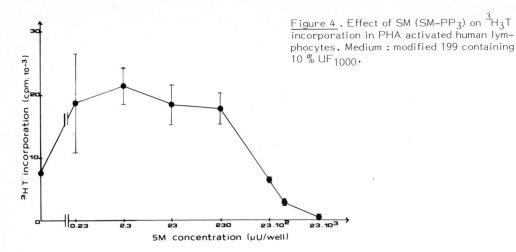

Figure 4 . Effect of SM (SM–PP$_3$) on ^{3}H$_3$T incorporation in PHA activated human lymphocytes. Medium : modified 199 containing 10 % UF$_{1000}$.

Table II . Incorporation ^{3}HT in PHA activated lymphocytes

$$R = \frac{\text{Incorporation with UF}_{1000} \ 10 \ \%}{\text{Incorporation with plasma} \ 20 \ \%} \times 100$$

		PHA Concentrations µg/ml							
		0		2,25		4,5		9	
Patient 1	Plasma 20 %	564	R	15516	R	39815	R	59269	R
	UF$_{1000}$ 5 %	590		4088		11438		48677	
	UF$_{1000}$ 10 %	537	95 %	23612	152 %	33376	84 %	51882	88 %
Patient 2	Plasma 20 %	659		27825		71629		83122	
	UF$_{1000}$ 5 %	168		2305		2349		71002	
	UF$_{1000}$ 10 %	289	44 %	13195	47 %	12811	18 %	20015	24 %
Patient 3	Plasma 20 %	306		35240		65899		79865	
	UF$_{1000}$ 5 %	264		440		21035			
	UF$_{1000}$ 10 %	246	80 %	8514	24 %	53053	81 %		

4. References

1. Murakami H., Masui H., Sato G.H. and col. (1982), Proc. Natl. Acad. Sci. USA, 79, 1158–1162.

2. Barnes D. and Sato G. (1980), Anal. Biochem. (1980), 102, 255–270.

3. Heulin M. H., Artur M., Malaprade D. and col. (1981), Biochem. Bioph. Res. Comm., 99, 644–653.

4. Straczek J. (1980), Purification de la somatomédine A humaine, Thèse de 3ème Cycle, NANCY.

5. Hall K. (1970), Acta Endocrinol., 63, 338–350.

Cell-Substratum Interactions

Role of Cell-Substratum Interactions in the Hormonal Control of Rat Prolactin Cells

Nicole Brunet[1], Denis Barritault[2], Danielle Gourdji[1], and Andrée Tixier-Vidal[1]

[1] Groupe de Neuroendocrinologie Cellulaire, Collège de France, F-75231 Paris Cedex 05, France
[2] Centre de Gérontologie, INSERM U.118, F-75016, Paris, France

INTRODUCTION

The importance of the extracellular matrix for cell proliferation and cell differentiation has been now established for several cell types (see rev. 5, 7, 9). However in the case of glandular anterior pituitary cells, this question is yet poorly documented. Until recently most attention has been given to the role of hormones, neurotransmitters, or neuropeptides in controlling the secretory activity of these cells. Whether these effects are dependent or not on the microenvironment of the glandular cells is still a matter of speculation.

In fact the organization of epithelial cell cords in the anterior pituitary tissue strongly suggests the possibility of various interactions, from cell to cell as well as between cells and basal lamina. Indeed the epithelial cell cords are composed of two cell types, the glandular cells and the follicular or stellate cells, the function of which is still unclear. These epithelial cords are continuously lined by a basement membrane which is itself facing the basement membrane of the capillary endothelium. The glandular cells display a discrete polarity, as revealed by the localization of most granule exocytosis along the basal lamina. However in contrast to the follicular cells, they are not linked by specialized junctions (main ref. 4, 14, 15). The analysis of the functional role of this microenvironment may be approached by various ways. Here we have examined the consequences on several features of prolactin cells of different culture substrata, using the serum free (SF) medium culture technology.

Two systems of rat anterior pituitary cells which secrete prolactin (PRL) have been used : GH3/B6 cells, a subclone of the GH3 strain which is derived from a rat pituitary somatomammotropic tumor (11) and their normal counterpart, primary cultures of rat anterior pituitary cells taken from adult animals. The first system represents an homogeneous population of prolactin cells whereas the second one retains the cellular heterogeneity of the anterior pituitary tissue.

When both systems are grown in serum supplemented (SS) medium (Ham F 10, 15% horse serum, 2.5% fetal calf serum) they firmly attach to the pastic of tissue culture dishes, either directly in the case of GH3/B6 cells (Fig. la)

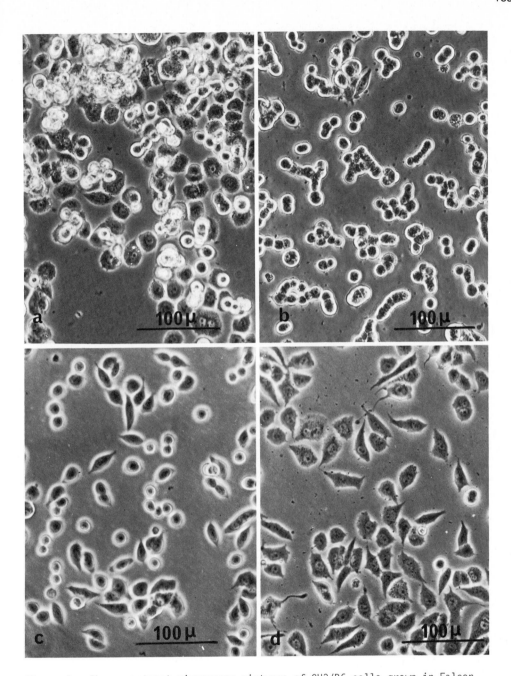

Figure 1. Phase contrast microscope pictures of GH3/B6 cells grown in Falcon tissue culture dishes for 24 hours in different conditions of seeding : a) SS medium on plastic, b) SFH3 medium on plastic, c) SFH3 medium following Pf coating of both dishes and cells, d) SFH3 medium onto BEC matrix.

or indirectly upon a basal sheet of fibroblasts (12). In both cases they secrete PRL and respond to potent stimulators of PRL secretion in vivo, in particular to a neuropeptide, thyroliberin (TRH) and to estradiol 17 β (E2) (see rev. 6, 10, 12).

We have previously found that when GH3 cells are subcultured and transferred from SS medium to a minimum SF medium they do not spread and loosely attach to the plastic substratum (2)(Fig. 1b). As compared to that previously established by Hayashi and Sato (8) this medium lacks several components which are potent regulators of PRL secretion, i.e TRH, triiodothyronine (T3), epidermal growth factor and fibroblast growth factor. It is here referred to as SFH1 (Ham's F12 - insulin, 10 μg/ml - transferrin, 5 μg/ml - parathyroid hormone, 0.5 ng/ml - penicillin 5 IU/ml streptomycin, 5 μg/ml). In some experiments, SFH1 medium has been supplemented with 10^{-7}M ethanolamine and 3×10^{-8}M selenium (referred to as SFH3). Here we compare several procedures to improve the attachment and spreading of GH3/B6 cells and their consequences on PRL secretion and cell proliferation. Moreover, we show that same methods are valid for both GH3/B6 cells and normal anterior pituitary cells cultured in absence of serum.

STUDIES ON GH3/B6 CELLS

When GH3/B6 cells are subcultured and transferred into SFH1 medium, although their basal PRL production decreases with time in culture, they remain responsive to TRH (ED 50 : 5×10^{-10}M)(2) and to E2 (ED 50 : 5×10^{-12}M) (Brunet, in preparation)(Fig. 2a). Moreover cell proliferation which is greatly reduced in SFH1, is stimulated by TRH (2) but not modified by E2 (Brunet, in preparation).

Four procedures were used to improve cell attachment. Two of them were found ineffective : fibronectin or serum coating (horse serum or fetal calf serum).

EFFECT OF P. FETUIN

Pedersen fetuin (Pf) added in solution to SFH1 (500 μg/ml) induces cell attachment as well as the spreading of some cells which take on a stellate or elongated shape (Fig. 1c). It also stimulates cell proliferation which however remains below that observed in SS medium (3). As shown in Fig. 2b, basal PRL production is increased in presence of Pf and the cell response to physiological doses of TRH and of E2 is maintained, but not amplified as compared to cells exposed to same doses in absence of Pf (3).

Since fetuin is an acidic glycoprotein and Pf is relatively heterogeneous, we investigated the possibility that it may act through binding to either the

TABLE I. Effect of culture conditions on GH3/B6 cell attachment. The % of adhesive cells has been determined by counting the cells which stick to the plastic after standardized pipeting. Cells were plated in 3.5mm Falcon tissue culture dishes (3×10^5 c./2ml). Dishes were coated with gelatin-L-polylysine-Pf as previously described (3). When indicated, cells were preincubated for 1 hr at room temperature in SFH3 + Pf and then washed with SFH3. For each dish we counted the number of cells detached by pipetting. The adhesive cells were collected after EDTA treatment and counted. Results are mean of triplicate ± SEM.

CULTURE CONDITIONS			TIME IN CULTURE AFTER PLATING					
Medium	dish coating	cell coating	1.5-2hrs	4 hrs	24 hrs	48 hrs	4 days	6 days
SS	-	-	11 ± 3	4 ± 4	10 ± 2	13 ± 2	15 ± 3	34 ± 4
SFH3	-	-	62 ± 9	19 ± 7	8 ± 3	1.5 ± 0.5	1.6 ± 0.4	1.3 ± 0.5
SFH3 +P fetuin	-	-	17 ± 4	15 ± 4	20 ± 6	13 ± 1	2.5 ± 0.5	3 ± 0
SFH3	P fetuin	-	36 ± 3	15 ± 6	27 ± 4	8 ± 1	1.5 ± 0.5	2 - 3
	P fetuin	P fetuin	47 ± 4	41 ± 5	49 ± 4	6 ± 2	3.5 ± 1	2.5 ± 0.5
	Gelatin + L-polylysine	-	43 ± 2	30 ± 5	4	-	5 ± 2	2 ± 0.1
	Gelatin + L-polylysine	P fetuin	47 ± 7	43 ± 3	31 ± 7	-	4 ± 0.5	4 ± 0.9
	Gelatin + L-polylysine + P fetuin	-	22 ± 2	25 ± 5	7 ± 4	-	4 ± 0.6	5 ± 0.8
	Gelatin + L-polylysine + P fetuin	P fetuin	52 ± 1	46 ± 5	45 ± 5	-	5 ± 0.3	9 ± 2.5
	BEC matrix	-	23 ± 7	25 ± 6	61 ± 3	-	41 ± 3	28 ± 4

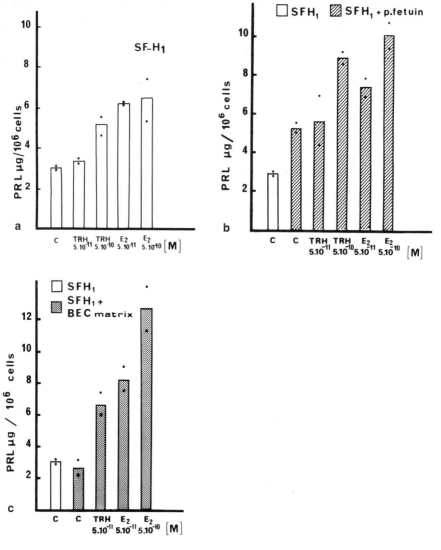

Figure 2. Effect on PRL production by GH3/B6 cells of physiological doses of TRH and of E2 added at seeding (3 x 10⁵ cells/2 ml of SFH1 medium). PRL content was measured by radioimmunoassay in medium collected from day 2 to day 4. Cells were seeded on plastic in the absence (2a) or presence of Pf (2b), or onto BEC matrix (2c). Mean and range of duplicates.

plastic or the cells, or both. We compared cell attachment in various conditions by counting the number of cells which resist to pipeting as a function of time in culture. Results are summarized in Table I. When cells are plated on plastic in SSM, they attach slowly but the % of attached cells increases with time in culture up to 6 days ; one should notice that due to active cell proliferation, newly divided cells most probably account for most of the non adhesive cells at 6 days. In contrast, after plating directly on plastic in SFH3, the cells attach quickly but very transiently since the % of adhesive cells is very low after 48 hours. Addition to SFH3 of Pf. in solution transiently improves cell attachment at least up to 48 hours. Coating the dishes with P. fetuin is ineffective, unless the cells are also preincubated with Pf. In that case, the % of adhesive cells is increased at least up to 24 hours. Moreover in the latter conditions the cells spread and take on the same elongated shape as in P fetuin supplemented medium. It may be concluded that as far as cell adhesiveness and cell shape are concerned, P fetuin is not necessary in solution and that it seems to mostly act through binding to the cell surface.

EFFECTS OF THE EXTRACELLULAR MATRIX OF BOVINE ENDOTHELIAL CORNEAL CELLS (BEC)

GH3/B6 cells have been subcultured and transferred in SFH3 in Falcon tissue culture dishes coated with BEC matrices according to Arruti and Courtois (1). A rapid and long lasting cell attachment is observed on this matrix (Table I). At the same time the cells spread very well but their shape is quite different from that observed in the presence of Pf (Fig. 1 d). After 4 days the cells begin to round up and to detach. It is therefore clear that BEC matrix is far more potent than Pf in inducing cell attachment and spreading.

Cell proliferation is not improved on BEC matrix. Moreover the proliferative effect of TRH + T3 is almost completely prevented (Fig. 3).

Basal PRL production is not modified on BEC matrix. In contrast, the PRL response to TRH and to estradiol is potentiated as compared to that of cells exposed to same hormones, in absence of BEC matrix (Fig. 2 c).

These results obtained with GH3/B6 cells show that cell proliferation, PRL secretion and hormone responsiveness are independently regulated by the substratum. Specific changes in cell shape concomitantly occur. However the exact link between cell shape, cell proliferation and secretory activity remains to be investigated.

PRIMARY CULTURES OF NORMAL PITUITARY CELLS

It was of great interest to compare the behaviour of normal pituitary cells to that of tumor derived cells regarding cell requirements for attachment, survival and secretory activity.

Normal anterior pituitary (AP) cells enzymatically dissociated from adult male rat pituitaries and seeded directly on plastic (Falcon or Limbro multiwell trays) in SFH1 do not attach and progressively die. Therefore we compared the effects of the two substrata which were previously found efficient for GH3/B6 cells.

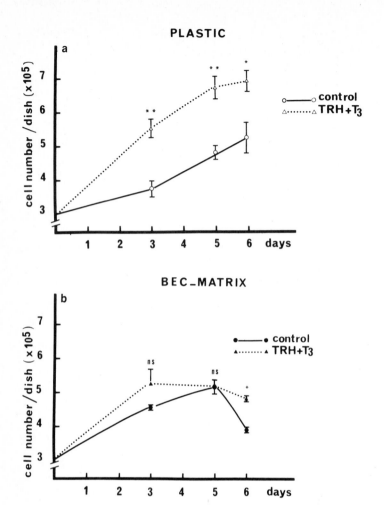

Figure 3. Proliferation of GH3/B6 cells seeded in SFH3 medium (3×10^5 cells/2 ml) either directly on plastic (3a) or onto BEC matrix (3b). TRH (2.5×10^{-9}M) and T3 (3×10^{-11}M) were added at seeding. Mean of triplicate $\pm$ SEM.

Statistical comparisons according to F test : $**$ P <0.01, $*$ P <0.05

EFFECTS OF P FETUIN COATING

AP cells seeded in SFH1 on plastic sequencially coated with gelatin, L-poly-lysine (M.W. 40.000-70.000) and Pf rapidly attach and progressively spread onto the substratum. Survival of numerous healthy looking immunostainable PRL cells is observed up to 7 days at least. Moreover fibroblast overgrowth is almost completely prevented (3) (Fig. 4 a).

The amount of PRL released into the medium in basal conditions increases with time in culture, at least up to 7 days. Moreover exposure to TRH (2.5×10^{-9}M)

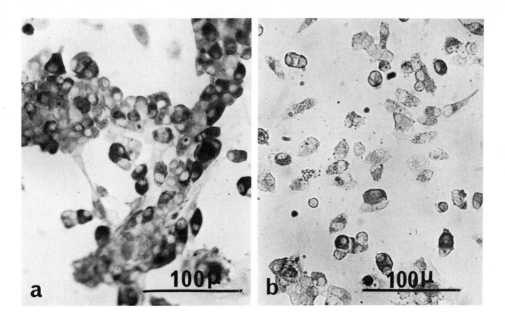

Figure 4. Light microscope picture of normal PRL cells grown for 7 days in SFH1 medium supplemented with selenium (3×10^{-8}M) and seeded on Limbro multiwell trays (2×10^5 cells/1 ml) precoated either with gelatine-L-polylysine-Pf (4a) or BEC matrix (4b). Cells have been immunostained with an anti-PRL serum according to Tougard et al (13)

from day 4 to day 6 induces an augmentation (130%) of PRL medium content. However the cells do not respond to E2 wich in addition counteract the effect of TRH (Fig. 5a). At the same time E2 provokes a cell rounding up (3).

EFFECTS OF BEC MATRIX

AP cells seeded in SFH1 on BEC matrix attach and spread within a few hours. Like onto Pf coating, almost no fibroblasts can be seen. Moreover the spreading of immunoreactive PRL cells is enhanced on BEC matrix as compared to Pf coating (Fig. 4 b).

The amount of PRL released into the medium in basal conditions increases with time in culture, although with a lower amplitude than for cells obtained from a same initial pool and seeded onto Pf coating (694 ng vs 1812 ng PRL/dish, from day 4 to day 6). Exposure to TRH (2.5×10^{-9}M) from day 4 to day 6 results in a 200% increase of PRL medium content. Moreover and in contrast to what is observed on Pf coating, addition of E2 at seeding (5×10^{-10}M) augments the PRL medium content and this effect is additive with that of TRH (Fig. 5 b).

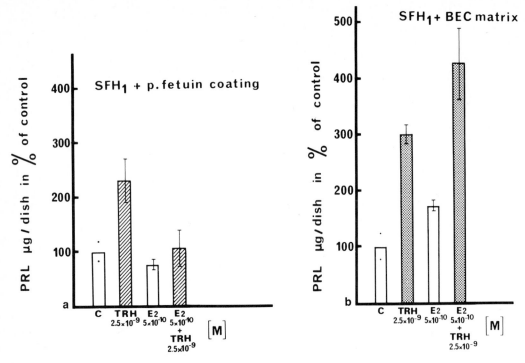

Figure 5. PRL response to TRH and E2 of normal AP cells seeded as described in Figure 4 legend : 5a, Pf coating - 5b, BEC matrix. PRL content was measured by radioimmunoassay in medium collected from day 4 to day 6. E2 was added at seeding and TRH was added at day 4. Mean of triplicates. Bars represent SEM.

CONCLUSION

Taken together the present findings strongly suggest that clonal tumor-derived GH3 PRL cells and normal PRL cells share common surface properties which are involved in the attachment of cells to macromolecular components fixed on rigid plastic surfaces.

Moreover it is clear that the two substrata that we have compared here interact, each in a specific manner, but similarly in both clonal and normal cells, on PRL secretion in response to specific stimuli. Interestingly enough, this can be correlated with modifications of cell shape which seem specific for a given substratum. As compared to Pf coating, BEC matrix seems to permit a better response to physiological regulators of PRL secretion and therefore to be closer from the normal in vivo situation. This is not surprising , at first sight, although the complete composition and structure of the BEC matrix is not completely known and that of the basement membrane of AP cells is still unknown. Further work using defined components of the basement membrane, such as collagen type IV or laminin

(9),are needed to progress in the understanding of mechanisms involved in these interactions as well as in the establishment of a chemically defined substratum.

SUMMARY

The effects of two cell substrata on cell attachment, cell spreading, cell proliferation and hormone secretion have been compared on two model systems of rat prolactin cells : clonal tumor-derived GH3/B6 cells and primary cultures of normal anterior pituitary cells.

When GH3/B6 cells grown in serum supplemented medium are subcultured and transferred to a chemically defined medium devoid of hormones known to regulate prolactin (PRL) in vivo (i.e TRH, T3 , EGF), they did not spread and were loosely attached but retained at least for a week the capacity to respond to thyroliberin (TRH) and to 17 β estradiol (E2).

Pedersen fetuin (P. fetuin), added in solution to SF H1 medium, improved cell attachment and spreading, cell proliferation and basal PRL secretion. However, the PRL response to TRH or to E2 was not modified. Coating the dishes and preincubating the cells with P. fetuin permitted a rapid but transient cell attachment. In comparison, plating GH3/B6 cells on endothelial corneal cell matrix (BEC) resulted in a rapid and long lasting attachment, together with cell spreading. However, cell proliferation was not improved. In contrast, the stimulation of PRL secretion by TRH or by E2 was greatly improved.

Normal rat PRL cells plated in SF H1 on uncoated plastic dishes did not attach and survived very poorly. Both P. fetuin coating and BEC matrix permitted attachment and spreading of these cells in absence of serum. This totally inhibited fibroblast development. On both substrata , basal PRL secretion increased in culture up to 7 days at least and TRH increased PRL secretion whereas E2 increased PRL secretion only on BEC matrix.

ACKNOWLEDGMENTS

We acknowledge the skilful technical assistance of Mrs R. Picart, E. Rosenbaum and Mr D. Grouselle,and C. Pennarun for the illustrations. This work was supported by grants from INSERM (118005) and CNRS (E.R. 89) to A. Tixier-Vidal, and from DGRST (81 L 0731) to Y. Courtois.

REFERENCES

1. Arruti, C., and Courtois, Y. 1982. Exp. Eye Res., 34 : 735-747.

2. Brunet, N., Rizzino, A., Gourdji, D., and Tixier-Vidal, A. 1981. J. Cell Physiol. 91 : 15-29.

3. Brunet, N., Gourdji, D., Tixier-Vidal, A. and Rizzino, A. 1982. In : "Growth of Cells in Hormonally Defined Media", Ed. by G. Sato, A. Pardee, and D. Sirbasku, Cold Spring Harbor Conferences on Cell Proliferation, vol. 9, pp. 169-177.

4. Farquhar, M.G. 1961. Angiology, 12 : 270-292.

5. Gospodarowicz, D., Cohen, D., and Fujii, D.K. 1982. In : "Growth of Cells in Hormonally Defined Media", Ed. by G. Sato, A. Pardee and D. Sirbasku. Cold Spring Harbor Conferences on Cell Proliferation, vol. 9, pp. 95-124.

6. Gourdji, D., Tougard, C., and Tixier-Vidal, A. 1982. in : "Frontiers in Neuroendocrinology", Ed. by W.F. Ganong, and L. Martini, Raven Press, N.Y., vol. 7, pp. 317-357.

7. Grotendorst, G.R., Kleinman, H.K., Rohrbach, D.H., Hewitt, A.T., Varner, H.H., Horigan, E.A., Hassell, J.R., Terranova, V.P., and Martin, G.R. 1982. In : "Growth of Cells in Hormonally Defined Media", Ed. by G. Sato, A. Pardee and D. Sirbasku. Cold Spring Harbor Conferences on Cell Proliferation, vol. 9, pp. 403-413.

8. Hayashi, I., Larner, J., and Sato, G. 1978. In Vitro, 14 : 23-30.

9. Kleinman, H.K., Klebe, R.J., and Martin, G.R. 1980. J. Cell Biol., 88 : 473-485.

10. Tashjian, A.H. Jr. 1979. Methods in Enzymology, 58 : 527-534.

11. Tashjian, A.H. Jr., Bancroft, F.C., and Levine, L. 1970. J. Cell Biol. 47,61-70.

12. Tixier-Vidal, A., Gourdji, D., and Tougard, C. 1975. Intern. Rev. Cytol., 41 : 173-239.

13. Tougard, C., Picart, R., and Tixier-Vidal, A. 1980. Am. J. Anat. 158 : 471-490.

14. Vila Porcile, E. 1972. Z. Zellforsch., 129 : 328-369.

15. Vila Porcile, E. and Olivier, L. 1980. In : "Synthesis and Release of Adeno-hypophyseal Hormones" Ed. by M. Jutisz and K.W.Mc Kerns, Plenum Press,pp.67-104.

Control by the Extracellular Environment of Differentiation Pathways in an Embryonal Carcinoma Cell Line

Michel Darmon

Département de Biologie Moléculaire, Institut Pasteur, 25, rue du Dr. Roux, F-75724 Paris Cedex 15, France

ABSTRACT. The embryonal carcinoma (EC) cell line 1003 forms multi-differentiated tumors when injected into syngeneic mice but is apparently nullipotential when grown in vitro in conventional media. Hormone-supplemented defined media were designed as an attempt to mimic in vivo conditions. Such media actually allowed 1003 cells to differentiate in vitro. The phenotypes eventually obtained depended upon the composition of the medium. Both diffusible factors and attachment factors were shown to control the differentiation of 1003 cells. The appearance of differentiated phenotypes was found to be due to induction - and not selection - phenomena. However, because of the impossibility to obtain clonal cultures of 1003 cells in serum-free media, experiments allowing to find out whether the extracellular environment exerts its effects on these cells at the level of determination or at the level of terminal differentiation could not be designed.

The teratocarcinoma of the mouse is a unique system to study in vitro some of the determination and differentiation events which occur during the embryogenesis of vertebrates (Jacob, 1978). The malignant multipotential stem cells of teratocarcinomas, called embryonal carcinoma cells (EC cells) have been shown to be able to loose their malignancy and to participate normally in embryonic development when grafted into mouse blastocysts (Brinster, 1974, Mintz and Illmensee 1975, Papaioannou *et al.* 1975). These dramatic experiments demonstrate that the fate of EC cells can be similar to that of the stem cells of the embryo if they encounter an appropriate environment. Such an epigenetic control may be thought to be achieved by direct cell-cell interactions and/or extracellular signals.

Recently, we have attempted to study the effect of the extracellular environment on teratocarcinoma differentiation by culturing EC cells in defined media. We have described a clonal EC cell line (1003) which forms multidifferentiated tumors in syngeneic hosts (see Fig. 1) but which remains undifferentiated when exponentially grown in

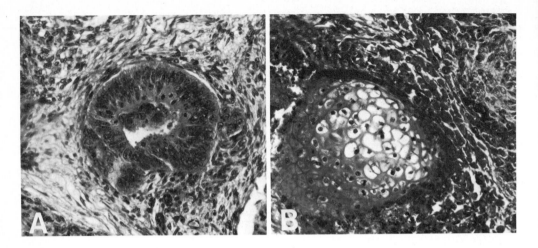

Fig. 1. Sections of a tumor formed by 1003 cells. (a) Neuroepithelial tubule. (b) Cartilage and mesenchymal tissue. Magnification X480. Staining : haematoxylin-eosin.

serum-containing media. When 1003 cells are grown in a serum-free defined medium containing insulin, transferrin and selenium, they obligatorily differentiate (Darmon *et al.* 1981) and, after 5 days of culture no EC cells may be rescued. The triggering of the differentiation process is not due to any specific component of the defined medium but to the deprivation of serum factors preventing differentiation. Actually, when serum is added to the defined medium at the time of plating, 1003 cells remain EC cells. Although serum-deprivation is sufficient to provoke the differentiation of 1003 cells, the nature of the differentiated phenotypes eventually obtained depends on the culture conditions. When fibronectin is used as an attachment factor 1003 cells grow for some generations in the defined medium while differentiating into neuro-epithelial cells, recognizable by their tendency to form rosettes and by the presence of veratridine-stimulatable sodium – channels (Darmon *et al.* 1981). Neuroepithelial cells subsequently transform into post-mitotic neurons. As terminal differentiation develops, vimentin filaments which are present in neuroepithelial cells are replaced by neurofilaments (Darmon *et al.*, in press). The 70 K neurofilament protein shows up at the stage of preneurons, so does the N6 nerve-specific cell-surface antigen (Darmon et al., 1982 a, b). The 200 K neurofilament protein appears later in mature neurons (Darmon et al., in press). Most neurons derived from 1003 are probably cholinergic as judged by the rather high activity of choline acetyl transferase (Darmon et al., 1982 c) which may be assayed in cell extracts

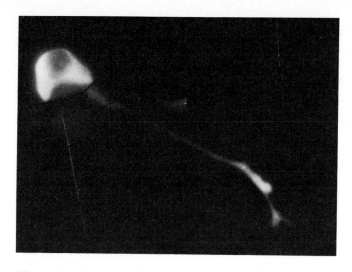

Fig. 2. Tyrosine-hydroxylase-positive neuron. Cells were fixed for
6 min in cold (- 20°C) methanol and were stained by indirect immunofluorescence with rabbit anti-tyrosine-hydroxylase antibodies. Rare
neurons (≃ 1/1000) are strongly positive ; they are always bigger than
other neurons (X1000).

(≃ 0.55 nmol Ach/h x mg protein). However, rare neurons (≃ 1 per 1000)
are catecholaminergic since they may be stained with an anti-tyrosine-
hydroxylase antibody (see Fig. 2).

When laminin was used as attachment factor instead of fibronectin, large patches of myotubes could be seen at the side of the neurons.
These myotubes could be stained with an antibody directed against embryonic muscular myosin (Darmon, in press).

When serum was added-back to serum-free cultures of 1003 prior
to neuronal differentiation (i.e. after 1-3 days) formation of neurons
did not occur, but most cells differentiated into embryonic mesenchymal
cells similar to the ones found at low frequency in serum-free cultures
(Darmon *et al*. 1981, 1982a, b ; Darmon and Serrero, in press). Mesenchymal cells produce embryonic mesenchymal tumors after injection into
syngeneic hosts.

These results show that after a certain time of serum-deprivation 1003 cells lose their EC characteristics (since they are not any
more able to yield an EC progeny) and become committed to differentiate.
Such committed cells can follow at least three pathways of differentiation : neuronal and muscular if serum-free conditions are maintained
throughout the experiment, mesenchymal if serum is readded. Contrary
to EC cells, committed cells bear the cell-surface NG2 antigen ; mesen-

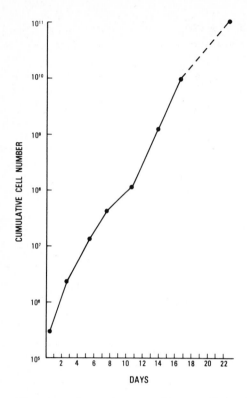

Fig. 3. Long term culture of 1003 cells in FGF-supplemented serum-free medium. 3×10^5 cells were plated on 60 mm dishes in a medium containing insulin, transferrin, selenium, fibronectin and 50 ng/ml pituitary FGF. When the culture reached confluence the cells were replated after dissociation with 1 mM EDTA in the same medium (4/5 fresh ; 1/5 conditionned). When the cumulative cell number reached 10^{10} cells ($\simeq$ 15 generations), the cells were replated either in the same serum-free medium, but without FGF supplement (dotted line) – the cells eventually differentiated into neurons – or in the same serum-free medium, supplemented with 15 % fetal calf serum – in that case most cells differentiated into mesenchymal cells ; some cells had an EC phenotype.

chymal cells retain the NG2 antigen, but this antigen is lost when neuroepithelial differentiation occurs (Darmon *et al.* 1982 a, b).

When 1003 cells were grown in serum-free medium (containing either fibronectin or laminin as attachment factors) supplemented with Fibroblast Growth Factor (50 ng/ml pituitary FGF or 500 ng/ml brain FGF) it was possible to subculture the cells for over 20 generations (Fig. 3) under an apparently undifferentiated phenotype. When such long-term cultures were replated in serum-free medium without FGF, growth slowed down, and most cells differentiated after a few generations into neuroepithelial and neuronal cells. However, these long term cultures differed from those performed in serum-containing medium : when serum was added to them the majority of the cells differentiated into mesenchymal cells although a few foci of EC morphology could be detected. Thus, it is likely that long-term cultures in serum-free medium supplemented with FGF are equivalent to 1-3 day-old cultures in unsupplemented serum-free medium.

When serum is added to serum-free cultures after neuronal differentiation has occurred, neurons degenerate, while the few fibroblast-like cells present in the culture start proliferating (Darmon *et al.* 1981). Such fibroblastic cells differ from embryonic mesenchymal cells by several properties : they form fibrosarcomas, do not bear the NG2 antigen and may be induced to differentiate into muscle cells or adipocytes after treatment with 5-azacytidine or dexamethasone, respectively (Darmon and Serrero, in press). Properties of embryonic mesenchymal cells and fibroblasts are stable after cloning (Darmon and Serrero, in press).

Table I summarizes the nature of the cell types obtained under various conditions and Table II lists some of the criteria used for their identification.

Results reported in this paper show unambiguously that the extracellular environment (diffusible factors and attachment factors) is able to control both the initiation of differentiation and the choice of differentiation pathways in cultures of an embryonal carcinoma cell line. Two important points must be discussed :

1) Are the phenotypic changes observed the result of the selection of rare differentiated cells preexisting in exponential cultures of 1003 or the result of an induction of differentiation triggered by

Table I. Effect of the extracellular environment on 1003 differentiation

CULTURE CONDITIONS	CELL TYPES
serum, exponential	EC
serum, confluent	EC + (endoderm)
serum-free, fibronectin	neurons + (embryonic mesenchyme)
serum-free, laminin	neurons + muscle + (embryonic mesenchyme)
serum-free, fibronectin or laminin, FGF	"non-EC"[*] + (EC)
serum-free, fibronectin or laminin, serum-readdition after 2 days	embryonic mesenchyme + (EC)
serum-free, fibronectin or laminin, serum-readdition after 12 days	fibroblasts + (degenerating neurons) $\pm$ muscle

[*] See Figure 4

( ) Indicate cell types being a minority

Table II. Identification of cell types

CELL TYPES	IDENTIFICATION CRITERIA
EC	Multi-differentiated tumors, ECMA-7 antigen,...
Endoderm cells	Prekeratin filaments, collagen type I
Neuroepithelium	Morphology, veratridine-stimulatable sodium channels, vimentin filaments
Neurons	N6 antigen, neurofilaments, veratridine-sensitive sodium channels, choline acetyl-transferase, (tyrosine hydroxylase)
Skeletal muscle	Morphology, embryonic myosin
Embryonic mesenchyme	Embryonic mesenchymal tumors, vimentin filaments, NG2 antigen
Fibroblasts	Fibrosarcomas, myogenesis after treatment with 5-Azacytidine, adipogenesis after treatment with dexamethasone

serum-deprivation ? This question was answered using immunofluorescent techniques (Darmon *et al*. 1982a, b ; Darmon, in press ; Darmon *et al*., in press) allowing to screen whole dishes of cells. No rare variants expressing antigens characteristic of differentiated cells could be found in exponential serum-containing cultures of 1003 cells. In con-fluent cultures in serum-containing medium however, some endoderm cells expressing keratin filaments and collagen I could be detected (Darmon *et al*., in press) but no other differentiated cells. It is thus clear that serum-deprivation INDUCES differentiation into neuroepithelium, muscle, mesenchyme, ...

2) Is the choice between alternative pathways of differentiation controlled by the environment at the level of determination or at the level of terminal differentiation ? It is tempting to speculate that serum-deprivation induces the formation of a unique multipotential cell type which is committed to differentiate but has not yet determined its choice. In that context, the choice may be thought to be controlled by attachment factors such as laminin or fibronectin, or by the re-addition of serum factors. These factors would then determine the proportion of the different cell types eventually obtained (Fig. 4 , model A). However it is also possible that serum-deprivation induces the formation of se-veral distinct precursors (neuroepithelial, mesenchymal, muscular...). In that context, the effect of attachment factors or serum factors would be due to preferential stimulation of terminal pathways of differentia-tion (Fig. 4 , model B). To make the difference between model A and mo-del B, it would be necessary to obtain clonal cultures of 1003 in the absence of serum in order to find out whether different conditions such

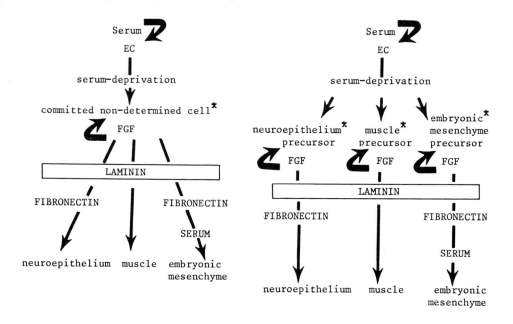

MODEL A   MODEL B

(★) In model A it is assumed that FGF stimulates the proliferation of a unique
     type of "non-EC" cells while in model B FGF is supposed to stimulate the
     proliferation of a cell population composed of various types of "non-EC"
     cells.

Fig. 4.   Alternative models for 1003 differentiation. Curved arrow indicate proliferation, straight arrows indicate differentiation.

as laminin vs fibronectin, serum re-added - or not - would alter, the
PROPORTION of the different cell types in clones of MIXED PHENOTYPES
(model A) or the NUMBER of PURE clones of each phenotype (model B). Up
to now it has been impossible to obtain serum-free cultures of 1003 at
densities lower than 5.10^2-10^3 cells/cm^2.

        Although we are still not able to determine at which develop-
mental stage extracellular factors control 1003 differentiation it is
clear that they are able to control both the initiation of the differentiation process and the nature of the phenotypes eventually obtained.
Further experiments are needed to unravel the physiological significance
of these results.

ACKNOWLEDGEMENTS.   The author wishes to thank Dr. R. Kemler for the gift
of ECMA 7 monoclonal antibodies, and Dr. D. Paulin for the gift of anti-
tyrosine hydroxylase antibodies. The author is grateful to Drs. F. Jacob,
H. Eisen and M.H. Buc-Caron for stimulating discussions.

REFERENCES

Brinster, R. : The effect of cells transferred into the mouse blastocyst on subsequent development. *J.Exp.Med. 140* : 1019-1056, 1974.

Darmon, M. : Laminin provides a better substrate than fibronectin for attachment, growth and differentiation of 1003 embryonal carcinoma cells. *In vitro*, in press.

Darmon, M., and Serrero, G. : Isolation of two different fibroblastic cell types from the embryonal carcinoma cell line 1003. Study of tumorigenic properties, surface antigens and differentiation responses to 5-Azacytidine and dexamethasone. *Cold Spring Harbor Conferences on Cell Proliferation 10*, in press.

Darmon, M., Bottenstein, J., and Sato, G. : Neural differentiation following culture of embryonal carcinoma cells in a serum-free defined medium. *Dev.Biol. 85* : 463-473, 1981.

Darmon, M., Stallcup, W., and Pittman, Q. : Induction of neural differentiation by serum-deprivation in cultures of the embryonal carcinoma cell line 1003. *Exp.Cell Res. 138* : 73-78, 1982a.

Darmon, M., Satllcup, W., Pittman, Q., and Sato, G. : Control of differentiation pathways by the extracellular environment in an embryonal carcinoma cell line. *Cold Spring Harbor Conferences on Cell Proliferation 9* : in press.

Darmon, M., Barret, A., Puymirat, J., and Faivre, A. : Cholinergic neurons and embryonic mesenchymal cells arise from the same population of precursor cells in cultures of embryonal carcinoma cells triggered to differentiate by serum-deprivation. *Biology of the Cell 45, (1)* : 10, 1982c.

Darmon, M., Buc-Caron, M.H., Paulin, D., and Jacob, F. : Control by the extracellular environment of differentiation pathways in 1003 embryonal carcinoma cells : study at the level of specific intermediate filaments. *EMBO Journal*, in press.

Jacob, F. : Mouse teratocarcinoma and mouse embryo. *Proc.R.Soc.Lond. B 201* : 249-270, 1978.

Mintz, B., and Illmensee, K. : Normal genetically mosaic mice produced from malignant terarocarcinoma cells. *Proc.Natl.Acad.Sci.U.S.A. 72* : 3585-3589, 1975.

Papaioannou, V., Mc Burney, M., Gardner, R., and Evans, M. : Fate of teratocarcinoma cells injected into early mouse embryos. *Nature 258* : 70-73, 1975.

Interaction of Metastatic and Non-Metastatic Tumor Lines with Aortic Endothelial Cell Monolayer and Their Underlying Basal Lamina

Volker Schirrmacher[1] and Israel Vlodavsky[2]

[1] Institut für Immunologie und Genetik, Deutsches Krebsforschungszentrum, D-6900 Heidelberg, FRG
[2] Department of Clinical Oncology, Hadassah University Hospital, Jerusalem, Israel

INTRODUCTION

A common and most important route for the dissemination of neoplastic cells within the body involves invasion and penetration of tumor cells into blood vessels and/or lymphatics (1-3). Following penetration of blood vessels, tumor cells are either carried away passively in the blood stream or remain at the site of vessel invasion where they proliferate and continue to shed emboli into the circulation (4). Tumor cells arrested in the capillary beds of different organs must then invade the endothelial cell lining and its underlying basal lamina in order to escape into the extravascular tissue and find a proper microenvironment where they can establish metastasis (1-3). Electron microscopic studies have shown local dissolution of the subendothelial basement membrane at its region of contact with invading tumor cells (5), thereby suggesting an enzymatic mechanism. Of particular significance are recent studies on the degradation of collagen type IV (6,7), fibronectin (8,9), laminin (10), and sulfated proteoglycans (8,9,11) by metastatic tumor cells because these macromolecules are the predominant structural constituents in basement membranes (8,12,13).

Blood borne tumor cells arrest, invasion and mediated solubilization of the subendothelial extracellular matrix (ECM) can be studied in vitro provided that both the tumor sublines and endothelial cells closely resemble their in vivo counterparts. Bovine aortic endothelial cells cultured in the presence of fibroblast growth factor (FGF) are most appropriate for this purpose because like in the in vivo situation they grow in two dimensions and exhibit both morpholigical and functional polarity (14). Most pertinent to the present study is a massive secretion of an underlying extracellular matrix (ECM) in a polar fashion and similar in organization and chemical composition (collagen type IV and V, heparan sulfate, laminin, fibronectin) to naturally occurring basal laminas (9,13-16). This matrix remains intact and firmly attached to the tissue culture plastic after denudation of the endothelial cell layer with Triton X-100.

In the present study we have used this highly characterized cell system as a model to study the interaction of tumor cells with the vessel wall. The tumor model system consisted of a low metastatic parental line (Eb) and a high metastatic spontaneous variant (ESb), both derived from a chemically induced T lymphoma (L 5178Y) of the DBA/2 mouse (17). These sublines are stable during in vitro cultivation and have been characterized with regard to caryotype (18), adhesive (19) and invasive capacity (20), immunogenicity (21), expression of tumor-antigens (22) and differentiation antigens (23). The two types of tumor cells were allowed to interact with intact or artificially wounded endothelial cell monolayer and with the underlying ECM when fully denuded of its endothelial cells. Tumor cell attachment was quantitated by counting the attached cells at various time intervals. Degradation of the ECM was analyzed by gel filtration or SDS polyacrylamide gel electrophoresis (PAGE) of labeled components released from the subendothelial ECM. The ECM was labeled either by lactoperoxidase catalyzed iodination or metabolically by $Na_2(^{35}S)O_4$. Technical details are described elsewhere (9).

RESULTS

1. Tumor cell attachment to the vascular endothelium and to the subendothelial extra cellular matrix (ECM)

The Eb and ESb lymphoma cells failed to attach to tissue culture plastic and grew in suspension mostly as single spheroidal cells (ESb) or small and loosely held cell aggregates (Eb). In contrast, both the high (ESb) and low (Eb) metastatic cells exhibited a firm cell attachment and flattening when seeded on top of the subendothelial ECM. Removal of the attached cells was not achieved by even a vigorous pipetting and required, like that of anchorage dependent cells, dissociation with trypsin (24). The kinetics of cell attachment was studied with ^{3}H-thymidine labeled Eb and ESb cells suspended in growth medium and added on top of either a confluent endothelial cell monolayer or directly on the underlying basal lamina denuded of its endothelial cells. As observed with other cell types (25,11) both the Eb and ESb lymphoma cells exhibited a much faster and firmer adhesion to the subendothelial ECM than to the apical surface of the endothelial cell layer. Thus, 30-40% of the seeded cells were firmly attached to the basal lamina within 10 min. as compared to only about 5% of either the Eb or ESb cells that were attached to the vascular endothelium at 3 h of incubation. There was no substantial difference between the Eb and ESb cells except at longer times (24-72 hrs.) where tumor cell detachment and aggregation occurred to a higher degree with the Eb than the ESb cells, particularly when plated on top of the vascular endothelium. In order to better resemble the in vivo situation of blood flow and sheer force, cell adhesion was studied also while gently shaking the culture dishes. Under this condition there was an almost complete inhibition of tumor cell adherence to the vascular endothelium as compared to a firm, albeit slower, attachment of both the Eb and ESb cells to the subendothelial ECM.

2. Tumor cell invasion through the vascular endothelium

The process of tumor cell invasion through the vascular endothelium was followed by phase and scanning electron micrographs taken at various times after seeding the tumor cells on top of a confluent endothelial cell monolayer. When visualized by phase microscopy, greater than 90% of the Eb cells appeared as single spheroids or forming small aggregates. In contrast, the ESb cells were mostly single and about 30% of the attached cells were seen to extend a cytoplasmic process between adjacent endothelial cells. These differences and the various modes of tumor cell invasion through the vascular endothelium were studied in greater detail by scanning electron microscopy (Fig. 1). At short incubation times (2-5h), more than 90% of either the Eb or ESb cells retained their spheroidal shape and less than 5% of the cells showed signs of penetration through the endothelial layer. At longer time intervals (6-24h), up to 40% of the attached ESb cells were seen at various stages of invasion (Fig. 1 B-D) as compared to about 10% of the Eb cells. Invasion of ESb cells was most frequently initiated by means of a cytoplasmic process indenting at junctions between adjoining endothelial cells. Tumor cell invasion then proceeded by streaming via the so formed gap with retration of endothelial cell borders in immediate contact with the invading cell. Less frequently, the ESb cells were seen to traverse across intact endothelial cells rather than at a site of junction. Lymphoma cells located underneath the vascular endothelium were seen at 32-48 h of incubation suggesting reformation of intercellular endothelial junctions so as to wall off the tumor cells from the exterior environment (24).
A marked difference between the low (Eb) and high (ESb) metastatic lymphoma cells was observed when the cells were plated in direct contact with the subendothelial ECM. Whereas the Eb cells mostly retained their spheroidal shape, the ESb cells adopted a more flattened morphology and 30-40% of the cells exhibited, within 5-24 h after seeding, an extension of pseudopods at least four times longer than the cell body (Fig. 1A).

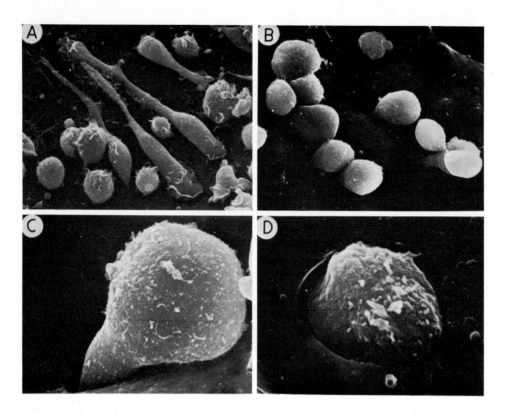

Fig. 1. Scanning electron micrographs of ESb lymphoma cells plated on top of a confluent endothelial cell monolayer (B-D) or on its underlying ECM. ESb cells (10^6 cells per 35 mm dish) were seeded and coincubated with the ECM or the endothelial cells for 8 h (A-C) or 24 h (D). They were then washed, fixed and processed for SEM. Extension of a long pseudopod (A), initial invasion by means of a cytoplasmic process (B,C) and subsequent penetration of the entire cell (D) was seen in 30-50% of the ESb cells. A 1350x; B 2100x; C 7200x; D 12600x.

It remains to be elucidated whether this extension of a cytoplasmic process facilitates tumor cell invasion through the endothelial lining and the subsequent degradation of the subendothelial ECM. Solubilization of the subendothelial ECM vicinal to edges of the cell body and pseudopods were often seen by scanning electron microscopy.

3. Tumor cell mediated solubilization of the subendothelial ECM
a) Degradation of iodinated ECM

To study whether the higher ability of the ESb lymphoma cells to invade the vascular endothelium was associated with a higher degradation of various components in the ECM, both the Eb and ESb cells were seeded on top of ECM which had been radiolabeled by lactoperoxidase catalyzed iodination. Serum-free culture medium was collected and replaced every day and the amount of TCA precipitable, ^{125}I-labeled material determined and analyzed by SDS-PAGE and autoradiography. By measuring either the total amount of ^{125}I-radioactivity released into the culture medium or the amount of TCA precipitable labeled material there was a higher activity associated with the ESb than with the Eb cells (9). The extent of Eb cell mediated release of iodinated material was, in most experiments, only slightly higher than that observed in control ECM coated dishes incubated with medium but no cells. Upon subjecting the culture media to slab gel electrophoresis it was found that regardless of the batch of iodinated ECM and lymphoma cells, a given volume of medium yielded a markedly higher intensity of bands when taken from cultures of ESb cells than from Eb cells. The nature of material released by the lymphoma cells from the ECM was analyzed by immunoprecipitation reactions with rabbit antisera directed against Fibronectin, Laminin or Collagen IV. Fibronectin appeared as the most prominent labeled protein released from the subendothelial matrix by the ESb cells. Because most of the lower molecular weight components also reacted with anti Fibronectin antibodies, this material is likely to represent split products of intact Fibronectin.

b) Degradation of sulfate containing proteoglycans

The ability of the Eb and ESb cells to degrade sulfated macromolecules in the ECM was studied by allowing the cells to interact with metabolically $(^{35}S)O_4^=$ - labeled ECM followed by gel filtration analysis of the degradation products released into the culture medium. In the absence of tumor cells, there was a spontaneous release of labeled material that consisted almost entirely (90%) of large molecular weight components. This material had an approximate molecular weight of $1-2\times10^6$ daltons since it comigrated with dextran blue (Mr= 2×10^6 daltons) on a Sepharose 2B column (Kav=0.53). A similar elution pattern was obtained when the nonmetastatic Eb cells were plated on top of the labeled ECM and the medium subjected to gel filtration on either Sepharose 2B or 4B columns. In contrast, plating the metastatic ESb cells in direct contact with the $(^{35}S)O_4^=$ - labeled ECM was associated with degradation of its sulfated proteoglycans into low molecular weight fragments. 80-90% of the released radioactivity was included when subjected to gel filtration on Sepharose 6B (Kav= 0.64) and Sepharose 4B (Kav=0.8). Based on Sephadex G-200 chromatography, the (^{35}S)-labeled fragments released by the metastatic ESb cells had a molecular weight of about 10,000 daltons. This pattern of degradation was not observed following treatment of the

$(^{35}S)O_4^=$ - labeled matrix with purified preparations of either trypsin, collagenase, hyaluronidase or elastase.

Precipitation studies with 1% cetyl piridinium chloride (CPC) revealed that greater than 90% of the $(^{35}S)O_4^=$ - radioactivity released in the absence or presence of lymphoma cells (either Eb or ESb) was precipitable, whereas that released by chondroitinase ABC was not. Therefore, even in the case of lymphoma cell mediated degradation, the released $(^{35}S)O_4^=$ - labeled glycosaminoglycan fragments were large enough for precipitation with CPC.

A correlation between tumor cell metastatic capacity and ability to degrade the subendothelial proteoglycans was also reported by Kramer and Nicolson (8). These investigators have shown that the low molecular weight $(^{35}S)O_4^=$-labeled fragment is almost entirely heparan sulfate. They also detected a unique endoglycosidase activity specific for heparan sulfate (26). Because heparan sulfate constitutes a major scaffolding proteoglycan of the subendothelial basal lamina and other extracellular matrixes, its preferential degradation by highly metastatic tumor cells may, in conjunction with solubilization of other matrix constituents facilitate tumor cell infiltration through blood vessels and tissues.

4. Sequential degradation of the subendothelial proteoglycans by enzymes secreted into the culture medium in presence or absence of serum-free medium

Further characterization of the degradation enzymes requires enzyme purification, a procedure which would be facilitated if the enzymes were released into culture supernatants. We therefore tested for the presence of glycosaminoglycan degradation activity in growth media conditioned by the lymphoma cells. Incubation of $(^{35}S)O_4^=$ - labeled ECM with medium collected from five day ESb cell cultures (ESb medium) yielded a low MW, $(^{35}S)O_4^=$ - labeled component similar to that released upon incubation of the ECM with ESb cells suspended in fresh medium. Furthermore, when the experiment was performed in a serum-free medium conditioned for three days by ESb cells (10^6 cells/ml) (Fig. 2), there was a 3-5 fold higher degradation activity than in a corresponding serum containing conditioned medium. In contrast, there was no release of low MW fragments by incubation with a serum-free or a serum containing medium preconditioned by Eb cells (Fig. 2). The ESb conditioned medium was therefore used in subsequent studies as a source for a soluble enzyme activity which may among other factors, facilitate tumor cell invasion and metastasis. The

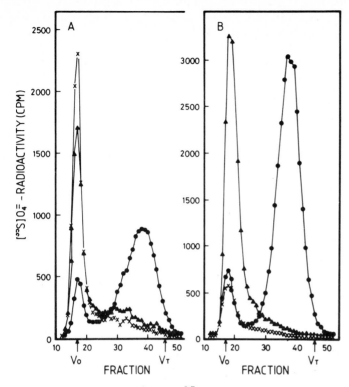

Fig. 2. Degradation of (^{35}S)O$_4^=$ - labeled ECM by serum containing (A) or
serum-free (B) media conditioned by Eb (▲) or ESb (●) cells. Respectively control media are included (x) to control for spontaneous release
of radioactivity. The culture medium consisted of RPMI-1640 with or without 10% FCS. Media collected after 48 h coincubation at 37ºC with the
labeled ECM were centrifuged and 0.6 ml aliquots subjected to gel filtration on Sepharose 4B columns. The excluded volume V_O was marked by
blue dextran and the total included volume V_t by phenol red.

Under serum-free conditions the spontaneous release of radioactivity
was reduced and the release of high molecular compounds by Eb conditioned medium and of low molecular compounds by ESb conditioned medium
increased.

ESb enzyme retained its activity after freezing and thawing or ultracen-
trifugation (100,000 xg, 1 h), but lost the activity after treatment for
3 min. at 95ºC. Its optimal pH was 6.2 and there was almost no activity
at pH 7.4. The high MW degradation products released upon incubation of
the ECM with Eb medium were precipitated by both 10% TCA and 1% CPC,
whereas the low MW component released by incubation with ESb medium was
precipitated by CPC but not TCA.

We could directly demonstrate that the Eb mediated high MW degradation
product can serve as a substrate for further degradation by the ESb
enzyme. Thus, addition of ESb medium to the high MW, (^{35}S)O$_4^=$ - labeled

material first released by incubation of the ECM with Eb medium yielded
the 10^4 daltons fragment, but there was no further degradation of the
high MW component upon a similar incubation with Eb medium. Release of
a low MW, $(^{35}S)O_4^=$ - labeled material was also observed after treating
the ECM with chondroitinase ABC, but unlike the ESb mediated degradation, the released radioactivity was not precipitated with 1% CPC.

Solubilization of the subendothelial basal lamina is likely to involve
multiple enzymes among which are a proteinase, collagenase type IV and
a recently identified endoglycosidase, all of which are capable of de-
grading under physiological conditions major structural constituents
of the ECM such as fibronectin, collagen type IV and heparan sulfate.
Our studies suggest that an endoglycosidase mediated solubilization of
the ECM glycosaminoglycans is preceded by a proteolytic activity present
in high and low metastatic tumor cells. It is possible that the degradative enzymes act like a cascade with one enzyme's product being the substrate for the next enzyme. Although these enzymes are secreted and
highly active in the culture medium, a firm tumor cell attachment to
either the vascular endothelium or the ECM seems to be required for
an efficient degradation of the subendothelial proteoglycans. This has
been suggested by showing that agitation of the culture dishes inhibited both tumor to endothelial cell attachment and subsequent release of
$(^{35}S)O_4^=$ - labeled degradation products. Furthermore, ESb medium placed
on top of a confluent endothelial cell layer released very small amounts
of $(^{35}S)O_4^=$ - labeled material as compared to when ESb cells were placed
on top of the endothelial cells. It is likely that ESb variant cells are
more invasive than the Eb parental lines because they (i) can better
penetrate the vascular endothelium, a property depending on cell motility, and (ii) exhibit a higher degradative acitivity once they are in
contact with the basal lamina.

SUMMARY

Cultured vascular endothelial cells which closely resemble their in vivo
counterpart, have been used as a model to study the interaction of blood
borne tumor cells with the vascular endothelium and its underlying basal
lamina; a) both high and low metastatic tumor cells exhibit a much faster
and firmer attachment to the subendothelial extracellular matrix (ECM)
than to the apical surface of the endothelial cell layer; b) under conditions of blood flow and sheer force, tumor cell arrest is expected to be
restricted to areas of exposed subendothelium such as found in cases of

endothelial damage and normal shedding; c) tumor cell invasion is most
often initiated by a cytoplasmic process indenting at junctions between
adjoining endothelial cells followed by regeneration of the endothelium
and sealing off the invasive cells from the exterior environment; d) the
proteoglycan scaffolding of the subendothelial ECM is degraded into high
and low molecular weight, sulfate containing, components. The latter are
released by means of a unique endoglycosidase like activity associated
with highly metastatic sublines of murine lymphoma and melanoma cells.

It is concluded that the protective role of the vascular endothelium is
fulfilled primarily by the nonadhesiveness of its luminal surface and
less by its forming an efficient barrier against tumor cell invasion.
The ability of highly metastatic tumor cells to degrade proteoglycans,
fibronectin, and other components of the subendothelial basal lamina,
facilitate their hematogenous dissemination and extravasation.

REFERENCES

1. Poste, G. and Fidler, I.J. The pathogenesis of cancer metastasis. Nature 283, 139-146 (1980).

2. Hart, I.R. and Fidler, I.J. Cancer invasion and metastasis. The Quarterly Review of Biology 55, 121-142 (1980).

3. Roos, E. and Dingemans, K.P. Mechanisms of metastasis. Biochim. Biophys.Acta 560, 135-166 (1979).

4. Warren, B.A., Chauvin, W.J. and Phillips, J. Blood-borne tumor emboli and their adherence to vessel walls. In: Cancer invasion metastasis: Biologic Mechanisms and Therapy. S.B. Day, et al. (eds). pp. 185-197, New York, Raven Press (1977).

5. Babai, F. Etude ultrastructurale sure la patogenie de l'invasion du muscle strie par des tumeurs transplantables. J.Ultrastr.Res. 56, 287-303 (1976).

6. Liotta, L.A., Abe, S., Gerhon-Robey, P. and Martin, G.R. Preferential digestion of basement membrane collagen by an enzyme derived from a metastatic murine tumor. Proc.Natl.Acad.Sci.USA 76, 2268-2272 (1979).

7. Liotta, L.A., Tryggvason, K., Garbisa, S., Hart, I.R., Foltz, C.M. and Shafie, S. Metastatic potential correlates with enzymatic degradation of basement membrane collagen. Nature 284, 65-66 (1980).

8. Kramer, R.H., Vogel, K.G. and Nicolson, G.L. Solubilization and degradation of subendothelial matrix glycoproteins and proteoglycans by metastatic tumor cells. J.Biol.Chem. 257, 2678-2686 (1982).

9. Vlodavsky, I., Fuks, Z., Ariav, Y., Altevogt, P. and Schirrmacher, V. Lymphoma cell mediated degradation of sulfated proteoglycans and fibronectin in the subendothelial extracellular matrix: Relationship to tumor cell metastasis. Submitted for publication.

10. Liotta, L.A., Goldfarb, R.H., Brundage, R., Siegal, G.P. and Garbisa, S. Effect of plasminogen activator (urokinase), plasmin, and thrombin on glycoprotein and collagenous components of basement membrane.

11. Vlodavsky, I., Ariav, Y., Atzmon, R. and Fuks, Z. Tumor cell attachment to the vascular endothelium and subsequent degradation of the subendothelial extracellular matrix. Exptl.Cell.Res. (1982) in press.

12. Hassell, J.R., Robey, P.G., Barrach, H.J., Wilczek, J., Rennard, S.I. and Martin, G.R. Isolation of a heparan sulfate containing proteoglycan from basement membrane. Proc.Natl.Acad.Sci.USA 77, 4494-4498 (1980).

13. Kefalides, N.A., Alper, R. and Clark, C.C. Biochemistry and metabolism of basement membranes. Int.Rev.Cytol. 61, 167-228 (1979).

14. Gospodarowicz, D., Vlodavsky, I., Greenburg, G., Alvarado, J., Johnson, L.R. and Moran, J. Studies on atherogenesis and corneal transplantation using cultured vascular and corneal endothelia. Rec.Prog.Horm.Res., 35, 375-448 (1979).

15. Gospodarowicsz, D., Greenburg, G., Foidart, J.M. and Savion, N. The production and localization of laminin in cultured vascular and corneal endothelial cells. J.Cell.Physiol. 107, 171-183 (1981).

16. Vlodavsky, I., Lui, G.M. and Gospodarowicz, D. Morphological appearance, growth behavior and migratory activity of human cells maintained on extracellular matrix versus plastic. Cell 19, 607-616 (1980).

17. Schirrmacher, V., Shantz, G., Clauer, K., Komitowski, D., Zimmermann, H.-P. and Lohmann-Matthes, M.L. Tumor metastases and cell-mediated immunity in a model system in DBA/2 mice. I. Tumor invasiveness in vitro and metastases formation in vivo. Int.J.Cancer 23, 233-244 (1979).

18. Dzarlieva, R., Schirrmacher, V. and Fusenig, N. Cytogenetic changes during tumor progression towards invasion, metastasis and immune escape in the Eb/ESb model system. Int.J.Cancer (1982) in press.

19. Schirrmacher, V., Cheingsong-Popov, R. and Arnheiter, H. Hepatocyte-tumor cell interaction in vitro. I. Conditions for rosette formation and inhibition by anti H-2 antibody. J.Exp.Med. 151, 984-989 (1980).

20. Lohmann-Matthes, M.-L., Schleich, A., Shantz, G. and Schirrmacher, V. Tumor metastases and cell-mediated immunity in a model system in DBA/2 mice. VII. Interaction of metastasizing and nonmetastasizing tumors with normal tissue in vitro. J.Natl.Cancer Inst. 64, 1413-1425 (1980).

21. Bosslet, K., Schirrmacher, V. and Shantz, G. Tumor metastases and cell-mediated immunity in a model system in DBA/2 mice. VI. Similar specificity patterns of protective anti-tumor immunity in vivo and of cytolytic T cells in vitro. Int.J.Cancer 24, 303-313 (1979).

22. Schirrmacher, V., Bosslet, K., Shantz, G., Clauer, K. and Hübsch, D. Tumor metastases and cell-mediated immunity in a model system in DBA/2 mice. IV. Antigenic differences between the parental tumor line and its metastasizing variant. Int.J.Cancer 23, 245-252 (1979).

23. Altevogt, P., Kurnick, J.T., Kimura, A.K., Bosslet, K. and Schirr-macher, V. Different expression of Lyt differentiation antigens and cell surface glycoproteins by a murine T lymphoma line and its high metastatic variant. Eur.J.Immunol. 12, 300-307 (1982).

24. Vlodavsky, I., Ariav, Y., Fuks, Z. and Schirrmacher, V. Lymphoma cell interaction with cultured vascular endothelial cells and with subendothelial basal lamina: attachment, invasion and morphological appearance. Submitted for publication.

25. Kramer, R.H., Gonzalez, R. and Nicolson, G.L. Metastatic tumor cells adhere preferentially to the extracellular matrix underlying vascular endothelial cells. Int.J.Cancer 26, 639-644 (1980).

26. Nakadjima, M., Inmura, T., Diferrante, D.T., Diferrante, N. and Nicolson, G.L. Rates of heparan sulfate degradation correlate with invasive and metastatic activities of B16 melanoma sublines. J.Cell.Biol. 91, 119a (1981).

Control of Behaviour and Growth by Imitating the Contact Environment

R. Wieser and G. Brunner

Institut für Immunologie, Johannes Gutenberg Universität, Obere Zahlbacher Str. 67, D-6500 Mainz, FRG

The behaviour of cells in vitro is the result of all the influences exerted by the actual microenvironment which, in a simplified form, is composed of two main compartments (Fig. 1): (i) the diffusive environment, (ii) the contact environment. These two compartments regulate the cell behaviour by distinct mechanisms induced by molecules which, beside being compartment-specific, differ in their mobility.

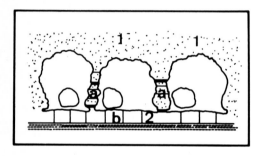

Fig. 1. The compartments of the cellular microenvironment:

1. Diffusive environment

2. Contact environment (a: cell-cell contacts; b: cell-substrate contacts

The diffusive environment comprises all those types of molecules that are freely diffusible, i.e. hormones, growth factors, vitamins, transport proteins, and nutrients (1). Generally these molecules induce the specific signal just by binding to specific receptors localized in the plasma membrane (2) or after the receptor-mediated endocytosis (3). The molecular mechanisms induced by these freely diffusible molecules must therefore be quite different from the action of the molecules composing the contact environment (Tab. I). These molecules are commonly in a fixed state either as the molecules generating the extracellular matrix or the basement membranes or by their insertion into the cell membrane. In the latter case a relatively high mobility is given in the plane of the plasma membrane.

An increasing body of experimental data suggests that such fundamental phenomena as growth homeostasis (5), cell differentiation (6), as well as embryogenesis (7), are regulated by the interaction of specific plasma membrane-localized molecules with substrate-localized molecules (cell-substratum interaction) (5) or with the plasma membrane molecules of neighboring cells (cell-cell interaction) (7). The molecular principle involved in these different regulation processes is still unknown, but evidence has accumulated that specific interactions of the cells with the contact environment are mediated by plasma membrane glycoproteins and surface lectins (9 - 11).

Table I.   Molecular components composing the contact environment
of mammalian cells

Cell-substrate contact	Cell-cell contact
* GAG	* Membrane glycoproteins
* Collagen	* Membrane lectins
* Fibronectin	* Membrane glycolipids
* Elastin	

In our contribution examples are given how a specifically imitated contact environment influences the morphological behaviour, the distribution of cell membrane molecules and the proliferation rate of GH_3-cells under serum-free, hormone-supplemented culture conditions.

MATERIALS AND METHODS

Chemicals, Media and Solutions: All chemicals and biochemicals were purchased from Sigma (Munich, FRG) unless stated otherwise. Fibroblast growth factor (FGF) was purchased from Collaborative Research (Paesel, Frankfurt, FRG); succinylated Concanavalin A (sCon A) was obtained from Polyscience (Paesel); ferritin, cationized ferritin and ferritin-labeled Concanavalin A (F-Con A) was obtained from Miles Laboratories; Phaseolus vulgaris lectin was purchased from Sigma and Difco. Trimethoxysilylpropyl-diethylenetriamine (TSTP) was obtained from Petrarch Systems (Levittown, PA, USA), $Na(^3H)_4B$ was obtained from NEN (Dreieich, FRG), (^3H)-thymidine was obtained from Amersham Buchler (Braunschweig, FRG).

Cell Culture: GH_3-cells were passaged routinely in 75 cm² flasks (Lux, Seromed, Munich, FRG) in a 1:1 mixture of Dulbecco's modified Eagle's medium (DMEM) and HAM F12 (F12), supplemented with trace elements (4) and serum (3% newborn calf serum (NCS) 5 % horse serum (HS), Gibco, Karlsruhe, FRG) and were cultivated at 37°C, 5% CO_2, and 95% humidity.

For the described experiments cells were cultured in serum-free, hormone-supplemented medium (DMEM/F12, supplemented with trace elements and 5 µg/ml insulin, 5 µg/ml transferrin, 1 ng/ml thyreotropin-releasing hormone, 5×10^{-10}M triiodothyronin, and 10 ng/ml fibroblast growth factor (Collaborative Research)).

Coating Procedure: The coating of plastic surfaces with proteins was performed as described in (12).

Covalent Coupling of Proteins to Derivatized Glass Dishes: Derivatization of glass dishes and coupling of proteins was performed according to (13).

Isolation of Surface Lectins, Mannose-Bearing and N-Acetylneuraminic Acid-Bearing Glycoproteins: Mannose-binding proteins (surface lectins) were isolated from GH_3-plasma membranes according to (14). Mannose-bearing and N-acetylneuraminic acid (NANA)-bearing glycoproteins were isolated from GH_3-cells by affinity chromatography using Con A-Sepharose and neuraminidase Sepharose (R. Wieser and G. Brunner, submitted), following a similar protocol as described for the isolation of mannose-binding proteins.

Isolation of GH_3-Plasma Membrane Proteins Interacting with Proteins Coated on Plastic Surfaces: The adsorption of the Con A and P.vulgaris lectins on polylysine-precoated plastic surfaces was done as described in (12). GH_3-cells were washed twice in PBS and adjusted to 1.5×10^6 cells/ml of hormone-supplemented DMEM/F12; 4 ml were added to one flask (50 ml, 25 cm²) and incubated for 2 hrs at 37°C with 5% CO_2. After decanting the medium, the adherent cells were washed briefly with PBS and sonicated in bidistilled water (20 ml) for 1 h at 4°C by a water-bath sonifier. The supernatant containing the cell debris was discarded, and the surfaces were washed twice with bi-distilled water in excess (50 ml), drained, and incubated with 0.5 ml of SDS buffer (20 mM Tris-HCl, 20 mM EDTA, 4.3% SDS, 5% β-mercaptoethanol, 10% saccharose, 5 pM pyronin G) per flask in the waterbath sonifier for 90 min at 60°C. This released the adsorbed lectins together with the plasma membrane molecules, which were bound when the GH_3-cells attached to the lectin-coated surface of the culture dish. After the desorption the material of several flasks was collected, concentrated by acetone precipitation, boiled for 10 min and electrophoresed in the system according to (15).

Cell Proliferation Test: The DNA-synthesis of GH_3-cells grown on coupled plasma membrane proteins was measured as described (R. Wieser and G. Brunner, submitted). Labeling of the sialic acid- and galactose residues of the glycomolecules was performed as in (16).

RESULTS

1. EARLY EVENTS

1.1 Interaction of GH_3-Cells with Substrate-Adsorbed Plant Lectins and Charged Polymers

1.1.1 Adsorption of Proteins on Plastic Surfaces: Early experiments on the influence of sugar-specific plant lectins and nonspecifically acting charged polymers were performed by applying a first coat of polylysine onto the polystyrene dish surface, followed by a coat of specific plant lectins. The use of polylysine as a first protein layer is a generally used method in cell culture experiments since - beside the efficiency of polylysine as cell-adhesion promoter (17) - it is believed that polylysine acts as a molecular adhesive.

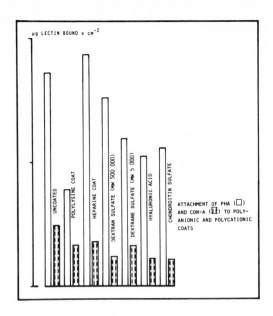

Fig. 2. Influence of precoated polymers on the adsorption of plant lectins

Intensive investigations in our laboratory (13, 18) on the behaviour of the protein layers under culture conditions showed, however, that (i) the precoating with polylysine results in an inhibition of the adsorption of the second protein to be added (Fig. 2). This inhibition depends on the one hand on the concentration of the adsorbed polylysine, and on the other hand on the nature of the charge of the polymers. (ii) The protein layers are unstable (Tab. II).

1.1.2 Phenotypic Behaviour of GH₃-Cells in Dependence of the Contact Environment:
When the GH₃-cells are cultured on dishes precoated with polylysine, followed by a coat of a specific plant lectins, the cells undergo marked morphological changes (Fig. 3). Depending on the sugar-specficity of the lectin the cells spread to different degrees within a period of 20 min after seeding in serum-free, hormone-supplemented medium. As shown in Fig. 4, succinylated Con A is most effective in promoting the spreading phase, whereas UEA and PHA are less effective. The induction of spreading sCon A

Table II.   Release of polymers from polystyrene surfaces

Treatment of culture dish	Phaseolus vulgaris		
	uncoated	polylysine precoated	polylysine uncoated
After 6 days (without medium change)	40	30	43
After 6 days (medium change on day 3)	65	73	n.d.

Values in percentage of the adsorbed total protein.

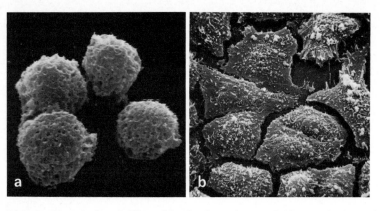

Fig. 3. Phenotype of GH₃-cells in dependence of the contact environment.
a) GH₃-cells on polylysine-coated culture dish.
b) GH₃-cells on polylysine/sCon A coated culture dish.
Magnification: a) = 2738 x, b) = 1140 x

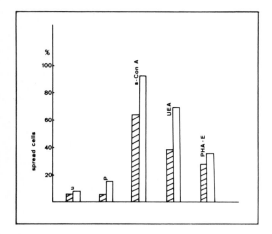

Fig. 4. Degree of spreading of GH₃-cells in dependence of the coated lectins and the diffusive environment. Blank columns: Hormone-supplemented DMEM/F12. Hatched columns: DMEM/F12.

is mannose-specific: the spreading can be inhibited (i) by saturation of the coated sCon A with mannan prior to the seeding of the cells and (ii) bei treating the cells with mannosidase (12). The spreading degree also depends on the diffusive environment. Firstly, under serum-supplemented conditions no differential effects of the lectins on the phenotypic behaviour of the cells can be observed. Secondly, the spreading process depends on the presence of hormones in the basal medium (Fig. 4). Further examinations of the hormonal factors which are essential for cell-spreading showed that insulin exerts nearly the same spreading-promoting as the whole hormone mixture (Fig. 5).

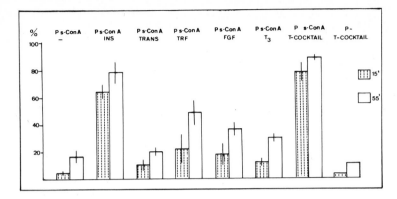

Fig. 5. Spreading efficiency of the single components of the hormone mixture

1.1.3 Molecular Changes in the Plasma Membrane induced by the Contact Environment:
The phenotypic changes induced by the interaction of the cells with a specific contact
environment occurs together with molecular alterations in the plasma membrane. If the
number of Con A receptors (mannose-bearing glycomolecules), expressed in the plasma
membrane in dependence of coated proteins, is determined (Fig. 6), three major principles can be stated: (i) cells grown in suspension have approximately half the number
of Con A receptors compared with cells grown on untreated culture dishes; (ii) a
positively charged contact environment (polylysine) further enhances the number of
Con A-receptors; (iii) coating the dishes with polylysine, followed by a coat of different concentrations of Con A increases the number of Con A-receptors at low Con A
concentrations, whereas high concentrations of Con A diminish the number of Con A-
binding sites.

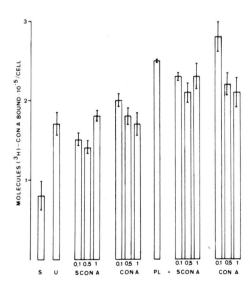

Fig. 6. Number of Con A-receptors on GH_3-
cells in dependence on the proteins coated
onto the culture surface.

S   =   suspended cells
U   = GH_3-cells grown on untreated plastic
        surfaces
PL =   Polylysine precoated culture surface.

0,1   concentrations of lectins
0,5   used for coating in mg
1

1.1.4 Protein Rearrangement induced by the Contact environment: In order to
clarify whether the observed differences in the number of Con A-binding sites are
due to a neoexpression or a rearrangement in the plane of the plasma membrane we
examined the glycoproteins which interacted with the coated proteins. The fluorographic
evaluation of the gels reveals three major principles involved in the rearrangement
of plasma membrane glycoproteins: The rearrangement depends (i) on the charge conditions on the cells [Fig. 7a: cells, neuraminidase-treated and labeled by the galactose-
oxidase-Na^{3}H$_4$B-method - no differences in the protein pattern of the molecules bound
to the different coats], (ii) on the charge conditions on the substrate [Fig. 7b,
marked differences of the protein pattern of the bound molecules are found when cells
are seeded on lectin coats with or without a polylysine precoat], (iii) on the sugar-
specificity of the coated lectins.

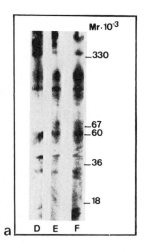
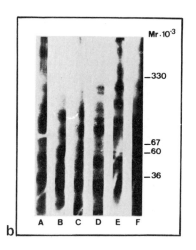

Fig. 7. Fluorography of the SDS gel electrophoretic pattern of GH$_3$ plasma membrane
proteins that interact with different proteins coated onto plastic surfaces.
7a: Neuraminidase-treated cells;   7b: untreated cells
A - C: Culture dishes without polylysine-precoat; D - F: Culture dishes with polylysine precoat; B, E : sCon A-coat; C, F : PHA-coat

The rearrangement is a specific, directed process. Using detergent extracts of
labeled cells or plasma membranes isolated thereof, instead of whole cells, up to
three times lower binding occurs. Furthermore, only minor differences can be observed
in dependence on the sugar-specificity of the lectins, whereas no differences can be
found when the lectins were coated on polylysine-treated or untreated surfaces.

2. LATE EVENTS

2.1 Interaction of GH₃-Cells with Covalently Coupled Endogenous Membrane Lectins and Glycoproteins

2.1.1 Covalent Binding of Proteins to Derivatized Glass Dishes: Since plant lectins influence the morphology and proliferation (19) of GH₃-cells, we tried to isolate molecules of the plasma membrane of GH₃-cells, which are able to influence the cell behaviour in a similar manner. The preceeding results suggest that mannose-related glycomolecules (mannose-specific lectins, mannose-bearing glycoproteins) are of importance in cell-substrate- and cell-cell interactions. Therefore, we isolated mannose-binding lectins and mannose-bearing glycoproteins. In addition we isolated NANA-bearing glycoproteins to cover a broad spectrum of different glycoproteins (Fig. 8).

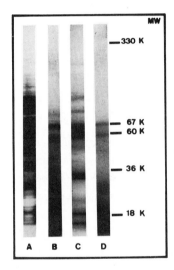

Fig. 8. SDS-gel-electrophoretic protein pattern of plasma membrane proteins isolated by affinity chromatography from Triton X-100 extract of GH₃-cells (A); B: NANA-bearing glycoproteins, C: Mannose-bearing glycoproteins, D: Mannose-binding proteins.

The isolated membrane molecules should be used as contact molecules to elucidate the involvement of membrane glycoproteins in the control of proliferation by cell-cell contacts.

As mentioned above, proteins, which are adsorbed to plastic surfaces are released to a great extent into the culture medium. These freely diffusible molecules bind to specific receptors located in the plasma membrane and are commonly internalized leading to molecular mechanisms which must be distinguished from those which are initiated by fixed molecules. Therefore, we developed a method (13) which allows to imitate "true" cell-cell contacts or cell-substrates by coupling proteins covalently to glass dishes. So, by the use of isolated components of biomatrices or basement membranes, cell-substrate interactions can be studied, whereas the use of plasma membrane proteins allows the imitation of cell-cell contacts.

Beside the advantage of this method in the firm binding of the proteins, an eight- to tenfold higher loading capacity is achieved.

2.1.2 Proliferation Inhibition by Isolated Membrane Molecules: Culturing GH₃-cells under serum-free, hormone-supplemented conditions for 40 hours on mannose-speci-

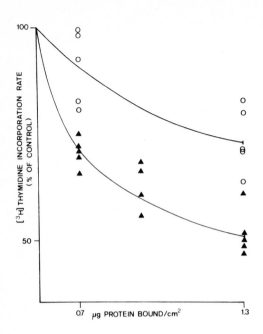

Fig. 9. (^{3}H)-thymidine incorporation rate into DNA depending on the concentration of NANA-bearing glycoproteins (▲) or mannose-binding lectins (o) coupled covalently to glass dishes and used as contact molecules.

fic membrane lectins and on NANA-bearing glycoproteins led to an inhibition of the proliferation rate in a concentration-dependent manner - as measured by thymidine incorporation into DNA (Fig. 9). The inhibition is of non-toxic manner and is observed only when these molecules are in a fixed state. If they are added to the hormone mixture in soluble form, the proliferation rate is not affected.

The inhibition exerted by the mannose-binding lectin can be abolished by treatment of the bound lectins with mannan prior to the addition of the cells. Due to the proliferation-stimulating activity of bound mannan in this assay it cannot be excluded that the reversion of inhibition is caused by mannan itself rather than by blocking the mannose-binding sites of the lectin.

Further controls for the specificity of the isolated compounds were made by coupling the proteins of the crude extracts, from which the specific molecules had been isolated. These protein mixtures have no influence on the incorporation of ^{3}H-thymidine or enhance the proliferation rate slightly.

If these experiments represent a true imitation of contact inhibition due to cell-cell contacts, then it should be assumed that the proliferation inhibition, shown in cells cultured on these membrane proteins, can be raised or lowered by varying the actual cell concentration. Compared with cells grown on glass dishes without coupled proteins, it is indeed shown that this inhibition is dependent on the actual cell density (Fig. 10). Interestingly, at the lowest density of cells grown on NANA-bearing glycoproteins a stimulation of DNA-synthesis is observed.

The incorporation of ^{3}H-thymidine into DNA decreases as a function of time after seeding the GH$_3$-cells on the coupled NANA-bearing glycoproteins (data not shown).

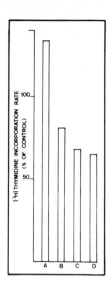

Fig. 10. (^{3}H)-thymidine incorporation rate of GH_3-cells as a function of cell density. NANA-bearing glycoproteins were coupled covalently to glass dishes at a concentration of 1 μg/cm^2. Cell densities: 2.5 x 10^4/ml (A); 5 x 10^4/ml (B); 1 x 10^5/ml (C); 2.5 x 10^5/ml (D).

DISCUSSION

Phenotypic Behaviour of GH_3-Cells: Cell adhesion and cell spreading is believed to be closely related to the control of growth (20). This correlation is aptly expressed in the term "anchorage-dependence of growth" which describes the inability of normal cells to grow unless they are attached to a substratum. Especially primary cells have unique demands on the treatment of the culture substrate (7) in order to proliferate actively. It is also known that specific components of a specific substratum, e.g. the basement membrane, are responsible for the support of cell proliferation but not for the cell attachment (21). On the other hand, the specific treatment of the substrate affects the responsiveness of cells to various hormones (22).

It is well known from a number of investigations (5, 7, 8, 23-25) that membrane-localized glycoproteins are involved in cell-substrate adhesion and cell-cell interactions. Since lectins are also found in the cell membrane of mammalian cells (14, 26) these sugar-specific molecules should be serious candidates for cell-cell and cell-substrate interactions by their binding to specific glycoproteins (23). In the in vivo situation either the plasma membrane-located glycoproteins (cell-cell interaction) or the molecules constituting the biomatrix (cell-substrate adhesion) must be seen as "contact molecules". By attaching these contact-specific molecules to culture surfaces the imitation of the respective cell-interactions should be possible. As a first approach in studying the glycomolecules involved in the contact interactions commercially available plant lectins were used as attachment molecules.

The experiments reported here suggest that mannose-specific glycomolecules localized in the plasma membrane of GH_3-cells are involved in the spreading process. This mannose-specificity is shown by the inhibition of spreading by (i) mannan-treat-

ment of sCon A, (ii) mannosidase-treatment of the GH$_3$-cells, and (iii) heat-denatura-
tion of sCon A. It is further shown that the spreading process depends on the initiation of specific metabolic pathways which, in GH$_3$-cells, are induced by insulin.
These metabolic pathways probably provide the energy for the spreading process (27).

   Rearrangement of Plasma Membrane Proteins: As a first response of cells to the
specific contact molecules a rearrangement of plasma membrane-localized molecules
(Fig. 11) must be postulated (29) as shown in the experiments. The extent and direction of the rearrangement depends on (i) the specificity of the contact molecules,
(ii) the charge condition on the cell plasma membrane and (iii) on the contact molecules. The rearrangement of plasma membrane proteins induced by polyvalent ligands
is a well known, though not yet functionally understood process. Apparently by the
rearrangement of the ligand-specific membrane proteins also a redistribution of li-
gand-unrelated proteins occurs (28). Probably the rearrangement leads to the formation of specific molecular distinct membrane areas (Fig. 12). The individual molecules of these areas are possibly stabilized by intermolecular bonds, e.g. by the
action of transglutaminases, whereas the whole areas are stabilized by their interaction with cytoskeletal elements. As a further step we suggest that, due to the
binding of the ligand to the receptor and the subsequent area formation, individual
molecule(s) of the receptor area undergo(es) conformational changes which make this/
these protein(s) susceptible for specific enzymes (e.g. protein kinases (30), proteases (31)). This first molecular derivative should be the "starting point " for the
specific intracellular message driving the cell into a specific proliferative and/or
differentiative direction.

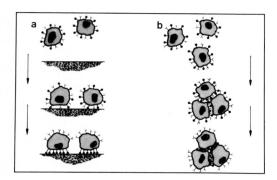

Fig. 11. Model of rearrangement of
membrane molecules suggested as a
first response of cells to cell-sub-
strate(s) or cell-cell contacts.

   Proliferation Control: The fact that plasma membrane-derived glycoproteins inhibit the proliferation rate of GH$_3$-cells to a high degree suggests that specific
cell-cell contacts are the main principle in the regulation of cell growth. The
evidence that the isolated components used are actually derived from the plasma membrane was provided by surface labeling techniques and by cell fractionation studies
(14).

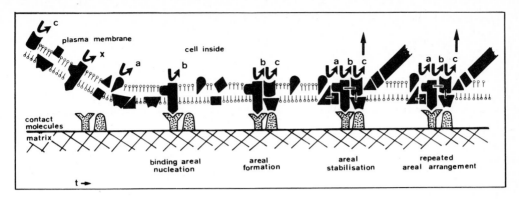

Fig. 12. Postulated molecular mechanisms in the plasma membrane induced by the contact environment.

In the past few years an increasing amount of experimental data suggests that membrane-localized glycoproteins are able to imitate the contact-dependent inhibition of growth (32 - 34). Calculations about the number of contacts required to inhibit the proliferation of GH_3-cells by 50% showed that 2×10^6 NANA-bearing glycoproteins interacting with one cell are necessary. This value is in good agreement with recently published observations showing that for a 50% inhibition of growth of BHK-cells by a brain-derived cell surface glycoprotein 5×10^6 bound molecules per cell are necessary (35).

The molecular nature of the compound(s) involved in the described contact-dependent growth control of GH_3-cells is not yet determined, nor are at the present time data available showing whether the active component resides in the protein or in the carbohydrate moiety of the molecule(s). However, it is assumed that the mechanism of the interaction of those substrate-bound carbohydrate-related proteins with the plasma membrane of the plated cells is of lectin-carbohydrate nature. It is likely that in the mammalian plasma membrane many proteins are localized which have lectin properties, regulating cell behaviour by interacting with carbohydrates of the cell membrane of the counterpart cell, as already mentioned by Hakomori et al. (23).

In conclusion, it is shown that

- the contact environment, whether cell-substrate- or cell-cell contacts, can be imitated by coupling endogenous plasma membrane molecules to the culture substrate.

- as a first response of the cell to an imitated contact environment a rearrangement of membrane proteins is observed.

- specific molecules isolated from the plasma membrane of GH_3-cells influence the proliferation behaviour in the sense of the "contact" inhibition of growth.

- the molecular mechanism of cell-cell contact-mediated growth control seems to be of lectin-carbohydrate nature.

ACKNOWLEDGEMENTS

The expert technical assistance of Ms Judith Becker and Mr Bernd Nitzgen is gratefully acknowledged. We thank Dr. G. Eisenbeis (Mainz) for instructions in scanning electron microscopy, and the Zoological Institute of the University Mainz for the permission to use the electron microscope Stereo Scan Mark 2A. The neuraminidase-Sepharose was kindly given to us by Drs. Kreilich and Ziegler (Institute for Biochemistry, University of Heidelberg).

This study was supported by the Deutsche Forschungsgemeinschaft (Br 703/5-3) and by the Stiftung Volkswagenwerk (Az I/35-736).

REFERENCES

1. Sporn, M.B. and Todaro, G.J. 1980. New Engl. J. Med. 19, 878.

2. Schreiber, A.B., Lax, I., Yarden, Y., Eshhar, Z., and Schlessinger, J. 1981. Proc. Natl. Acad. Sci. USA 78, 7535.
   Verlander, M.S., Venter, J.C., Goodman, M., Kaplan, N.O., and Saks, B. 1976. Proc. Natl. Acad. Sci. USA 73, 1009.

3. Pastan, Y.H. and Willingham, M.C. 1981. Ann. Rev. Physiol. 43, 239.

4. Hutchings, S.E. and Sato, G.H. 1978. Proc. Natl. Acad, Sci. USA 75, 801.

5. Frazier, W. and Glaser, L. 1979. Ann. Rev. Biochem. 48, 491.

6. Reid, L. 1983. Proc. of the First Eur. Conf. on Serum-Free Cell Culture. Springer Verlag, Heidelberg.

7. Moscona, A.A. 1974. In: The Cell Surface in Development (Moscona, A.A., ed.) John Wiley & Sons, pp 67 - 99.

8. Gospodarowicz,D., Vlodavsky, J., Greenburg, G. and Johnson, L.K. 1979. In: Hormones and Cell Culture (Sato, G.H. and Ross, R., eds.) Cold Spring Harbor Laboratory, pp 561-592.

9. Novogrodsky, A. and Ashwell, G. 1977. Proc. Natl. Acad. Sci. USA 74, 676.

10. Olden, K., Parent, J.B., and White, S.L. 1982. Biochim- Biophys. Acta 650, 209.

11. Barondes, S. 1981. Ann. Rev. Biochemistry 50, 207.

12. Brunner, G. 1982. Cell Tissue Res. 224, 553.

13. Brunner, G., Nitzgen, B., Speth, V., Wieser, R. (1982). In: Growth of Cells in Hormonally Defined Media (Sato, G.H., Pardee, A., Sirbasku, D., eds.). Cold Spring Harbor Laboratory, New York, Vol. 9, in press.

14. Wieser, R., Golecki, J.R., and Brunner, G. 1981. Biochim. Biophys. Acta 648, 275.

15. Laemmli, U.K. 1970. Nature (London) 227, 680.

16. Gahmberg, C.G. and Andersson, L.C. 1977. J. Biol. Chem. 252, 5888.

17. Mazia, D., Schatten, G., and Sale, W. 1975. J. Cell. Biol. 66, 198.

18. Wieser, R. and Brunner, G. 1983. submitted

19. Brunner, G. and Wieser, R. 1982. Eur. J. Cell. Biol. 24, 4.

20. Folkman, J. and Moscona, A. 1978. Nature 273, 345.

21. Greenburg, G. and Gospodarowicz. 1982. Exp. Cell. Res. 140, 1.

22. Salomon, D.S., Liotta, L.A., and Kidwell, W.R. 1981. Proc. Natl. Acad. Sci. USA 78, 382.

23. Hakomori, S., Gahmberg, C.G., Laine, R. and Kijimoto, S. 1979. In: Control of Proliferation in Animal Cells (Clarkson, B. and Baserga, R., eds.). Cold Spring Harbor Laboratory, pp 461-472.

24. Roseman, S. 1979. In: The Cell Surface in Development (Moscona, A., ed.). John Wiley & Sons, New York, pp 255 - 271.

25. Mannino, R.J. and Burger, M.M. 1975. Nature 256, 19.

26. Monsigny, M., Kieda, C., Roche, A.C. 1979. Biol. Cellulaire 33, 289.

27. Grinnell, F. 1978. Int. Rev. Cytol. 53, 65.

28. Raz, A. and Bucana, C. 1980. Biochim. Biophys. Acta 597, 615.

29. Cuatrecasas, P. 1975. In: Cell Membranes (Weissmann, G and Claiborne, R., eds.) HP Publishing Co. Inc., New York, pp 184 .

30. Cohen, S., Fava, R.A. and Sawyer, S.T. 1982. Proc. Natl. Acad. Sci. USA 79, 6237.

31. Seals, J.R. and Czech, M.P. 1980. J. Biol. Chem. 255. 6529.

32. Raben, D., Lieberman, M.A., and Glaser, L. 1981. J. Cell. Physiol. 108, 35.

33. Kawakami, H. and Terayama, H. 1981. Biochim. Biophys. Acta 646, 161.

34. Petersen, S.W. and Lerch, V. 1981. J. Cell Biol. 91, 116.

35. Kinders, R.J. and Johnson, T.C. 1982. Biochem, J. 206, 527.

Neural Cells

Cells of the Peripheral Nervous System; Requirements for Expression of Function in Tissue Culture

R. P. Bunge, D. J. Carey, D. Higgins, C. Eldridge, and D. Roufa
Department of Anatomy and Neurobiology, Washington University School of Medicine,
St. Louis, MO 63110, USA

Utilizing mixtures of cell types, complex media, and a collagen substratum, it is possible to obtain a remarkable degree of functional expression in nerve tissue in culture, including myelination, synaptogenesis and histotypic organization (for review see Bunge, 1975; Crain, 1976 and Fischbach and Nelson, 1977). In order to gain an understanding of the contribution of individual cell types to specific functions, and to delineate the precise nutritional and environmental requirements for these functions, it is necessary to define media and substratum components and to study pure cell populations. Furthermore, because certain cell functions are only observed when cell types are cocultured, it is necessary to study cell types when separated and after recombination. In this chapter we briefly describe recent experience with this approach to the study of autonomic and sensory neurons, and of Schwann cells, in the peripheral nervous system. The chapter is primarily a review of work from our laboratory; space does not allow a general review.

Separation of Cell Types from the Peripheral Nervous System

Several approaches have been devised for the preparation of specific neuronal types in pure populations from both sensory and autonomic ganglia. Removal or suppression of the nonneuronal populations may be accomplished by the use of antimitotic agents (Wood, 1976), by selective adhesion to specific surfaces (McCarthy and Partlow, 1976a) or by adjustments of media components (Manthorpe et al., 1980; Patterson and Chun, 1974), among others. In our laboratory populations of Schwann cells are obtained from embryonic sensory ganglia explants (freed of fibroblasts by brief treatment with antimitotic agents) grown for several weeks on a collagen substratum to provide an extensive outgrowth of axons populated by Schwann cells. Removal of the centrally located explant, with consequent axon loss, leaves an outgrowth zone containing a pure Schwann cell population (Wood, 1976). Alternately, Schwann cells may be prepared by dissociating segments of neonatal rat sciatic nerve after trypsin treatment, and briefly subjecting the mixed cell population thus obtained to an antimitotic agent (Brockes et al., 1979). This kills many of the more rapidly proliferating fibroblasts; the remainder are subjected to complement mediated cell lysis after reacting with the thy-1 antigen. An essentially pure population of Schwann cells remains after this treatment.

For the preparation of essentially pure neuronal populations in explants more extensive antimitotic treatment of the culture is required (Wood, 1976); if the neurons are placed in dissociated culture rather less antimitotic treatment removes essentially all nonneuronal cells (Wood et al., 1980). Having separated pure populations of neurons and Schwann cells it is possible to recombine these using cells from different sources. Thus, Cornbrooks et al. (1982b) have reported that Schwann cells obtained from the genetic mutant, dystrophic, express a similar defect in function in culture (faulty basal lamina formation) whether relating to normal axons or axons from the dystrophic mouse.

It should be noted that in addition to establishing that pure poulations of a single cell type have been obtained, attention must also be given to the stage of development expressed by the cell at the time it is taken for culture. Certain cells can be shown to express different properties on different days of embryonic development. The initial growth rate of superior cervical ganglion neurons (on a substrate of reconstituted rat tail collagen) is relatively slow if taken from a 15 day embryo, maximal if taken from a neonatal animal, and slower again if taken from a more adult animal (Argiro and Johnson, 1982). This expression of different growth characteristics appears to be similarly expressed as the tissue "ages" in culture. Thus, a 15 day ganglion kept in culture for 6 days exhibits growth rates similar to a ganglion freshly explanted from a 21 day fetus. Thus, attention to both purity of cell type and state of initial maturation is desirable.

It should also be noted that certain cell functions are expressed only when cells are recombined with different cell types. Dorsal root ganglion neurons in pure culture do not form synapses upon themselves, but will synapse with spinal cord neurons in coculture (see Crain, 1976). The Schwann cell in isolation in culture undergoes relatively little proliferation, but when cocultured with neurons it is stimulated to proliferate (McCarthy and Partlow, 1976b ; Salzer and Bunge, 1980; Wood and Bunge, 1975). Direct contact between axon and Schwann cell is required for this stimultion (Salzer et al., 1980). With maturation the cultured Schwann cell becomes surrounded by a conspicuous basal lamina; this component does not form unless contact with an axon is established (M. Bunge et al., 1980; 1982). The Schwann cell also requires continuing contact with axons capable of inducing myelination in order to express myelin specific components (Mirsky et al., 1980).

Defining the Substratum

Peripheral nerve tissue in culture presents a dramatic example of the dependence of certain steps in cellular differentiation on contact with specific substratum components. Certain neurons survive but fail to extend neurites unless provided with specific substratum constituents (e.g., Collins, 1980). Schwann cells grown under conditions in which they do not establish or fail to retain contact with the usual collagen substratum fail to complete differentiation even though provided with normally functional axons and a fully supplemented medium (Bunge and Bunge, 1978). The dependence of axonal growth on substratum and cellular factors in the immediate vicinity of the axons is well known (for review see Varon and Adler, 1981).

A recent study by Roufa et al. (1982a,b) demonstrated that relatively minor variations in the collagen substratum influenced the ability of non-neuronal cells to grow from explants in company with neurite outgrowth. On collagen prepared to provide a more three dimensional substratum migration of non-neuronal cells from the ganglion was inhibited and neurites extended directly on the collagen. Use of a more two dimensional collagen substratum allowed investigation of the influence of the non-neuronal cells on the outgrowing neurites, for on this substratum they accompanied the outgrowing neurites. Both the extent and pattern of neurite outgrowth were changed in the presence of non-neuronal cells, and these changes appeared to reflect differences in the type of non-neuronal cells growing from ganglia taken from embryos and different ages. They concluded that use of different substrata may alter non-neuronal cell behavior which in turn influences neuritic growth.

Defining the Medium

In general it appears that establishing the optimal medium for the expression of specific cell function will require separate studies for each cell type of interest, with attention to the developmental stage of the cell at the time of culture initiation. Data are available for autonomic ganglion neurons and Schwann cells from peripheral tissue grown in defined media; defined media for astrocytes are discussed elsewhere in this volume.

Our own laboratory has not undertaken extensive attempts to design culture media but has gained considerable experience with growing primary cells in serum-free culture medium designed by others for use with neuronal cell lines. The medium designated N2 by Bottenstein and Sato (1979) was formulated to promote the proliferation of a rat neuroblastoma line. A list of other neuronal cell lines which proliferate well in this medium is given by Bottenstein (1982). The medium consists of a 1:1 mixture of Dulbecco's modified Eagle's and Ham's F12 medium, supplemented with insulin, transferrin, progesterone, putrescine, sodium selenite and nerve growth factor. This medium was also tested on cells from several central nervous system regions (for review see Bottenstein, 1982) and on dissociated chick dorsal root ganglion neurons (Bottenstein et al., 1980). This initial work stressed neurite growth and cell survival and proliferation in defined medium. Our observations have concentrated on questions of the extent of cellular differentiation when cultures are maintained for extended periods in defined medium.

Autonomic Neuron Function in Defined Medium

When neonatal rat superior cervical ganglion neurons are placed in culture (either on explants or in the dissociated state) these normally adrenergic neurons, in time, begin to express cholinergic (as well as certain retained adrenergic) properties (for review see Bunge et al., 1978; Patterson 1978). Expression of cholinergic function is observed when these neurons are cocultured with certain other cell types (e.g, heart cells; Patterson 1978) or grown in medium containing both serum and embryo extract (Johnson et al., 1980). The neuron under these conditions often becomes "dual function" (Furshpan et al, 1976; Higgins and Burton, 1982) in that it expresses both adrenergic and cholinergic properties. Because the neuron expresses acetylcholine receptors it has the capability, if it releases acetylcholine, of providing chemical synaptic input to sibling neurons in the same culture dish, and to itself (Furshpan et al., 1976). Induction of the cholinergic traits has been shown to occur if the cultured neurons are exposed to conditioned medium from heart cells in culture (Patterson, 1978); the identity of the inducing component(s) is under study. An unanswered question in this work is why this neuron in culture develops cholinergic properties, while the majority of superior cervical ganglion neurons do not develop this property in vivo. Interestingly, a small number of neurons in adrenergic autonomic ganglion supplying sweat glands express cholinergic function in vivo; Landis and Keefe (1980) have recently shown that these neurons display adrenergic characteristics early in development.

The use of defined medium in culturing this neuronal type might be expected to preclude cholinergic development, in that it would eliminate inducing agents from the medium, and this has proved to be the case (Iacovitti et al., 1982). Culturing neonatal rat superior cervical ganglion principal neurons on collagen substratum with the defined medium, N2 (containing nerve growth factor) of Bottenstein and Sato (1979), these workers reported that extended periods of neuronal survival were possible in the complete absence of nonneuronal cells. Under these conditions, these neurons continued to express, in modified form, certain of their expected adrenergic properties, including the development of tyrosine hydroxlase and dopamine-β-hydroxylase activities, small stores of endogenous norepinephrine, synaptic vesicles with dense cores, and tyrosine hydroxylase-immunoreactive staining properties. They did not develop detectable levels of choline acetyltransferase.

Higgins and Burton (1982) studied the electrophysiological properties of sympathetic neurons maintained in N2. Intracellular recordings obtained between the 16th and 98th day in vitro showed that these neurons could generate substantial (up to 90 mV) action potentials in response to depolarizing current injections; these responses were dependent on tetrodotoxin-sensitive Na^+ channels, cobalt-sensitive Ca^{++} channels and tetraethylammonium-sensitive K^+ channels. Action potentials were often followed by prominent, long hyperpolarizing afterpotentials (10-15 mV, 150 msec); the duration of these long afterpotentials was reduced in the presence of Co^{++}. In addition, it was observed that acetylcholine, but not norepinephrine, depolarized these neurons by a hexamethonium-sensitive mechanism. These data indicate that, when maintained in a chemically-defined medium, sympathetic neurons of rat fetuses express many of the basic membrane properties observed in neurons of superior cervical ganglia recently removed from adult rats (McAfee and Yarowsky, 1979). Indeed, since dorsal root ganglion neurons (R. Bunge et al., 1982) spinal cord neurons (Habets et al., 1981) neuroblastoma cells (Bottenstein and Sato, 1979) and heart cells (D. Higgins, unpublished observations) grown in N2 are capable of generating action potentials, it is possible that this medium will be found to provide sufficient support to a wide variety of excitable cells to allow them to express differentiated electrical properties (see also Bottenstein, 1982).

Although neurons of the embryonic superior cervical ganglion that have been maintained in N2 express many traits appropriate to their sympathetic and adrenergic heritage, these neurons also differ from their counterparts in vivo. When intra-cellular cellular recordings were obtained from pairs of neighboring sympathetic neurons in N2, Higgins and Burton (1982) observed that synaptic interactions were frequent (up to 60% of all pairs tested) at all times in vitro. At many synapses, both hyperpolarizing and depolarizing DC potential changes spread from one neuron to another. At other synapses, the spread of DC potential changes oculd not be direct-ly demonstrated; however, interactions at such synapses were not inhibited by antag-onists of several neurotransmitters, by elevation of the $Mg^{++}Ca^{++}$ ratio, or by the addition of Co^{++}. Thus, most, if not all, of synaptic interactions among sympa-thetic neurons in N2 medium were electrotonic; such electrical synapses were not observed among dorsal root ganglion neurons maintained in the same medium. Thus, as late as the 21st embryonic day, not only the choice of neurotransmitter, but also the mode of transmission has not been irrevocably determined in sympathetic neurons.

Schwann Cell Function in Defined Medium

Manthorpe et al. (1980) reported that mouse dorsal root ganglia and their accompanying Schwann cells could be maintained in defined medium. Schwann cell proliferation in response to neuronal presence was reported but these cultures were not carried long enough to assess Schwann cell functions such as ensheathment and myelination. Subsequently, Moya et al. (1980) reported that Schwann cells maintained in coculture with sensory neurons for extended periods underwent extensive proliferation but failed to differentiate (ensheath small axons and myelinate larger axons and form basal lamina). In order to obtain full Schwann cell function it was necessary to supplement the defined media with both serum and embryo extract. Under these conditions axon ensheathment, myelination and basal lamina production in relation to Schwann cell surfaces begin within several days (Figs. 1 and 2). The culture system used in these experiments is particularly useful for it allows poising the culture in defined medium and then, with media supplementation, progression to myelination within one week. The poised culture will remain in a "hold" condition for several weeks, fully populated by Schwann cells unable to complete differentiation.

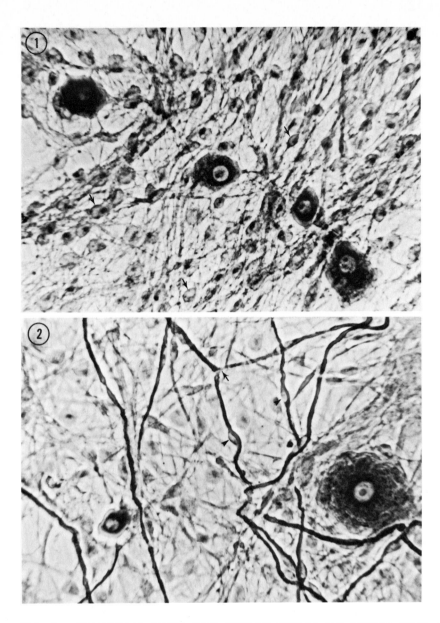

Fig. 1. Dissociated dorsal root ganglion neurons and Schwann cells maintained in
the defined medium N2 (see text). The culture is first established in serum supplemented medium to allow neuronal maturation; during this period the fibroblast population is eliminated with antimitotic agents. After shifting to serum-free medium
substantial Schwann cell proliferation has occurred but Schwann cell differentiation
(ensheathment of small axons and myelination of larger axons) has not occurred. On
electron microscopic examination no extracellular matrix materials are seen in these
cultures. The nuclei of individual Schwann cells are indicated at the arrows. This
and all subsequent light micrographs are Sudan black stains after aldehyde fixation. Phase X495. Fig. 2. A culture prepared as in Fig. 1, 10 days after
supplementing the medium with serum and embryo extract. Myelin segments are stained
black; several myelin-related Schwann cell nuclei are indicated by arrowheads. A
point of branching of a myelinated fiber is indicated by the arrow. Phase. X495.

In their study of Schwann cell secretory activity, conducted on pure Schwann cell populations in culture, Carey and Bunge (1981) extended the above observations to determine whether Schwann cells in defined medium were deficient in secretory activity. Comparing cultures maintained on defined medium with sibling cultures supplemented for two days with serum and embryo extract, they reported a 4-fold increase in secretory activity with supplementation of the N2 medium.

Schwann cells under normal conditions (i.e. in supplemented medium in the presence of neurons) synthesize and secrete an extracellular matrix consisting of a basal lamina and a fibrillar reticular lamina. This matrix is known to contain collagen (types I, III, IV and V), as well as the glycoproteins laminin and fibronectin (M. Bunge et al., 1980; Carey et al., in preparation; Cornbrooks et al., 1982a). As mentioned above, Schwann cells grown in the presence of neurons in defined medium fail to assemble a morphologically visible basal lamina. When the secretion of extracellular matrix components by Schwann cells in defined medium was examined biochemically it was observed that no pepsin resistant collagen was secreted (Carey and Bunge, unpublished). In contrast, laminin was detected in the medium of these cultures. The expression of laminin by Schwann cells in defined medium is also indicated by immunofluorescent studies with anti-laminin antibodies (Cornbrooks et al., 1982a). Subsequent experiments revealed that of the additions to defined medium which are required for full Schwann cell development, serum, but not embryo extract, corrects the secretion deficiency, and dialyzed serum is nearly as effective in promoting Schwann cell secretion as is complete serum. In a survey of purified hormones and other additives for ability to restore normal Schwann cell secretion only the vitamin ascorbic acid has shown any activity. When cultures of Schwann cells and neurons are fed the usual defined medium supplemented with 50 μg/ml ascorbate, a co-factor required for collagen hydroxylation reactions, collagen secretion is enhanced (Carey, Eldridge and Bunge, unpublished). In addition, the secretion of several non-collagenous proteins is also increased. After several days of feeding Schwann cell-neuron cultures ascorbate supplemented defined medium daily some Schwann cells begin myelin formation (Figs. 3 and 4.) (Eldridge and Bunge, unpublished). Electron microscopic analysis of such cultures reveals areas in which the basal lamina and reticular lamina have begun to form. These areas of extracellular matrix formation correspond to those regions where myelination of axons by Schwann cells is occurring (Eldridge, Williams and Bunge, unpublished). This result supports the idea that extracellular matrix formation in cultures is a necessary prerequisite for subsequent normal Schwann cell development, and furthermore indicates that a fully defined medium for expresion of normal Schwann cell function may be within reach.

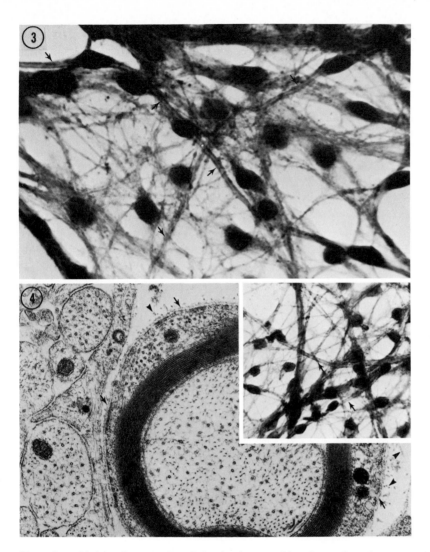

Fig. 3. Light micrograph of beginning myelin formation in a culture containing sensory neurons and Schwann cells 4 days after supplementing defined medium with serum and embryo extract. Myelin sheaths, indicated by arrows, have begun to form throughout this culture. Schwann cells not related to the myelin segments are associated with small, unmyelinated nerve fibers. Sister cultures, maintained in N2 medium, show little or no myelination, even after several additional weeks in culture. X800. Fig. 4. Myelin formation in defined medium supplemented with ascorbate. N2 medium was supplemented with 50 µgr/ml ascorbate and the culture refed daily. Some myelin has begun to form, and is visible at the light microscopic level, as early as 4 days after ascorbate supplementation (inset; arrows). Electron microscopy of a culture fixed after 9 days of supplementation shows that in areas of myelin formation extracellular matrix materials, including basal lamina (at arrows) and small collagen fibrils (at arrowheads), are beginning to form. Electron micrograph X38,500; inset X275.

Conclusions

This brief chapter discusses selected results on the use of defined medium with primary cells on the nervous system in tissue culture. Because the types of cultures discussed are in many instances postmitotic the defined media serve not for the study of controls of proliferation but for the study of controls in differentiation. Thus, two examples are provided in which the expression of specific cellular traits are regulated by media components. In the first example, an adrenergic neuron is shown to express a selected repertoire of adrenergic characteristics in defined medium as well as to show unusual electrotonic junction formation. This same neuron in supplemented medium would express cholinergic traits. In a second example, Schwann cell function is shown to be retarded in defined medium. In this case the defined medium offers the opportunity to search for media components necessary for the Schwann cell functions of ensheathment and myelination. Thus, the use of defined medium with postmitotic cells has proven useful in delineating the controls on cellular differentiation in the nervous system.

Acknowledgments

Work in the authors' laboratory is supported by NIH grants NS 09923, NS 14416 and National Multiple Sclerosis grant RG 1118. Training support was provided by NIH grant NS 07071 (C.E., D.H., D.R) and by the Muscular Dystrophy Association (D.J.C.).

References

Argiro, V. and Johnson, M.I. 1982 Patterns and kinetics of neurite extension from sympathetic neurons in culture are age dependent. J. Neurosci. 2: 503-512.

Bottenstein, J.E. 1982 Growth requirements of neural cells in vitro. In: Advances in Cellular Neurobiology (in press).

Bottenstein, J.E. and Sato, G.H. 1979 Growth of a rat neuroblastoma cell line in serum-free supplemented medium. Proc. Natl. Acad. Sci. U.S.A. 76: 514-517.

Bottenstein, J., Skaper, S., Varon, S. and Sato, G. 1980 Selective survival of neurons from chick embryo sensory ganglionic dissociates utilizing serum-free supplemented medium. Exptl. Cell Res. 125: 183-190.

Brockes, J.P., Fields, K.L. and Raff, M.C. 1979 Studies on cultured rat Schwann cells. I. Establishment of purified populations from cultures of peripheral nerve. Brain Research 165: 105-118.

Bunge, M.B., Williams, A.K. and Wood, P.M. 1982 Neuron-Schwann cell interaction in basal lamina formation. Dev. Biol. 92: 449-460.

Bunge, M.B., Williams, A.K., Wood, P.M., Uitto, J. and Jeffrey, J.J. 1980 Comparison of nerve cell and nerve cell plus Schwann cell cultures, with particular emphasis on basal lamina and collagen formation. J. Cell Biol., 84: 184-202.

Bunge, R.P. 1975 Changing uses of nerve tissue culture 1950-1975. In: The Nervous System, D.B. Tower, ed., Raven Press, New York, pp. 31-42.

Bunge, R.P., and Bunge, M.B. 1978 Evidence that contact with connective tissue matrix is required for normal interaction between Schwann cells and nerve fibers. J. Cell Biol., 78: 943-950.

Bunge, R.P., Bunge, M.B., Carey, D.J., Cornbrooks, C.J., Higgins, D.H., Johnson, M.I., Iacovitti, L., Kleinschmidt, D.C., Moya, F. and Wood, P. 1982 Functional expression in primary nerve tissue cultures maintained in defined medium. Cold Spring Harbor Conferences on Cell Proliferation. 9: 1017-1031.

Bunge, R.P., Johnson, M. and Ross, C.D. 1978 Nature and nurture in the development of the autonomic neuron. Science 199: 1409-1416.

Carey, D.J. and Bunge, R.P. 1981 Factors influencing the release of proteins in cultured Schwann cells. J. Cell Biol. 91: 666-672.

Collins, F. 1980 Neurite outgrowth induced by the substrate associated material from nonneuronal cells. Develop. Biol. 79: 247-252.

Cornbrooks, C., Carey, D., Timpl, R., McDonald, J. and Bunge, R. 1982a Immunohisto-chemical visualization of fibronectin and laminin in adult rat peripheral nerve and peripheral nerve cells in culture. Soc. Neurosci. Abstr. 8: 240.

Cornbrooks, C.J., Mithen, F., Cochran, J.M. and Bunge, R.P. 1982b Factors affecting Schwann cell basal lamina formationin cultures of dorsal root ganglia from mice with muscular dystrophy. Dev. Brain Res. (in press).

Crain, S. 1976. Neurophysiologic Studies in Tissue Culture. Raven Press, New York.

Fischbach, G.D. and Nelson, P.G. 1977 Cell culture in neurobiology. In: Handbook of Neurophysiology, E. Kandel, ed., pp. 719-774.

Furshpan E.J., MacLeish P.R., O'Lague P.H. and Potter D.D. 1976 Chemical transmission between sympathetic neurons and cardiac myocytes developing in microcultures: Evidence for cholinergic, adrenergic, and dual-function neurons. Proc. Natl. Acad. Sci. U.S.A. 76: 4225-4229.

Habets A.M.M.C., Baker R.E., Brenner E. and Romijn H. 1981 Chemically defined medium enhances bioelectric activity in mouse spinal cord-dorsal root ganglion cultures. Neurosci. Lett. 22: 51-56.

Higgins D. and Burton H. 1982 Electrotonic synapses are formed by fetal rat sympathetic neurons maintained in a chemically-defined culture medium. Neuroscience 7: 2241-2253.

Iacovitti L., Johnson M.I., Joh T.H., and Bunge R.P. 1982 Biochemical and morphological characterization of sympathetic neurons grown in chemically defined medium. Neuroscience 7: 2225-2240.

Johnson M.I., Ross C.D., Meyers E., Spitznagel L. and Bunge R.P. 1980 Morphological and biochemical studies on the development of cholinergic properties in cultured sympathetic neurons. I. J. Cell Biol. 84: 680-691.

Landis,S.C. and Keefe, D. 1980 Development of cholinergic sympathetic innervation of eccrine sweatglands in rat footpad. Soc. Neurosci. Abstr. 6: 379.

Manthorpe, M., S. Skaper and Varon, S. 1980. Purification of mouse Schwann cells using neurite-induced proliferation in serum-free monolayer culture. Brain Res., 196: 467-482.

McAfee, D.A. and Yarowsky, P.J. 1979 Calcium-dependent potentials in the mammalian sympathetic neurone. J. Physiol. 290: 507-523.

McCarthy, K. and Partlow, L. 1976a Preparation of pure neuronal and non-neuronal cultures from embryonic chick sympathetic ganglia: a new method based on both differential cell adhesiveness and the formation of homotypic neuronal aggregates. Brain Res. 114: 391-414.

McCarthy, K. and Partlow, L., 1976b Neuronal stimulation of [^{3}H] thymidine incorporation by primary cultures of highly purified non-neuronal cells, Brain Res. 114: 415-426.

Mirsky, R., Winter, J., Abney, E., Pruss, R., Gavrilovic, J. and Raff, M. 1980 Myelin specific proteins and glycolipids in rat Schwann cells and oligodendro-cytes in culture. J. Cell Biol. 84: 483-494.

Moya, F., Bunge, M. and Bunge, R. 1980 Schwann cells proliferate but fail to differentiate in defined medium, Proc. Natl. Acad. Sci. (U.S.A.) 77: 6902-6906.

Patterson P.H. 1978 Environmental determination of autonomic neurotransmitter functions. Ann. Rev. Neurosci. 1: 1-17.

Patterson, P.H. and Chun, L.L.Y. 1974 The influence of non-neuronal cells on catecholamine and acetylcholine synthesis and accumulation in cultures of dissociated sympathetic neurons. Proc. Natl. Acad. Sci. U.S.A. 71: 3607-3610.

Roufa, D.G., Johnson, M.I. and Bunge, M.B. 1982a Influence of ganglion age, non-neuronal cells and substratum in neurite outgrowth in culture. (submitted for publication).

Roufa, D., Cornbrooks, C., Johnson, M. and Bunge, M. 1982b Preparation of homogenous populations of immature Schwann cells from early embryonic sympathetic ganglia. Soc. Neurosci. Abstr. 8: 240.

Salzer, J.L. and Bunge, R.P. 1980 Studies of Schwann cell proliferation. I. An analysis in tissue culture of proliferation during development, Wallerian degeneration and direct injury, J. Cell Biol., 84: 739-752.

Salzer, J.L., Bunge, R.P. and Glaser, L.   1980   Studies of Schwann cell proliferation: III.   Evidence for the surface localization of the neurite mitogen.   J. Cell Biol. 84: 767-778.

Varon, S. and Adler, R. 1980 Nerve growth factors and control of nerve growth. Curr. Topics. Develop. Biol. 16: 207-252.

Wood, P.M. 1976 Separation of functional Schwann cells and neurons from normal peripheral nerve tissue. Brain Res. 115: 361-375.

Wood, P.M. and Bunge, R.P. 1975 Evidence that sensory axons are mitogenic for Schwann cells. Nature 256: 662-664.

Wood, P., Okada, E. and Bunge, R. 1980 . The use of networks of dissociated rat dorsal root ganglion neurons to induce myelination by oligodendrocytes in culture. Brain Research, 196: 247-252.

Selection and Cultivation of Astrocytes at Different Developmental Stages

Günther Fischer

Institut für Neurobiologie, Universität Heidelberg, Im Neuenheimer Feld 504, D-6900 Heidelberg, FRG

INTRODUCTION

Important aims in neurobiology are to understand the processes which determine the differentiation of neural cells in brain tissue; of primary interest is that of the main neural cell types neurons, astrocytes and oligodendrocytes. One may assume that signals via direct cell-cell contact and interactions of cells with the extracellular matrix are important as well as signals via diffusible factors like hormones, growth or differentiation factors. Because such complex signals can often not be readily studied in detail in intact tissue, cell cultures have been utilized to follow differentiation of cells in less complex systems. The best experimental control of the cellular environment (contact environment and composition of diffusible factors) is thought to be possible in monolayer cultures. Therefore, an idealized experiment would be to start with a homogenous population of precursor cells of one of the main neural cell types which will become fully differentiated cells after a series of defined manipulations concerning cell contact environment, growth and differentiation factors, hormonal and nutritional requirements.

Attempts have been made in recent years to enrich the main neural cell types of vertebrates including methods like density gradient centrifugation (1-3), selection by immunological methods (3, 4), by differential cell adhesion (5-7), and by growth in chemically defined serum-free media (see for example 8-13). Although remarkable progress was made in the enrichment of neurons (e.g. 9), oligodendrocytes (4), astrocytes (10, 13), and Schwann cells (see Bunge et al. in this volume), in no case could undifferentiated stem cells for the main neural cell types be enriched by these methods. One important reason may be that cellular markers are not available which would allow an easy identification of stem cells.

Regarding astrocytes, some progress was made in this respect with the development of antibodies which can distinguish different developmental stages of these cells (14-17). For example glial fibrillary acidic (GFA) protein which is a constituent of intermediate type filaments can be recognized specifically in astrocytes by the use of specific antibodies (16). Vimentin which is also a constituent of intermediate type filaments is co-expressed in GFA protein positive astrocytes. However, it was found that vimentin is expressed earlier in development than GFA protein in mice (14, 15). Therefore, vimentin positive astrocytes which do not yet express GFA protein are thought to be precursor cells for GFA protein positive astrocytes. They are termed more immature astrocytes in the following paper in contrast to more mature ones which express both markers, vimentin and GFA protein. However, vimentin is also present in other cells like ependymal cells, fibroblasts and fibroblast-like cells (14). Therefore a positive identification of more immature astrocytes with vimentin alone is not possible. The expression of other cell-type specific markers (for instance the fibroblast-specific marker fibronectin (18)) has to be ruled out. In addition, one has to show that presumptive precursor cells can express astrocyte specific properties (like GFA protein) under appropriate conditions.

Until recently the enrichment of astrocytes was restricted to more mature cells by the use of serum containing media. Even when embryonic brain tissue was used for the preparation of cells in which GFA protein is hardly or not expressed (19) more mature astrocytes became the dominant cells within a rather short time. Therefore one had to assume that factors are present in serum which favour the maturation of astrocytes at least in the sense of expression of GFA protein as a step in differentiation. However, with the use of serum-free media a cell population could be enriched which fulfilled the criteria of being more immature astrocytes (10). The cells were homogenous in respect to the expression of vimentin and the absence of cell-type specific markers for fibroblasts, oligodendrocytes and neurons. Moreover they could be induced to express GFA protein.

In the following paper some aspects of the selection of these more immature astrocytes are presented together with some aspects of their differentiation.

MATERIALS AND METHODS

Cell preparation and cell cultures (10)

Single cell suspensions from 2-day-old C57B1/6J mouse cerebellum were prepared by a combination of trypsin and mechanical dissociation in the presence of DNase. Cell numbers were determined with a Coulter counter. Cells were plated at a density of 1×10^5 cells on poly-L-lysine coated glass coverslips with three glass coverslips (16 mm Ø) per 35 mm Ø Petri dish and cultivated in 1 ml of a chemically defined serum-free medium (medium A) which consisted of BME-Earle's supplemented with 1 mg/ml fatty acid-free bovine serum albumin, 10 µg/ml insulin, 10 µg/ml hyaluronic acid, 0.1 mg/ml transferrin, 1 ug/ml trypsin inhibitor aprotinin, 10 nM EGF (purified as described previously (20) more than 99% pure as judged by SDS-PAGE) and in addition, 30 nM selenium, 0.25% glucose and 2 mM glutamine. As antibiotics, 100 U/ml penicillin and 135 µg/ml streptomycin were added.

The medium was renewed completely 24 hrs after plating or subcultivation of cells and subsequently every 3 - 4 days. In control experiments, cells were cultivated in BME-Earle's containing 10% horse serum or 10% fetal calf serum and supplemented with glucose, glutamine and antibiotics as described for medium A or in another defined medium consisting of BME-Earle's with 1 mg/ml bovine serum albumin, 10 µg/ml insulin, 0.1 mg/ml transferrin, 1 µg/ml trypsin inhibitor aprotinin and 0.1 nM L-thyroxin and 30 nM selenium, 0.25% glucose, 2 mM glutamine and penicillin as well as streptomycin as mentioned above. This medium was originally developed for the survival of cerebellar neurons (9).

Subcultivation of cells was performed by an incubaton step with 0.05% trypsin and 0.1 mM EDTA in phosphate-buffered saline (PBS), pH 7.0, for 1 - 2 min at room temperature as described (10). Cells were plated in medium A on poly-L-lysine coated glass coverslips at a density of 1×10^5 cells per coverslip with three coverslips per Petri dish.

Immunocytochemical staining

To stain the cells, antibodies against vimentin and GFA protein were used in an indirect double immunofluorescence labeling procedure (14). Guinea-pig antiserum against vimentin and rabbit antiserum against GFA protein were used as first antibodies. Fluorescein isothiocyanate-conjugated goat anti-guinea pig immunoglobulins (FITC-GAG, Antibodies Incorporated, via Paesel, Frankfurt, F.R.G.) and tetramethyl-rhodamine isothiocyanate-conjugated goat anti-rabbit immunoglobulins (TRITC-GAR, Nordic Immunology, via Byk Mallinckrodt, Dietzenbach-Steinberg, F.R.G.) as second antibodies. In control experiments, cultures were stained with antibodies against galactocerebrosides (21), L1 antigen (22) and fibronectin (18) which are specific for oligodendrocytes, neurons and fibroblasts, respectively.

^{3}H-thymidine incorporation

Cells were incubated for 3 1/2 hrs with 2 μCi/ml ^{3}H-thymidine in the appropriate medium. Trichloracetic acid (TCA) precipitable material was measured as described (23).

Determination of cell numbers

Cells were removed from the glass coverslips as for subcultivation. They were resuspended as a single cell suspension in 1 ml of trypsin inhibitor solution (1 mg/ml in BME-Earle's) by pipetting. Cell numbers were determined in an aliquot of 50 - 500 μl with a Coulter counter as described previously (24).

RESULTS AND DISCUSSION

Cultivation of early postnatal mouse cerebellum in serum containing media

Cell preparations of brain tissue are normally composed of various amounts of the main neural cell types neurons, oligodendrocytes and astrocytes together with minor cell populations like fibroblasts and others. Astrocytes often are only a minor subpopulation, as for example in cell preparations from early postnatal mouse cerebellum (Tab. 1). The distribution of different cell types was determined by the use of cell-type specific antibodies which recognize GFA protein in astrocytes (16), galactocerebrosides in oligodendrocytes (21), L1 antigen in neurons (22) and fibronectin in fibroblasts and fibroblast-like cells (18). It can be seen that after one day in vitro (DIV) neurons dominate by far, followed by more mature astrocytes which express vimentin and GFA protein (14). The more immature astrocytes express vimentin but not other cell type specific markers like fibronectin or galactocerebrosides (10). These more immature astrocytes represent about 1-2% of all cells after 1 DIV and it is an open question if there are any of them left after 12 DIV. If so their proportion has to be very small. The by far dominating cells after 12 DIV are more mature astrocytes which can therefore be easily enriched by cultivating cells of early postnatal mouse cerebellum (but also from other brain areas) in serum-

Table 1

Composition of monolayer cultures of 6-day-old mouse cerebellum after 1 and 14 days in vitro (DIV) cultivated in medium containing 10% horse serum.

	% of cells	
cell types	1 DIV	14 DIV
neurons	90	1 - 5
more mature astrocytes vim ⊕ GFA ⊕	5 - 8	85 - 90
more immature astrocytes vim ⊕	1 - 2	< 1
other cell types fibroblasts oligodendrocytes ependymal cells	1 - 2	10 - 15

2.5×10^5 cells were plated per glass coverslip. Cell composition was determined after immunocytochemical staining of the cultures with cell type specific antibodies. Expression of vimentin (vim ⊕) and GFA protein (GFA ⊕) is indicated.

supplemented media. Similar results are obtained when fetal calf serum is used instead of horse serum.

Growth requirements for more immature astrocytes

To enrich more immature astrocytes, serum was replaced by different mixtures of hormones, growth factors and other constituents. Epidermal growth factor (EGF) was among the growth factors tested for it could be shown that the proliferation of some astrocytes in primary cultures of mouse cerebellum could be stimulated by EGF (23). The series of selection experiments ended up with medium A containing fatty-acid free bovine serum albumin, EGF, transferrin, insulin, hyaluronic acid and selenium as main constituents (10).

When cells of early postnatal mouse cerebellum were cultivated with this medium, the cell density increased very rapidly. To identify proliferating cells the cultures were characterized by the use of cell type specific antibodies with double-immunostaining techniques. It became obvious that a particular cell type proliferated which expressed vimentin but not GFA protein, fibronectin, galactocerebrosides, or L1 antigen. Therefore it became very likely that the proliferating cells were more immature astrocytes. As shown later on this could be demonstrated conclusively, for these cells could express GFA protein under appropriate conditions.

The question then arose as to which constituents of medium A were necessary for the proliferation of the more immature astrocytes. This was investigated by omitting each component of medium A leaving the other constituents unchanged in respect to composition and concentration. When either EGF or transferrin were omitted from the medium the cell density did not increase with time in culture (see Fig. 1 C,D). In the

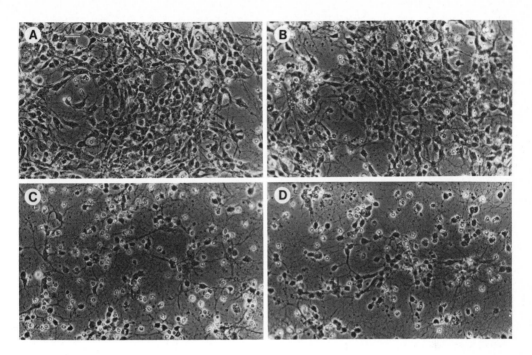

Fig. 1. Comparison of mouse cerebellar cells grown for 7 days in different defined
    media: (A) cells grown in medium A; (B) medium A lacking insulin; (C) medium
A lacking EGF; (D) medium A lacking transferrin. Representative areas of the cultures
are shown. Bar represents 20 μm.

absence of insulin the increase in cell density was significantly lower than in medium
A (see Fig. 1 A,B). Immunostaining of the cultures after 7 DIV revealed that more
immature astrocytes were present in the absence of insulin but not detectable in the
absence of either EGF or transferrin.

   These results could be verified when the rate of ^{3}H-thymidine incorporation was
measured as an equivalent of DNA synthesis and cell proliferation. In the absence of
either EGF or transferrin the rate of ^{3}H-thymidine incorporation decreased very
rapidly from the initially measurable base value to background levels (see Fig. 2)
whereas in the absence of insulin the increase in the rate of ^{3}H-thymidine incorporation was much lower compared to the values measured for medium A. In a series of
similar experiments it was found that bovine serum albumin had a similar but smaller
effect than insulin and that hyaluronic acid and selenium had only very small effects
on the proliferation of astrocytes.

   Therefore it could be assumed that EGF in combination with transferrin is abso-
lutely necessary for the proliferation of more immature astrocytes and that insulin
and bovine serum albumin have additional stimulatory effects. This could be shown
conclusively in a further series of experiments (25).

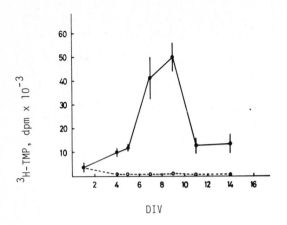

Fig. 2. ^{3}H-thymidine (^{3}H-TMP) incorporation in mouse cerebellar cultures in dependence of the time in cultures. Cells are grown in medium A ●——● or in the absence of either EGF or transferrin ○---○. Each point represents the mean of triplicate values with standard deviation.

When the number of cells was determined in relationship to time in culture, a several fold increase over the initially present cell number was measured (Fig. 3). Since most of the cells after about 12 DIV were more immature astrocytes (∼ 90%), which represented only a subpopulation of cells (1 - 2%) at 1 DIV, this increase in cell number corresponds to a dramatic proliferation of the more immature astrocytes in medium A.

However, the proliferation of the more immature astrocytes in medium A is not a process which goes on continously and this behaviour is common for non-transformed cells. After about 10 to 11 days a drop in the rate of ^{3}H-thymidine incorporation could be measured (Fig. 2). At this stage the more immature astrocytes formed a dense monolayer with spots of multilayer cell clusters. It seems possible that the low rate of ^{3}H-thymidine incorporation at this time reflects a contact inhibition in growth. At later cultivation periods the formation of cell debris could be seen

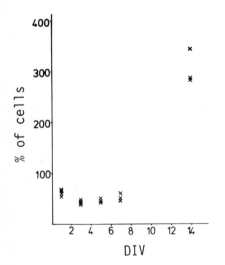

Fig. 3. Proliferation of cells from 6-day-old mouse cerebellum cultivated in medium A. After various DIV (abscissa) the cell number on single glass coverslips was determined in triplicate values as described. 100% represents the number of cells seeded per coverslip (2,5 x 10^5).

because part of the more immature astrocytes died. The reason for the death of part
of the cells is not clear at the moment. A possible explanation would be that the
more immature astrocytes can only run through a limited number of cell cycles before
they have to differentiate. When the appropriate factors for the differentiation are
not present the cells may die at this stage. Described growth or differentiation
factors for astrocytes (see for example 26, 27) may then be necessary for the survival and differentiation of the more immature astrocytes.

Establishment of homogenous cultures of more immature astrocytes

Although a high and selective enrichment of more immature astrocytes was found in
medium A, other cells (estimated to be < 10%) were still present after 10 - 12 DIV
including more mature astrocytes, some oligodendrocytes, and neurons. The more
mature astrocytes seemed to survive but not to proliferate in medium A because their
density in representative microscopic fields did not increase. A subcultivation
procedure was attempted to get rid of other cell types and thus obtain homogenous
populations of the more immature astrocytes.

When the cultures were stained 3 days after subcultivation with double-immunostaining techniques for fibroblasts, oligodendrocytes, neurons, and more mature astrocytes using cell-type specific antibodies against markers like fibronectin, galactocerebrosides, L1 antigen, and GFA protein, respectively, the overall contamination
with other cell types besides more immature astrocytes was about 1% or lower. By far
most of the contaminating cells were more mature astrocytes ($\sim$80%).

This revealed that with a combination **of selective** growth conditions for more
immature astrocytes combined with a subcultivation step highly pure cultures of
more immature astrocytes could be obtained.

When the growth requirements for more immature astrocytes were studied in secondary
cultures similar results were obtained as in primary cultures. In the absence of
either EGF or transferrin the rate of ^{3}H-thymidine incorporation decreased very
rapidly and a high percentage of the more immature astrocytes died within a few days.
These effects were smaller in the absence of either insulin or bovine serum albumin.
Thus, the same components appear to be important for the growth and survival of
more immature astrocytes in primary and secondary cultures. It further seems unlikely that other cell types gave an additional support as long as the more immature
astrocytes proliferated in primary cultures. In addition the growth behaviour of the
more immature astrocytes was comparable in primary and secondary cultures. After
subcultivation, an increase in the rate of DNA synthesis could be seen in the first
few days, followed by a decrease (see Fig. 6). Again the cells proliferated to form
a dense monolayer in the first few days. Afterwards they formed cell clumps and
part of the cells died. Later on surviving cells spread on the substratum and proliferated to form again a dense monolayer. This latter behaviour corresponded with the
new increase of the rate of ^{3}H-thymidine incorporation. As in primary cultures it

seems to be possible that the appropriate differentiation factors may be missed by the cells when the cell density and the number of cell cycles have reached critical values.

Although EGF plays a dominant role for the proliferation and survival of more immature astrocytes as shown above and for the proliferation of a subpopulation of more mature astrocytes in vitro (23), its role under in vivo conditions for the proliferation of astrocytes is not proven unless its presence in brain is shown during time periods important for the proliferation of astrocytes. It may be that not EGF but EGF-like molecules effect survival and proliferation of astrocytes since these are known to be present in embryonic brain tissue (28).

Induction of astrocyte specific properties - expression of GFA protein

The immunostaining experiments indicated that it was very likely that the cells selected by proliferation in medium A were more immature astrocytes. Since it is known that in serum containing medium more mature astrocytes and not more immature ones (in respect to the expression of vimentin and GFA protein as markers) dominate by far it was tried to induce the expression of GFA protein in the more immature astrocytes by cultivating them further on in serum containing medium. Different time intervals after this switch to serum-containing medium the cultures were stained for vimentin and GFA protein in a double immunostaining procedure.

When medium A was replaced by BME-Earle's containing either 10% horse serum or 10% fetal calf serum (FCS) the more immature astrocytes (Fig. 4) changed their morphology within one day. In areas of low cell density the cells became more epitheloid and about 70% expressed GFA protein within one day. After three days nearly all cells had become GFA protein positive (Fig. 5). Three and seven days after the switch to serum containing media the homogeneity of the cultures were checked by immunostaining methods. Again cell type specific antibodies against fibronectin, galactocerebrosides, and L1 antigen were used. It was found that significantly less than 1% of all cells were other cells besides astrocytes (namely fibroblasts and oligodendrocytes). With these experiments it became very unlikely that precursor cells for other cell types like fibroblasts, oligodendrocytes, or neurons are enriched together with the more immature astrocytes in substantial numbers.

It is obvious, however, that not all cells are stained with identical intensities, by antibodies directed against GFA protein (see Fig. 5). Part of the cells were stained very strongly,some only weakly and others with intensities in between. However, a clear filamentous type of staining could be seen in nearly all cells.

It was shown with the experiments described above that more immature astrocytes could differentiate to become more mature ones (in respect to expression of GFA protein) under appropriate culture conditions. It was unclear, however, if proliferation steps were necessary for this differentiation. The measurement of the rate

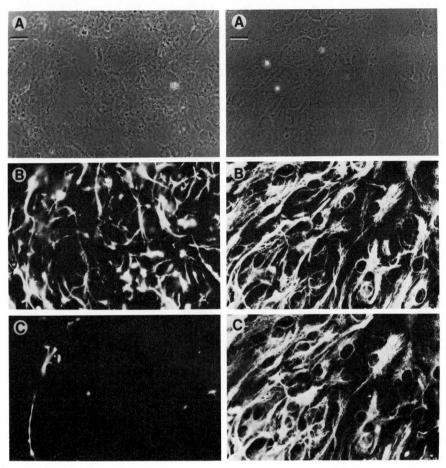

Fig. 4   Fig. 5

Fig. 4. Staining of secondary cultures of mouse cerebellar cells three days after subcultivation. Cells were further grown in defined medium A and stained for vimentin (B) and GFA protein (C); (A) represents the same microscopic field as shown in (B) and (C); bar represents 20 µm.

Fig. 5. Staining of secondary cultures of mouse cerebellar cells three days after replacement of defined medium A by medium containing 10% horse serum. Cells were stained for vimentin (B) and GFA protein (C); (A) represents the same microscopic field as shown in (B) and (C); bar represents 20 µm.

of ^{3}H-thymidine incorporation revealed that the switch from medium A to serum containing media induced a very rapid decrease in DNA synthesis. This effect was more pronounced when the medium contained FCS instead of horse serum (Fig. 6).

It became likely from these experiments in combination with the finding that the number of cells did not increase significantly when medium A was replaced by serum containing media (29) that the majority of the more immature astrocytes do   not need to proliferate to become more mature astrocytes; it can be further ruled out

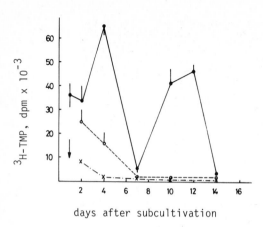

Fig. 6. ^{3}H-thymidine (^{3}H-TMP) incorporation in secondary cultures of
mouse cerebellar cells selected by
growth for 12 days in medium A. Cells
were further grown in medium A ($\bullet$—$\bullet$)
or medium A was replaced one day
after subcultivation by medium
supplemented with either 10% horse
serum (o---o) or 10% fetal calf serum
(x–·–x). Each point represents the
mean of triplicate values with
standard deviation.

that a small subpopulation of precursor cells present among the cells growing exclusively in medium A will proliferate in serum containing media to become the
dominating cells within a 1 - 3 days period.

It was then tried if this differentiation of the more immature astrocytes could
also be induced in other culture media. Since astrocytes did survive but obviously
not proliferate in a defined medium developed for the survival of neurons (9) this
medium was used for similar switch experiments as described above. One day after
subcultivation medium A was replaced by the other defined medium and 12 days later
the cultures were stained for vimentin and GFA protein (Fig. 7). It was found that
all surviving cells expressed both markers. Although the majority of the more
immature astrocytes did not survive the change in cultivation conditions in these
experiments (exact numbers can not be given at present), the number of surviving
cells is by far larger than the number of more mature astrocytes already present
before the medium is changed. It is therefore very likely that some more immature
astrocytes have differentiated to become more mature ones also under these conditions.

It would be interesting to know if the surviving cells under the latter conditions
differ in some respect from those which do not survive the switch in culture conditions. Although the cells selected by cultivation in medium A are homogenous in
respect to the expression of a variety of markers (positive for vimentin but negative
for GFA protein, fibronectin, galactocerebrosides, L1 antigen) it is unclear if they
are heterogenous in respect to other criteria (see for example 17). A heterogeneity
in respect to other markers, which would indicate different subpopulations of
astrocytes among the more immature ones selected in medium A, may then easily explain
the difference in survival.

Reversibility of the expression of GFA protein

The question then arose if the differentiation of more immature astrocytes to become
more mature ones is a reversible process. The following series of experiments

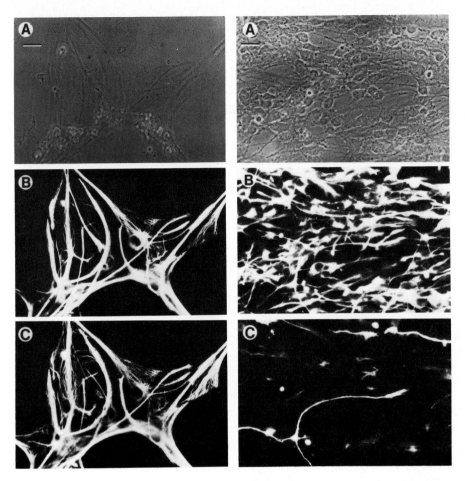

Fig. 7   Fig. 8

Fig. 7. Staining of secondary cultures of mouse cerebellar cells 12 days after replacement of medium A by a defined medium selected for the survival of neurons. Cells
were stained for vimentin (B) and GFA protein (C); (A) represents the same microscopic
field as shown in (B) and (C); bar represents 20 μm.

Fig. 8. Staining of secondary cultures of mouse cerebellar cells. One day after subcultivation medium A was replaced by medium containing 10% horse serum. 8 days later
serum containing medium was replaced again by medium A. 7 days later the cells were
stained for vimentin (B) and GFA protein (C);(A) represents the same microscopic field
as shown in (B) and (C); bar represents 20 μm.

addresses this question. Again, one day after subcultivation, medium A was replaced
by BME-Earle's containing 10% horse serum. Three days (or in another experiment 8
days) later, ther serum containing medium was again replaced by medium A. One week
after this second switch the cultures were stained with a double immunostaining
procedure for vimentin and GFA protein. In both cases more immature astrocytes were
again the dominating cells one week after the second switch. Data are given for cells
which remained for 8 days in serum containing medium (Fig. 8).

However, a significant number of cells remained GFA protein positive although their density in representative microscopic fields decreased in comparison to cultures kept in serum containing media. On the basis of these experiments one can assume that more mature astrocytes (at least part of them) can become again more immature ones under appropriate conditions. This loss in expression of GFA protein, which may reflect in some way a "dedifferentiation" of astrocytes, seems to be dependent on a proliferation step. This becomes likely by experiments which showed that after the switch from serum containing medium to medium A the rate of DNA synthesis (measured by ^{3}H-thymidine incorporation) increased rapidly (Fig. 9).

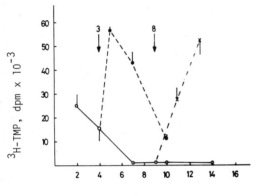

Fig. 9. ^{3}H-thymidine (^{3}H-TMP) incorporation in secondary cultures of mouse cerebellum. One day after subcultivation defined medium A was replaced by medium containing 10% horse serum (o——o); 3 days later (●---●) or 8 days later (x---x)serum containing medium was replaced again by defined medium A. Each point represents the mean of triplicate values with standard deviation.

days after subcultivation

Simultaneously the total cell density in representative microscopic fields' increased. However, exact numbers are not available at present.

Although these experiments have made it likely that a "dedifferentiation" of astrocytes can occur under appropriate conditions the final proof may however be based on experiments where clonal techniques are used in combination with different growth conditions to follow this described phenomenon on a single cell basis rather than on the basis of mass cultures.

The mass cultures described here are however a very useful system to study a certain aspect of the differentiation of astrocytes with detailed biochemical methods - namely the expression of GFA protein together with other changes occuring at the same time.

Acknowledgements

The excellent technical assistance of Christa Raab is gratefully acknowledged. I thank Dr. M. Schachner for support and helpful discussions and Dr. C. Lagenaur for comments on the manuscript. I thank Drs. A. Bignami (Boston, USA) and Dr. W. W. Franke (Heidelberg, F.R.G.) for the gift of antibodies against GFA protein and vimentin, respectively. This work was supported by Deutsche Forschungsgemeinschaft (Scha 185/5, 185/8-2 and Fi 327/1-1).

REFERENCES

1 Poduslo, S.E. and Norton, W.T. (1972). J. Neurochem. 19: 727-736

2 Snyder, D.S., Raine, C.S., Faroog, M., and Norton, W.T. (1980) J. Neurochem. 35: 1614-1620

3 Campbell, G.LeM., Schachner,M. and Shannon,S.O. (1977) Brain Res. 127: 69-86

4 Meier, D.H., Lagenaur, C., and Schachner, M. (1982) J. Neurosci. Res. 7: 119-134

5 Varon, S. and Raiborn, Jr. C.W. (1969) Brain Res. 12: 180-199

6 Barde, Y.A., Edgar, D., and Thoenen, H. (1980) Proc. Nat. Acad. Sci. USA 77: 1199-1203

7 McCarthy, K.D. and DeVellis, J. (1980) J. Cell Biol. 85: 890-902

8 Brunner, G., Lang, K., Wolfe, R.A., McClure, D.B., and Sato, G.H. (1981) Develop. Brain Res. 2: 563-575

9 Fischer, G. (1982) Neurosci. Lett. 28: 325-329

10 Fischer, G., Leutz, A., and Schachner, M. (1982) Neurosci. Lett. 29: 297-302

11 Betz, H. and Müller, K. (1982) Exp. Cell Res. 138: 297-302

12 Wakade, A.R., Edgar, D., and Thoenen, H. (1982) Exp. Cell Res. 140: 71-78

13 Morrison, R.S. and DeVellis, J. (1981) Proc. Nat. Acad. Sci. USA 78: 7205-7209

14 Schnitzer, J., Franke, W.W., and Schachner, M. (1981) J. Cell Biol. 90: 435-447

15 Dahl, D., Rueger, D.C., Bignami, A., Weber, K., and Osborn, M. (1981) Eur. J. Cell Biol. 24: 191-196

16 Bignami, A., Dahl, D., and Rueger, D.C. (1980) Advanc. Neurobiol. 1: 285-310

17 Schachner, M. (1982) J. Neurochem. 39: 1-8

18 Schachner, M., Schoonmaker, G., and Hynes, R.O. (1978) Brain Res. 158: 149-158

19 Raju, T., Bignami, A., and Dahl, D. (1981) Dev. Biol. 85: 344-357

20 Savage, R.C., Jr. and Cohen, S. (1972) J. Biol. Chem. 247: 7609-7611

21 Raff, M.C., Mirsky, R., Fields, K.L., Lisak, R.P., Dorfman, S.H., Silberberg, D.H., Gregson, N.A., Liebowitz, S., and Kennedy, M. (1978) Nature 274: 813-816

22 Rathjen, F. and Schachner, M. (1983) EMBO J., in press

23 Leutz, A. and Schachner, M. (1981) Cell Tissue Res. 220: 393-404

24 Fischer, G. and Schachner, M. (1982) Exp. Cell Res. 139: 285-296

25 Fischer, G., in preparation

26 Lim, R. (1980) Curr. Top. Dev. Biol. 16: 305-322

27 Weibel, W., Pettmann, B., Daune, G., Labourdette, G., and Sensenbrenner, M., this volume

28 Nexø, E., Hollenberg, M.D., Figueroa, A., and Pratt, R.M. (1980) Proc. Nat. Acad. Sci. USA $\underline{77}$: 2782-2785

29 Fischer, G., in preparation

Cholinergic Differentiation
in Serum-Free Aggregating Fetal Brain Cells

P. Honegger and B. Güntert
Institut de Physiologie, Université de Lausanne, CH-1011 Lausanne, Switzerland

INTRODUCTION

Several years ago we have reported the successful culture of fetal rat brain cells in a serum-free chemically defined medium using aggregating cell culture techniques (24). A comparison of serum-free cultures with their counterparts grown in the presence of fetal calf serum revealed certain morphological and biochemical differences, most notably a diminished developmental increase in choline acetyltransferase (CAT) activity, presumably due to a delayed maturation of cholinergic neurons (24). Therefore, we have examined different ways to optimize culture conditions in chemically defined media. A general improvement in longterm culture could be achieved by modifying the media composition according to the metabolic requirements of the cells (25,26). In addition, we have found factors which specifically stimulate the development of cholinergic neurons, particularly in cultures derived from fetal rat telencephalon : triiodothyronine (T_3) greatly enhances the developmental increase in CAT activity (22); nerve growth factor (NGF) (23), and elevated potassium ion (K^+) concentrations (21) further stimulate CAT irreversibly. The present report shows that the stimulation of cholinergic differentiation by both NGF and K^+ is controlled by T_3, whereas the increase in CAT activity produced by a macromolecular fraction isolated from media conditioned by brain cells is independent of T_3.

METHODS AND MATERIAL

Cell culture
Aggregating cell cultures of fetal (15 days gestation) rat (Wistar, Madörin, Füllinsdorf) telencephalon were prepared and grown in chemi-

cally defined media as before (23). The mechanically dissociated (27) cells (3 x 10^7 cells/flask) were incubated under constant gyratory agitation (70 rpm) in serum-free medium at 37°C, in an atmosphere of 10 % CO_2/ 90 % humidified air. Media were changed (exchange of 5 ml) every 3 days (unless stated otherwise) until day 14, and every other day thereafter. Within the first week, the rotation speed was gradually increased to 80 rpm.

The complete serum-free growth medium consisted of Dulbecco's Modified Eagle Medium (DMEM, no pyruvate, high glucose, Gibco cat. no. 320-1965), supplemented with : 1 µg/ml human transferrin (Sigma); 5 µg/ml crystalline bovine insulin (Sigma); 30 nM 3,3',5-triiodothyronine (Sigma); 20 nM hydrocortisone-21-phosphate (Sigma); 1.36 µg/ml vitamin B$_{12}$ (Sigma); 1 µg/ml biotin (Sigma); 10 µg/ml DL-α-tocopherol (Sigma); 5 µg/ml retinol (Fluka); 1 mM choline chloride (Sigma); 10 µM L-carnitine (Supelco); 10 µM linoleic acid (Sigma); 1 µM lipoic acid (Sigma); trace elements as before (26); 25 µg/ml gentamicin (Seromed).

Purified astrocyte monolayer cultures were prepared according to Morrison and De Vellis (36). The mechanically dissociated (27) cells of newborn rat brain cortex (3 x 10^7 cells/flask of 75 cm^2) were first grown in DMEM containing 10 % fetal calf serum (FCS, Gibco). After 10 days the oligodendrocytes were removed by vigorous shaking, and the remaining astrocytes replated (2 x 10^6 cells/flask of 75 cm^2) in DMEM containing 10 % FCS. After 7 days, the cultures were washed with serum-free medium and continued to grow in defined medium (same media composition as for aggregating cell culture). The conditioned media were collected after 7 days in defined medium.

Preparation of a macromolecular extract from conditioned media

All manipulations were done at 4°C. To pooled media (1.5-2 l) ammonium sulfate powder was added slowly up to 90 % saturation. The resulting precipitate was isolated by centrifugation (20 min, 40'000 g), dissolved in a small volume of 0.9 % NaCl containing 0.25 mM Hepes buffer pH 7.5, dialyzed against the same solution (in Spectrapor bags, molecular weight cutoff 6'000-8'000), and sterilized by membrane filtration (Gelman Acrodisc, 0.2 μm pores).

Analytical methods

Choline acetyltransferase (EC 2.3.1.6.) activity was assayed by a radiometric method as before (23).

Protein was determined according to Lowry et al. (33) using bovine serum albumin as standard. Statistical comparisons were made using the Student's *t*-test. P values > 0.05 were considered not significant.

Chemicals

All chemicals were of the highest purity available. NGF (2.5 S-NGF) and 2.5 S-NGF antiserum (rabbit) were purchased from Collaborative Research, Waltham, Mass. The IgG fraction of the antiserum was prepared according to Levy and Sober (30). Rabbit IgG, and β-lactoglobulin were obtained from Miles Laboratories, Milano.

RESULTS

Stimulation of CAT by NGF and elevated K^+ : dependency on T_3.

Aggregating cell cultures of fetal rat telencephalon were grown for 12 days either in the absence or in the presence of T_3 (30 nM), and treated from day 2 with : a) NGF (5 ng/ml); b) KCl (30 mM); or c) NGF plus KCl. The results (Table 1) show that in T_3-deficient cultures neither NGF nor K^+ influenced the specific activity (s.a.) of CAT. In contrast, cultures grown in the presence of T_3 showed significantly increased levels of CAT s.a. after treatment with either NGF or elevated K^+. The simultaneous addition of NGF and KCl did not produce an additive effect (Table 1), suggesting the involvement of a common molecular mechanism of stimulation.

Table 1. Stimulation of CAT in aggregating cell cultures of fetal rat
telencephalon by NGF and elevated K^+ concentrations :
dependency on T_3

Treatment[a]	CAT specific activity[b] (pmole/min·mg protein)	
	T_3-deficient	T_3-supplemented[a]
Untereated controls	38.1 ± 1.5	61.0 ± 1.8
NGF (5 ng/ml)	37.0 ± 1.9	94.6 ± 2.4*
KCl (30 mM)	38.1 ± 1.2	96.4 ± 2.5*
NGF + KCl	40.3 ± 1.8	100.7 ± 3.7*

[a] Treatments with NGF and KCl were started on culture day 2. NGF was
added daily; K^+ concentrations were increased to 30 mM by exchanging
a medium aliquot with the same volume of an osmolar solution of KCl
(180 mM), on culture days 2; 5; 8; and 11. T_3-supplemented media
contained 30 nM T_3 from the beginning (day 0).

[b] Data are the mean (±SEM) of 8 cultures assayed on day 12

* Significant increase compared to controls ($P < 0.0005$)

Stimulation of CAT by endogenous factors

We have observed recently (34) that aggregating cultures of fetal rat
brain release a great variety of newly synthesized proteins into the
growth medium, and that the pattern of accumulated proteins changed
with progressing cellular differentiation *in vitro*. Therefore, we have
investigated a possible auto-conditioning of these cultures.

Aggregating cell cultures of fetal rat telencephalon were grown for
12 days under prevention of media auto-conditioning by changing the
media every day (instead of every 3 days). As shown in Table 2, CAT
s.a. of these cultures was significantly reduced, whereas glutamic

Table 2. Influence of media auto-conditioning on CAT activity in
aggregating cell cultures of fetal rat telencephalon

Treatment[a]	CAT specific activity[b] (%)
Controls (media changes every 3rd day)	100 ± 4
NGF (5 ng/ml)	184 ± 5*
NGF + anti-NGF IgG	100 ± 1
Anti-NGF IgG	92 ± 5
Normal rabbit IgG	112 ± 6
Media changes every day	68 ± 2**

[a] Treatments were started on day 2. NGF and IgG (bound to Protein A-Sepharose) were added daily. All cultures were grown in the presence of 30 nM T_3.

[b] Data are the mean (±SEM) of 4 cultures assayed on day 12. The mean specific activity of the controls was 50.6 ± 1.9 pmole/min·mg protein.

* Significant increase compared to controls ($P < 0.001$)

** Significant decrease compared to controls ($P < 0.005$)

acid decarboxylase s.a. (not shown) remained unchanged. Cultures grown in the presence of anti-NGF IgG bound to Protein A Sepharose in quantities sufficient to neutralize 5 ng/ml NGF showed no change in CAT s.a. (Table 2), suggesting that the endogenous factor(s) stimulating CAT were not recognized by the antibodies to NGF.

In order to further investigate the formation and release of factors stimulating the maturation of cholinergic brain neurons *in vitro*, a macromolecular fraction was isolated by ammonium sulfate (90 %)

Table 3. Stimulation of CAT in aggregating cell cultures of fetal rat telencephalon by a macromolecular fraction extracted from conditioned media.

Treatment[a]	Days in vitro	CAT specific activity[b] (pmole/min·mg protein)	
		T_3-deficient	T_3-supplemented
Untreated controls	12	21.2 ± 3.0	38.8 ± 3.3
	19	31.2 ± 3.2	111.7 ± 8.0
Conditioned media extract	12	38.6 ± 3.3*	66.2 ± 4.2**
	19	110.6 ± 2.2***	209.4 ± 13.1***

[a] Daily treatments (beginning on day 2) with an aliquot (2.8 µg protein/ml) of a macromolecular fraction from conditioned media of aggregating fetal rat telencephalon cells.

[b] Data are the mean (±SEM) of 4 cultures assayed on day 12 and day 19 respectively.

The significant increases compared to controls are marked
* $(P < 0.01)$; **$(P < 0.0025)$; and *** $(P < 0.0005)$

precipitation from pooled conditioned media of aggregating telencephalon cell cultures, and tested for its biological activity. As shown in Table 3, the addition of the conditioned media fraction to aggregating cells of fetal rat telencephalon caused a significant increase in CAT s.a., both on day 12 and day 19. In contrast to NGF and elevated K^+, the macromolecular fraction stimulated CAT both in the presence and in the absence of T_3. This effect appeared to be specific, since the addition of comparable amounts of β-lactoglobulin (Table 4) or albumin (not shown), proteins which stimulate CAT at high concentrations, were ineffective. It could also be excluded that the stimulation of the macromolecular fraction was due to transferrin (the only

Table 4. Influence of various protein treatments on CAT activity in aggregating cell cultures of fetal rat telencephalon.

Treatment[a]	CAT specific activity[b] (%)
Untreated controls	100 ± 5
Conditioned media extract of aggregating telencephalon cells (2.8 µg protein/ml)	153 ± 11*
Conditioned media extract of astrocyte monolayer cultures (1.5 µg protein/ml)	133 ± 6*
Transferrin (10 µg/ml)	89 ± 3
β-Lactoglobulin (2.8 µg/ml)	85 ± 13
β-Lactoglobulin (750 µg/ml)	140 ± 9*

[a] Daily treatments beginning on day 2. All cultures were grown in the absence of T_3.

[b] Data are the mean (±SEM) of 4 cultures assayed on day 12. The mean specific activity of the controls was 25.1 ± 1.3 pmole/min·mg protein.

* Significant increase compared to controls ($P < 0.025$).

protein essential for the serum-free culture) since elevated transferrin media concentrations (up to 10-fold) did not cause an increase in CAT s.a. (Table 4).

A macromolecular fraction prepared from conditioned media of serum-free astrocyte cultures also stimulated CAT (Table 4), indicating that astrocytes are able to synthesize and release factor(s) stimulating cholinergic brain neurons.

DISCUSSION

Stimulation of CAT by NGF and elevated K$^+$

The finding that both NGF and elevated K$^+$ enhance the development of
CAT in a similar irreversible, T$_3$-dependent way suggests that they
stimulate the differentiation of cholinergic telencephalon neurons
by a common molecular mechanism. There are several recent findings
in the literature indicating similarities in the action of NGF and
elevated K$^+$: 1) depolarizing concentrations of K$^+$ and NGF can induce
transmembranal ion fluxes in PC 12 pheochromocytoma cells (7,40), as
well as in spinal sensory and sympathetic ganglion neurons (44).
However, we have found no effect of T$_3$ on both the Na$^+$, K$^+$-ATPase
activity and the ouabain-sensitive uptake of Rb$^+$ (a tracer for K$^+$) on
culture day 5, when T$_3$-treated cultures showed already a significant
increase in CAT (not shown). This suggests that the Na$^+$, K$^+$-pump was
not the limiting step for the action of NGF and K$^+$. 2) Analogous to
the well documented stimulation by NGF of the survival and differentiation of sympathetic and sensory neurons (e.g., refs. 17,29),
elevated K$^+$ concentrations enhance the survival and/or differentiation of chick embryo sympathetic ganglia explants (39), as well as of
dissociated cultures of chick, mouse, and human dorsal root ganglion
neurons (8, 42), chick parasympathetic neurons (5), and chick cholinergic retina neurons (6). 3) The rate of RNA and protein synthesis
is stimulated by elevated extracellular K$^+$ in brain slices (32), and
by NGF in PC 12 cells in direct relationship with neurite formation
(16). Interestingly, thyroid hormones have been shown to modulate
protein biosynthesis at a pretranslational level (43), and to stimulate primarily the growth of pre- and postsynaptic elements (28). It
has been proposed that thyroid hormones regulate the biosynthesis
of microtubule proteins essential for microtubule assembly and neurite growth (14). It is therefore conceivable that in aggregating
telencephalon cell cultures NGF and elevated K$^+$ enhance the differentiation of cholinergic neurons by stimulating the formation and/or
assembly of microtubule proteins.

Stimulation of CAT by endogenous factors different from NGF

The stimulation of CAT in aggregating fetal telencephalon cells by a macromolecular fraction from conditioned media was independent of T_3, and therefore distinguishable from the action of NGF and K^+. There are many reports in the literature indicating the existence of neurotrophic factors distinct from NGF. Such factors, stimulating the *in vitro* survival and/or differentiation of peripheral neurons (1,3,4,9,10,13,18,37,38), spinal cord motoneurons (12,15,19), or neuronal cell lines (2,13,20,35), have been detected in various tissues (1,13,15), as well as in conditioned media of both primary cell cultures (4,9,10,15,18-20,37,38) and established cell lines (2,3,20,34,38). As yet, little is known about the sensitivity of brain neurons to neurotrophic factors. It has been suggested that glial cells support the survival and/or differentiation of brain neurons (45), and neurotrophic activity has been found also in brain tissues or brain cells (11,13,31,41). The present results indicate that the maturation of (at least some) cholinergic telencephalon neurons is influenced by two different types of neurotrophic factors : 1) NGF or a NGF-like factor, and 2) a macromolecular factor synthesized and released by astrocytes (and perhaps also other brain cells). In view of the recent finding (11) of two hippocampal factors accelerating neurite growth, one NGF-like stimulating sympathetic neurons, and another, not blocked by antiserum to NGF, stimulating parasympathetic neurons, the present results support the idea that these neurotrophic factors have a physiological significance in the brain.

ACKNOWLEDGEMENTS

We wish to thank Ms. Sonia Gattesco for excellent technical assistance, and Dr. Mukut Sharma, Department of Biochemistry, University of Baroda, for his help to culture purified astrocytes. This work was supported by the Swiss National Foundation for Scientific Research (grant no. 3. 641. 80).

REFERENCES

1. ADLER R, LANDA KB, MANTHORPE M, VARON S (1979) Cholinergic neurotrophic factors: intraocular distribution of trophic activity for ciliary neurons. Science 204:1434-1436

2. ARENANDER AT, DE VELLIS J (1981) Glial-released proteins III. Influence on neuronal morphological differentiation. Brain Res 224:117-127

3. BARDE YA, LINDSAY RM, MONARD D, THOENEN H (1978) New factor released by cultured glioma cells supporting survival and growth of sensory neurones. Nature 274:818

4. BENNETT MR, NURCOMBE V (1979) The survival and development of cholinergic neurons in skeletal muscle conditioned media. Brain Res 173:543-548

5. BENNETT MR, WHITE W (1979) The survival and development of cholinergic neurons in potassium-enriched media. Brain Res 173:549-553

6. BETZ H (1981) Choline acetyltransferase activity in chick retina cultures: effect of membrane depolarizing agents. Brain Res 223:190-194

7. BOONSTRA J, VAN DER SAAG PT, MOOLENAAR WH, DE LAAT SW (1981) Rapid effects of nerve growth factor on the Na^+,K^+-pump in rat pheochromocytoma cells. Exp Cell Res 131:452-455

8. CHALAZONITIS A, FISCHBACH GD (1980) Elevated potassium induces morphological differentiation of dorsal root ganglionic neurons in dissociated cell culture. Dev Biol 78:173-183

9. COLLINS F (1978) Induction of neurite outgrowth by a conditioned medium factor bound to the culture substratum. Proc Natl Acad Sci USA 75:5210-5213

10. COUGHLIN MD, BLOOM EM, BLACK IB (1981) Characterization of a neuronal growth factor from mouse heart-cell-conditioned medium. Dev Biol 82:56-68

11. CRUTCHER KA, COLLINS F (1982) In vitro evidence for two distinct hippocampal growth factors: basis of neuronal plasticity? Science 217:67-68

12. DRIBIN LB, BARRETT JN (1980) Conditioned medium enhances neuritic outgrowth from rat spinal cord explants. Dev Biol 74:184-195

13. EDGAR D, BARDE YA, THOENEN H (1979) Induction of fibre outgrowth and choline acetyltransferase in PC 12 pheochromocytoma cells by conditioned media from glial cells and organ extracts. Exp Cell Res 121:353-361

14. FELLOUS A, LENNON AM, FRANCON J, NUNEZ J (1979) Thyroid hormone and neurotubule assembly in vitro during brain development. Eur J Biochem 101:365-376

15. GODFREY EW, SCHRIER BK, NELSON PG (1980) Source and target cell specificities of a conditioned medium factor that increases choline acetyltransferase activity in cultured spinal cord cells. Dev Biol 77:403-418

16. GUNNING PW, LANDRETH GE, LAYER P, IGNATIUS M, SHOOTER EM (1981) Nerve growth factor-induced differentiation of PC 12 cells: evaluation of changes in RNA and DNA metabolism. J Neurosci 1:368-379

17. HARPER GP, THOENEN H (1980) Nerve growth factor: biological signi-ficance, measurement, and distribution. J Neurochem 34:5-16

18. HELFAND SL, RIOPELLE RJ, WESSELS NK (1978) Nonequivalence of con-ditioned medium and nerve growth factor for sympathetic, parasym-pathetic, and sensory neurons. Exp Cell Res 113:39-45

19 HENDERSON CE, HUCHET M, CHANGEUX J-P (1981) Neurite outgrowth from embryonic chicken spinal neurons is promoted by media conditioned by muscle cells. Proc Natl Acad Sci USA 78:2625-2629

20. HEUMANN R, ÖCALAN M, HAMPRECHT B (1979) Factors from glial cells regulate choline acetyltransferase and tyrosine hydroxylase activi-ties in a hybrid-hybrid cell line. FEBS Lett 107:37-41

21. HONEGGER P (1982) NGF-sensitive brain neurons in culture. In: SCHLUMPF M, LICHTENSTEIGER W (eds) Drugs and Hormones in Brain De-velopment. Monographs in Neural Sciences (COHEN MM, series ed) S Karger, Basel, in press

22. HONEGGER P, LENOIR D (1980) Triiodothyronine enhancement of neuro-nal differentiation in aggregating fetal rat brain cells cultured in a chemically defined medium. Brain Res 199:425-434

23. HONEGGER P, LENOIR D (1982) Nerve growth factor (NGF) stimulation of cholinergic telencephalic neurons in aggregating cell cultures. Dev Brain Res 3:229-238

24. HONEGGER P, LENOIR D, FAVROD P (1979) Growth and differentiation of aggregating fetal brain cells in a serum-free, defined medium. Nature 282:305-308

25. HONEGGER P, LENOIR D, GÜNTERT B (1982) Aggregating brain cell cul-ture: which nutritional medium is "physiologic" ? Naunyn-Schmiede-berg's Arch Pharmacol 321:R11

26. HONEGGER P, MATTHIEU J-M (1980) Myelination of aggregating fetal rat brain cell cultures grown in a chemically defined medium. In: BAUMANN N (ed) Neurological Mutations Affecting Myelination, INSERM Symposium Nr 14, Elsevier/North-Holland Biomedical Press, pp 481-488

27. HONEGGER P, RICHELSON E (1976) Biochemical differentiation of me-chanically dissociated mammalian brain in aggregating cell culture. Brain Res 109:335-354

28. LAUDER JM (1978) Effects of early hypo- and hyperthyroidism on de-velopment of rat cerebellar cortex IV. The parallel fibers. Brain Res 142:25-39

29. LEVI-MONTALCINI R, ANGELETTI PU (1968) Nerve growth factor. Physiol Rev 48: 534-569

30. LEVY HB, SOBER HA (1960) A simple chromatographic method for pre-paration of gamma globulin. Proc Soc Exp Biol 103:250-252

31. LINDSAY RM (1982) Adult rat brain astrocytes support survival of both NGF-dependent and NGF-insensitive neurones. Nature 282:80-82

32. LIPTON P, HEIMBACH C (1977) The effect of extracellular potassium concentration on protein synthesis in guinea-pig hippocampal slices. J Neurochem 28:1347-1354

33. LOWRY OH, ROSEBROUGH NJ, FARR AL, RANDALL RJ (1951) Protein measurement with the Foli-phenol reagent. J Biol Chem 193:265-275

34. MARCHAND CM-F, MOOSER V, HONEGGER P (1981) Developmental changes in extracellular proteins in serum-free brain cell culture. Proc 8th Int Meeting of ISN, Nottingham, p 71

35. MONARD D, SOLOMON F, RENTSCH M, GYSIN R (1973) Glia-induced morphological differentiation in neuroblastoma cells. Proc Natl Acad Sci USA 70:1894-1897

36. MORRISON RS, DE VELLIS J (1981) Growth of purified astrocytes in a chemically defined medium. Proc Natl Acad Sci USA 78:7205-7209

37. NISHI R, BERG DK (1979) Survival and development of ciliary ganglion neurones grown alone in cell culture. Nature 277:232-234

38. PATTERSON PH, CHUN LLY (1977) The induction of acetylcholine synthesis in primary cultures of dissociated rat sympathetic neurons I. Effects of conditioned medium. Dev Biol 56:263-280

39. PHILLIPSON OT, SANDLER M (1975) The influence of nerve growth factor, potassium depolarization and dibutyryl (cyclic) adenosine 3', 5'-monophosphate on explant cultures of chick embryo sympathetic ganglia. Brain Res 90:273-281

40. SCHUBERT D, LaCORBIERE M, WHITLOCK C, STALLCUP W (1978) Alterations in the surface properties of cells responsive to nerve growth factor. Nature 273:718-723

41. SCHURCH-RATHGEB Y, MONARD D (1978) Brain development influences the appearance of glial factor-like activity in rat brain primary cultures. Nature 273:308-309

42. SCOTT BS (1977) The effect of elevated potassium on the time course of neuron survival in cultures of dissociated dorsal root ganglion. J Cell Physiol 91:305-316

43. SEELIG S, LIAW C, TOWLE HC, OPPENHEIMER JH (1981) Thyroid hormone attenuates and augments hepatic gene expression at a pretranslational level. Proc Natl Acad Sci USA 78:4733-4737

44. SKAPER SD, VARON S (1980) Properties of the sodium extrusion mechanism controlled by nerve growth factor in chick embryo dorsal root ganglionic cells. J Neurochem 34:1654-1660

45. TOUZET N, SENSENBRENNER M (1978) Stimulatory role of glial cells on the differentiation of dissociated chick embryo encephalon cells. Dev Neurosci 1:159-163

DNA Synthesis in Nuclei and Mitochondria Purified from Serum-Free or Supplemented Glial Cell Cultures

R. Avola[1], D. Curti[2], B. Lombardo[1], P. Ragonese[1], M. Renis[3], and G. Ricceri[1]

[1] Institute of Biochemistry, Faculty of Medicine, University of Catania, Italy
[2] Institute of Pharmacoloy, Faculty of Sciences, University of Pavia, Italy
[3] Mental Hospital of Bisceglie, Bari, Italy

ABSTRACT

Nuclear and mitochondrial DNA synthesis in serum-free or supplement-ed rat glial cell cultures at different days after plating was studied. Furthermore in mitochondria purified from cells grown in basal nutrient medium some enzymatic activities related to energy transduction (citrate synthase, malate dehydrogenase, total NADH-cytochrome c reductase, cytochrome oxidase and glutamate dehydrogenase) were measured. [Methyl-^{3}H] thymidine was added at different days after plating to the serum-supplemented and to the serum-free culture media. During the period tested the specific activity of total, nuclear and mitochondrial DNA decreased from 8 DIV to 21 DIV and increased at 30 DIV in the serum-supplemented glial cell cultures; on the contrary, it decreased from 15 DIV up to 32 DIV in the serum-free cultures. The specific activity of nuclear DNA was always higher than that of mitochondrial DNA. In the serum-supplemented cultures the specific activity of the above mentioned mitochondrial enzymes increased from 8 DIV up to 21 DIV, and decreased at 30 DIV.

INTRODUCTION

Cells dissociated from 2 days old rat cerebral hemispheres and grown in basal nutrient medium at high concentration on plastic surface of Petri dishes (Ø 100 mm) develop into a mixed population of glial cell culture (1), composed of at least three morphologically different cell types. The predominant cell type consists of astroglial cells, which form a monolayer. The second cell type, rarely observed, consists of ependymal cells. The third type consists of small cells, scattered upon the astroglial layer, which were identified as oligodendroglial cells by ultrastructural and histochemical criteria (2).

The neuroblasts degenerate rapidly during the two first weeks and after 14 days in vitro (DIV), the cell layer is mainly composed of flat polygonal shaped cells. At 21 DIV most cells develop a slightly fibrous aspect. Ultrastructural and biochemical studies showed the presence of gliofilaments and glial fibrillary acidic (GFA) protein as well as S-100 protein in these cells, indicating the astroglial nature of these cultures (2).

The aim of the present study was to investigate some biochemical characteristics of serum-free or supplemented rat glial cell cultures during their maturation and differentiation with particular regard to nuclear and mitochondrial DNA synthesis and to some enzymatic acti-vities related to energy transduction [citrate synthase (EC 4.1.3.7), malate dehydrogenase (EC 1.1.1.32), total NADH-cytochrome c reductase

(EC 1.6.99.3), cytochrome oxidase (EC 1.9.3.1) and glutamate dehydrogenase (EC 1.4.1.3)].

MATERIALS AND METHODS

Glial cell cultures, prepared as described by Booher and Sensenbrenner (1) were incubated at 37°C in a humidified 5% CO_2-95% air atmosphere. The nutrient medium consisted of Dulbecco's modification of Eagle's minimum essential medium (DMEM; GIBCO), supplemented by 10% fetal calf serum (GIBCO). The serum-free glial cell cultures were grown in a chemically defined medium for 72 hr before labeling. The serum-free supplemented (SFS) medium, modified by Bottenstein and Sato (3) contained: 5 µg insulin/ml, 100 µg transferrin (human)/ml, 2×10^{-8} M progesterone, 10^{-4} putrescine, 10^{-12} M 17-ß-estradiol and 3×10^{-8} M sodium selenite. [Methyl-^{3}H] thymidine (5 µCi/ml, spec. act. 2 Ci/mmol) was added at different days after plating (8,14,21,30 DIV) to the serum-supplemented and (15,22,32 DIV) to the serum-free culture media. After two hours of incubation (time established in preliminary kinetic experiments) at 37°C, the medium was removed, the cells were washed with cold 0.9% NaCl, harvested and homogenized. The separation and purification of nuclei and mitochondria, the extraction of DNA and its specific activity determination were accomplished as previously described (4). In the mitochondria purified from cells grown in basal nutrient medium the specific activity of the following enzymes was measured by spectrophotometric methods: citrate synthase, malate dehydrogenase, total NADH-cytochrome c reductase, cytochrome oxidase and glutamate dehydrogenase.

RESULTS AND CONCLUSIONS

The results show that in the serum-supplemented glial cell cultures during the period tested the specific activity of total DNA as well as of nuclear and mitochondrial DNA decreases from 8 DIV up to 21 DIV and increases at 30 DIV (Fig. 1). On the contrary, in the serum-free

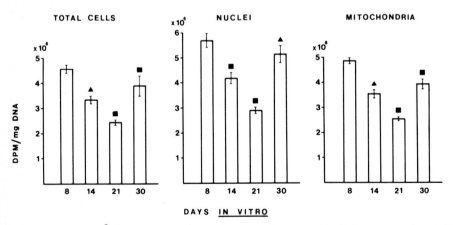

Fig. 1. [Methyl-^{3}H] thymidine (5 µCi/ml of culture medium) incorporation into DNA of homogenate, nuclei and mitochondria from serum-supplemented glial cell cultures at different days after plating. The results are expressed as specific radioactivity (dpm/mg DNA). Each value is the mean of 4 determinations from three different experiments ±S.E.M. Significance by Student's t test is referred to the difference of each age from the previous one: ■ P<0.01; ▲ P<0.001.

glial cell cultures thymidine incorporation into total, nuclear and mitochondrial DNA decreases from 15 DIV up to 32 DIV (Fig. 2). These results indicate that the rate of glial cell multiplication in these cultures is progressively decreasing up to the third week after plat-

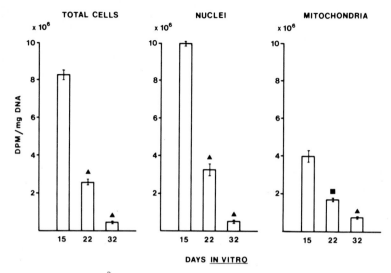

Fig. 2. [Methyl-^{3}H] thymidine (5 µCi/ml of serum free culture medium) incorporation into DNA of homogenate, nuclei and mitochondria from serum-free (for 72 h) rat glial cell cultures at different days after plating. The results are expressed as specific radioactivity (dpm/mg DNA). Each value is the mean of 4 determinations from three experiments ±S.E.M. Significance by Student's t test is referred to the difference of each age from the previous one: ■ P<0.01, ▲ P<0.001.

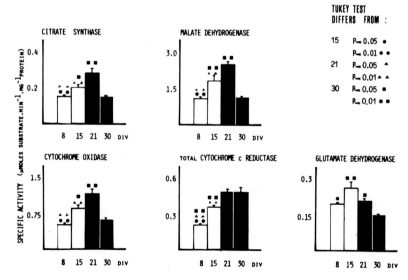

Fig. 3. Mitochondrial enzymatic activities related to energy transduction in serum-supplemented glial cell cultures, at different days after plating. The results are expressed as specific activity (µmoles substrate min^{-1}, mg^{-1} protein). The data were submitted to the anova and subsequently to the Tukey tests for the statistical analysis

ing. The increased specific activity of DNA at 30 DIV in the serum-supplemented glial cell cultures, might be due to oligodendroglial cell multiplication in these experimental conditions. On the contrary, the continuous decrease of DNA specific activity in the serum-free glial cell cultures up to 32 DIV might depend on the lack of some growth factors present in the serum, which are required for oligodendrocyte maturation and differentiation after four weeks in culture. Moreover, the specific activity of nuclear DNA is always higher than that of mitochondrial DNA in both culture systems as already observed in developing rat brain (4).

The specific activity of the above mentioned mitochondrial enzymes in the serum-supplemented cultures significantly increases from the 8th up to the 21st day in culture and then significantly decreases at 30 DIV except for total NADH-cytochrome c reductase which shows no difference between 21 and 30 DIV and for glutamate dehydrogenase which starts to decline after 15 DIV (Fig. 3). The modifications of the enzymatic activities found in the present study indicate some maturation phenomena correlated with the energy metabolism of glial cells in culture.

ACKNOWLEDGEMENT

This work was accomplished by financial support from C.N.R. (Italy). D. Blarasin, A. Costa and C. Desiderio are gratefully acknowledged for their skillful assistance.

REFERENCES

1) Booher J., Sensenbrenner M. - Neurobiology, 1972, 2, 97-105.
2) Sensenbrenner M., Devilliers G., Bock E., Porte A. - Differentiation, 1980, 17, 51-61.
3) Bottenstein J.E., Sato G.H.- Proc.Natl.Acad.Sci.USA,1979,76,514-517.
4) Giuffrida A.M., Gadaleta M.N., Serra I., Renis M., Geremia E., Del Prete G., Saccone C. - Neurochem. Res., 1979, 4, 37-52.

Guanylate Cyclase Activators Hemin and Sodium Nitroprusside Stimulate the Growth of Transformed Cells in Serum-Free Medium

P. Basset, J. Zwiller, G. Ulrich, and M. O. Revel

Centre de Neurochimie du CNRS, 5, Rue Blaise Pascal, F-67084 Strasbourg Cedex, France

ABSTRACT

Hemin and sodium nitroprusside, which strongly activate purified guanylate cyclase *in vitro*, were also found to stimulate leukemic, glioma and neuroblastoma cells to divide in serum-free medium. The involvement of guanylate cyclase activation in the proliferative response to hemin and sodium nitroprusside is discussed.

1. Introduction

Despite extensive investigation, little evidence has been produced concerning a role of cGMP in the regulation of the growth of normal and transformed cells [1,2]. The possibility that cGMP serves as a positive signal to cell growth has been suggested notably for lymphocytes and fibroblasts in which cGMP levels increase after stimulation with mitogenic agents [3]. We have recently demonstrated that hemin and sodium nitroprusside, which strongly activate purified guanylate cyclase *in vitro*, are also able to stimulate glioma and neuroblastoma cells to divide in serum-free medium [4]. We report here that comparable results are obtained with mouse leukemic L1210 cells. The involvement of guanylate cyclase activation and the possible role of iron in these growth stimulations of transformed cells are discussed.

2. Materials and Methods

L1210 leukemic cells were grown in flasks (4.5×10^5 cells per 25 cm^2 Falcon culture flask) in RPMI 1640 under standard conditions in the presence of either 10 % fetal calf serum (FCS) or of guanylate cyclase activators added at day 0 of culture. C6 glioma cells and N1E-115 neuroblastoma cells were cultured as previously reported [4].

3. Results

The growth promotion measured by the increase in cell number induced by either hemin (10^{-6} M) or sodium nitroprusside (10^{-5} M) is shown in Fig. 1. The growth observed after 4 days of culture were identical with both compounds and represented 20-25 % of that obtained under comparable culture conditions in the presence of 10 % FCS. In Table 1, the growth stimulations obtained for L1210 leukemic cells, N1E-115 neuro-

220

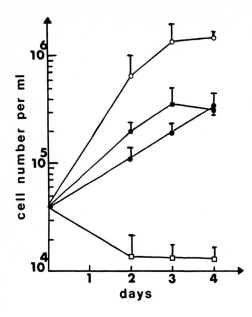

Fig. 1. Effect of hemin and sodium nitroprusside on the growth of L1210 leukemic
cells. □ Without serum; O with 10 % FCS;
● 10⁻⁶ hemin; ■ 10⁻⁵ sodium nitroprusside.
Each point represents the mean ± SD of
the cell number in 4 flasks.

Table 1. Comparative growth stimulations
of some transformed cell lines by hemin
and sodium nitroprusside

Cells	Hemin	Nitroprusside	Serum
L1210[a]	23	22	106
N1E-115[b]	16	6	140
C6[c]	16	17	30

[a] 10^{-6} hemin, 10^{-5} nitroprusside (day 4);
[b] 10^{-6} hemin, 10^{-6} nitroprusside (day 10);
[c] 10^{-7} hemin, 10^{-5} nitroprusside (day 10).
Growth stimulations are expressed as the
ratio between the cell number in the presence of guanylate activators or FCS and
the cell number in absence of activators
or FCS.

blastoma cells and C6 glioma cells with either hemin or sodium nitroprusside are compared. In contrast, these compounds did not stimulate normal cells, including 3T3
fibroblasts, to divide. Other guanylate cyclase activators, sodium azide and hydroxylamine, were also tested on C6 glioma and L1210 leukemic cells. Growth promotion was
only observed with hydroxylamine (10^{-4} M) which elicited a growth stimulation of 2 at
day 8 for C6 glioma cells.

4. Discussion

While the mitogenic action of hemin and sodium nitroprusside on transformed
cells seems a general phenomenon, their mechanism of action in the cell remains to be
established. It is generally accepted that nitroprusside activates guanylate cyclase
by forming nitric oxide (NO) [5] and that heme acts by forming a ligand with NO [6].
We have suggested that the *in vivo* activation of guanylate cyclase could be involved
in the mitogenic action of these compounds, since a similar synergism between hemin
and sodium nitroprusside was observed for C6 glioma cell growth promotion and for the
stimulation of purified guanylate cyclase activity [4].

To examine this hypothesis, we tested other NO forming products such as sodium
azide and hydroxylamine, which are also known to activate guanylate cyclase. The
fact that these compounds were not able to promote cell growth as did sodium nitro-

prusside might be due to the tissue ability to metabolize azide and hydroxylamine, since these compounds, in contrast with sodium nitroprusside, are known to require enzymic transformation in order to stimulate guanylate cyclase [5,7]. However, this result might also indicate that the mitogenic action of sodium nitroprusside is not related to its ability to form NO. Since sodium nitroprusside and hemin are both iron-containing compounds, their mitogenic properties might be related to iron supply as iron is known to play a key role in cell proliferation [8,9]. Nevertheless guanylate cyclase itself could be involved in cell growth elicited by iron. Iron could catalyze the *in vivo* formation of the OH radical which is known to be a potent activator of guanylate cyclase activity [10]. Iron could also stimulate heme synthesis and thus guanylate cyclase activity, if heme played a role in the physiologic activation of the enzyme as has been suggested [6,11,12].

Our results indicate that hemin and sodium nitroprusside are mitogens for transformed cells but not for normal cells. Further investigations are needed to define how these compounds act in the cell and if their action is related to their ability to stimulate guanylate cyclase.

5.   References

1. Goldberg, N.O. and Haddox, M.K. (1977) *Ann. Rev. Biochem. 46*, 823-896.
2. DeRubertis, F.R. and Craven, P.A. (1980) *Adv. Cyclic Nucleot. Res. 12*, 97-109.
3. Coffrey, R.G., Hadden, E.M., Lopez, C. and Hadden, J.W. (1978) *Adv. Cyclic Nucleot. Res. 9*, 661-676.
4. Zwiller, J., Basset, P., Ulrich, G. and Mandel, P. (1982) *Exp. Cell Res.*, in press.
5. Arnold, W.P., Mittal, C.K., Katsuki, S. and Murad, F. (1977) *Proc. Natl. Acad. Sci. 74*, 3203-3207.
6. Craven, P.A. and DeRubertis, F.R. (1978) *J. Biol. Chem. 253*, 8433-8443.
7. Craven, P.A., DeRubertis, F.R. and Pratt, D.W. (1979) *J. Biol. Chem. 254*, 8213-8222.
8. Barnes, D. and Sato, G. (1980) *Anal. Biochem. 102*, 255-270.
9. Novogrodsky, A., Ravid, A., Glaser, T., Rubin, A.L. and Stenzel, K.H. (1982) *Exp. Cell Res. 139*, 419-422.
10. Mittal, C.K. and Murad, F. (1977) *Proc. Natl. Acad. Sci. 74*, 4360-4364.
11. Gerzer, R., Hofmann, F. and Schultz, G. (1981) *Eur. J. Biochem. 116*, 479-486.
12. Ignarro, L.J., Degnan, J.N., Baricos, W.H., Kadowitz, P.J. and Wolin, M.S. (1982) *Biochim. Biophys. Acta 718*, 49-59.

Tracing the Astroglial Cell-Lineage in Vitro by Modification of the Microenvironmental Conditions

Klaus Lang and Gerd Brunner

Institut für Immunologie, Obere Zahlbacher Str. 67, D-6500 Mainz, FRG

Since the introduction of serum-free, hormone-supplemented media many research reports have shown that it is possible to select one defined cell-type out of a heterogeneously composed organ dissociate. In this paper we will show that not only cell-types can be selectively cultivated, but also different variants of one cell-type (in this case the astrocyte) can be grown selectively and, furthermore, these variants can be interchanged by modification of the medium conditions.

Brains of newborn Wistar-Furth rats of one or two days of age were removed and disintegrated, using a combined mechanical and enzymatical procedure (1). The resulting cell suspension was washed and the cells were seeded directly into serum-free medium on polylysine-coated 3.5 cm dishes at a density of $5 \cdot 10^5$ cells/dish. Basal medium was a 1:1 mixture of Dulbecco's modified Eagle's medium and Ham's F12, supplemented with trace elements, glucose, and antibiotics. Medium was changed on day 1, 3, 6 after plating and subsequently every 4 days. Two kinds of experiments were performed: _selection experiments_: cells were maintained under the same medium conditions over the whole culture period; _switching experiments_: cells were selected in one medium for at least two weeks, then the cultures were washed, and another medium was added. After four days a second switch could be performed. Cultures were maintained for longer than four months.

Medium C_0, derived from C_6-medium which was originally developed for the serum-free cultivation of C_6-glioma cells (2), consists of insulin (2 µg/ml), transferrin (5 µg/ml) and Gimmel-factor (10 µg/ml) (3). This medium supports the selection and proliferation of the first variant of astroglial cells: _primitive astroglial cells_ (No.1 in the fig.). Their morphology and contact behaviour is similar to that of C_6-glioma cells. They also show a high proliferation activity. Like all the other cells described in this report they are positive to immunostaining against the astroglial-specific 10 nm-filament-protein GFAP (glial fibrillary acidic protein (4).

Another medium, which was termed B_9, allows the selection of _astrocytes_ with numerous long and branched processes (No.3 in the fig.). They do not proliferate. Medium B_9 consists of: insulin (5 µg/ml), transferrin (100 µg/ml), selenium ($3 \cdot 10^{-8}$M), thyroglobulin (100 µg/ml), T_3 (0.03

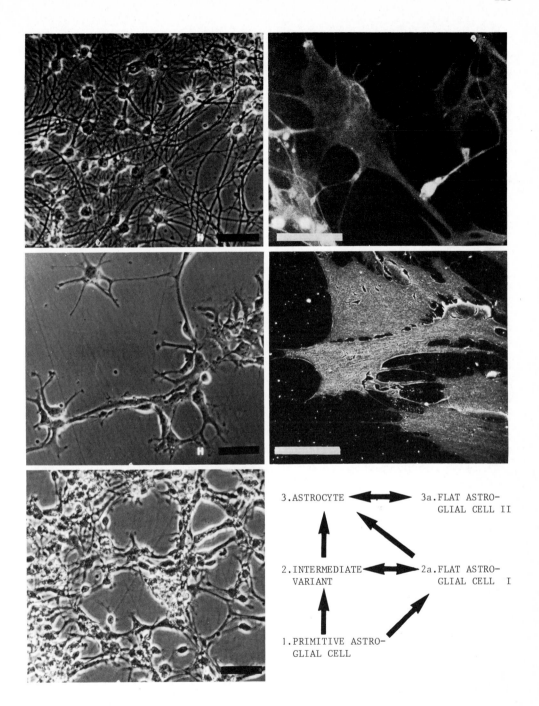

The 5 variants of astroglial cells and the possibilities of changing
one variant into another. 1-3:phase contrast. 2a:Scanning EM and 3a:
immunofluorescence staining against GFAP;an astrocyte is shown which
is switching into a flat cell.Both characters are visible.
Barrs represent 50 μm.

nM), and estradiol (10 ng/ml). The same results can be obtained with the improved medium B27 which contains: insulin (5 μg/ml), transferrin (100 μg/ml), and thyroglobulin (10 μg/ml).

Two other media were obtained by combining the factors prominent in C_0- and B_9-medium: B_{19} (B_9-medium + Gimmel-factor) and B_{23} (C_0-medium + thyroglobulin). In B_{19}-medium another variant of astroglial cells is selected: the *intermediate variant* (No.2 in the fig.). Its morphology is similar to that of the primitive astroglial cells, but the processes are more numerous and longer. Moreover, they do not proliferate. In medium B_{23} astrocytes are selected. These data show that Gimmel-factor acts as a differentiation-inhibiting factor and thyroglobulin as a maturation-factor to astroglial cells. Whether the effects of thyroglobulin are due to T_3 or T_4 remains to be tested.

These three variants of astroglial cells, found in selection-experiments in serum-free medium, can be transformed into a fourth variant of astroglia: the *flat astroglial cell* (No. 2a, 3a in the fig.). These flat fibroblast-like cells have previously often been denominated astroblasts. Flat astroglial cells show up rapidly when, after a selection time of at least two weeks in serum-free media, cultures of primitive, intermediate, or mature astroglial cells are transferred to medium containing 10 % newborn calf serum.

Moreover, primitive and intermediate astroglial cells can be changed to astrocytes in medium B_9 or B_{27}, and primitive cells can be switched to intermediate ones by using medium B_{19}. These events are irreversible. Flat cells can be switched back to intermediate astroglial cells, but only if the cells had not been in the astrocyte-phase before. In this case flat astroglial cells can only be converted into astrocytes. This finding suggests that flat astroglial cells have to be divided into two groups with the same morphology, but with biochemical differences. The possibilities of converting the different variants of astroglial cells are indicated in the figure.

The behaviour of subcultivated cells is identical to that of their primary counterparts.

Our experiments show that the serum-free cell culture initiates new potentials for the in vitro exploration of cell lineages.

This work was supported by the Stiftung Volkswagenwerk.

References

1) Brunner, G., Lang, K., Wolfe, R.A., McClure, D.B., Sato, G.H.:Dev. Brain Res. 2, (1981) 563 – 575.
2) Wolfe, R.A., Sato, G.H., McClure, D.B.: J. Cell Biol. 87 (1980) 434–441.
3) McClure, D.B., Ohasa, S., Sato, G.H.: J. Cell Physiol. 107 (1981) 195 – 207.
4) Bignami, A., Eng, L.F., Dahl, D., Uyeda, C.T.: Brain Res. 43 (1972) 429 – 435.

Growth of Perfused and Nonperfused Neuronal Cell Lines in Serum Deprived Medium

A. L. Peterson and E. Walum

Unit of Neurochemistry and Neurotoxicology, University of Stockholm, Enköpingsvägen 126, S-172 46 Sundbyberg, Sweden

ABSTRACT

Growth of four neuronal cell lines cultured in serum deprived medium utilizing traditional and perfusion culturing techniques were studied. Changing from serum supplemented medium to medium deprived of serum in traditional cultures, resulted in a cessation of cellular proliferation, as well as a decrease in cellular viability. In perfusion cells retained their viability and continued to proliferate until confluency.

1.   Introduction

Traditional cell culture techniques with periodic changes of growth medium represents a closed system in which nutrient levels decrease and metabolic endproducts accumulate (1). A steady state system, more relevant to the in vivo situation, can be achieved by utilizing perfusion techniques (2).

We have perviously found that culturing of the neuronal cell lines neuroblastoma C1300 clones N1E115 and N18 and gliomas C6 and 138MG, in perfusion in serum supplemented medium causes dramatic changes with respect to both growth characteristics and the degree of morphological differentiation as compared to traditional culturing (3). It is known that serum deprivation induce morphological and biochemical differentiation in cultures of neuroblastoma and glioma cells (4, 5), and that these alterations are followed by a stop in cellular proliferation. We have in this work tested, whether the improvement in culture conditions obtained by using a perfusion technique, would alter these responses of serum deprivation. A new in disco perfusion technique which permits the perfusion of standard plastic culture dishes was utilized (3).

2.   Materials and methods

Stock cultures. Glioma C6 and glioma 138MG, neuroblastoma C1300 cells clones N1E115 and N18 were grown in Costar plastic flasks in Ham's F10 medium, supplemented with 9 % newborn calf serum and 4 % fetal calf serum. The medium contained 100 units of penicillin and 50 ug streptomycin per ml. Cultures were kept in an incubator at $37^O C$ in a humidified atmosphere of 5 % CO_2 in air. Medium was changed twice a week and sub-cultures were made using 0.25 trypsin in a phosphate-buffered salt-solution.

Perfusion technique. The perfusion technique used in this work has previously been described in detail (3). It is based on the use of a perfusion block (pat.nr. 8101564-4, PCT/SE82/00050, Fig 1) which permits the perfusion of cell cultures in disco.

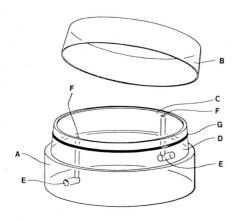

Fig. 1. Perfusion-block:
(A) Perfusion-block in poly-carbonate plastic, (B) plastic culture dish, (C) turned coun-ter-sink, (D) cone with an outer diameter equal to the inner diameter of the plastic culture dish, (E) in- and out-let, with luer connections, (F) in- and outlet at the peri-feri of the countersink, (G) rubber O-ring.

Experimental cultures. For the present experiments cells were plated into Falcon 60 mm tissue culture dishes, at a density of $2.4x10^4$ cells/cm^2. After four days of in-cubation in serum supplemented medium, one set of cultures were introduced into the perfusion system. Recirculating perfusion were then carried out with 50 ml medium de-prived of serum, at a rate of 0.3 ml/min. Nonperfused cultures were washed and in-cubated in serum deprived or serum containing medium respectively. Both perfused and nonperfused cultures were incubated for another four days. Cell numbers were deter-mined at day four and day eight in a Coulter Counter Model B.

Chemicals. Ham's F10 medium, fetal calf serum, newborn calfserum, antibiotics and trypsin were purchased from Flow Laboratories Ltd, Irvine, Scotland.

3.   Results

Results obtained in cultures, perfused (P) and nonperfused (NP), in medium de-prived of serum, as well as controlcultures grown in medium supplemented with serum (NSP) are summarized in Table 1.

Table 1. Growth of perfused (P) and nonperfused (NP) neuronal cell lines, cultured for four days in medium without serum. SP denotes cell densities at start of perfusion and NPS the number of cells in nonperfused serum containing controls. Cell numbers are expressed as 10^3 cells/cm^2 $\pm$ SD. Numbers of experiments are indicated in brackets.

Cell line	SP	NPS	NP	P
C6	156 ± 33 (5)	272 ± 30 (5)	184 ± 10 (5)	340 ± 37 (6)
138MG	53 ± 4 (6)	103 ± 13 (5)	71 ± 10 (5)	70 ± 7 (6)
N18	92 ± 4 (6)	118 ± 5 (5)	27 ± 10 (5)	127 ± 36 (6)
N1E115	32 ± 5 (8)	35 ± 1 (3)	18 ± 3 (4)	56 ± 4 (5)

A dramatic decrease in cellular viability could be seen in the NP neuroblastoma cells. Cell densities decreased to 50 % and 30 % of the initial cell number (SP) for N1E115 and N18 respectively. In P cultures of the two cell lines the viability was retained. In addition, a significant increase (90 %) in cell number as compared to initial values (SP) was seen in P N1E115 cultures. This indicates a maintained proliferative capacity in serum free medium. In NP cultures of the glioma cell lines C6 and 138MG no loss in viability was observed. On the contrary a slight increase in cell number (18 % and 34 % respectively) was registered. The growth of C6 cells was further increased in perfusion, whereas 138MG cells were unresponsive (Table 1).

4.   Discussion

Culturing the neuroblastoma cells under steady state condition (P) resulted in a retained viability. Serveral physical and chemical factors are likely to have contributed. However, it is unlikely that a more effective oxygenation was responsible. Since neuroblastoma cells have been shown to be largely independent on oxidative metabolism for maintaining growth and viability (6, 7), it appears plausible that increased nutrient supply and removal of metabolic end products were of greater importance. The marked difference in viability between P and NP cultures of neuroblastoma cells as well as the differences in response to NP conditions between glioma and neuroblastoma cells might thus be explained as follows: Neuroblastoma cells in contrast to glioma cells are known to have a deficient antioxidative capacity (8) including low activities of glutathione peroxidase (9). Neuroblastoma cells cultured in defined medium require the addition of selenium, known to induce glutathione peroxidase activities in these cells (10), to the medium for maintained viability and growth (11). It may therefore be argued that serum free culturing of neuroblastoma cells increases the demands for an antioxidative capacity. Accordingly the decrease

in cellular viability in NP serum free cultures may be attributed to radical formation in cells and media. Consequently cells cultured in perfusion might be protected
from oxidative stress, by the washing away and dilution of reactive metabolites.

With the exception of the glioma cell line 138MG, all cell densities were found
to be higher in P than NP cultures. It is interesting to note that densities in both
P and NP 138MG cultures correspond to the density at confluency (12). Furthermore,
teoretical estimations of densities at confluency for glioma C6 and neuroblastoma
N18 correspond to the maximal densities reached in P cultures. Thus it seems that
steady state conditions allow these cell lines to maintain their proliferative activity until confluency in serum free medium. Based on the present experiments, it it
not possible to explain mechanisms behind this observation. However. it is a general
opinion that both neuroblastoma and glioma cells in culture express many normalized
properties (4, 12). The stop in cell division at confluency therefore could be a re-
miniscent of the density dependent inhibition of growth observed in cultures of normal cells (13).

REFERENCES

1. Kruse P.F.Jr in: Growth, nutrition and metabolism of cells in culture. Rothblat
   G.M. ed. Vol. 2. New York: Academic Press: 1972:11-66.
2. Patterson M.K.Jr. Perfusion and mass culture systems. Tissue culture association:
   1976:243-249.
3. Peterson A.L. and Walum E. In Vitro (submitted).
4. Schubert D. Neurobiology 4:376-387:1974.
5. Walum E., Nissen C., Hertz L. and Edström A. J.Neurochem. 23:881-883:1974.
6. Walum E. and Peterson A.L. Acute toxic action of chemicals in cultures of mouse
   neuroblastoma C.1300 cells (in preparation).
7. Erkell L.J. in: Differentiation of cultured neuroblastoma cells: physico-chemical
   aspects. Thesis, University of Gothenburg, Sweden: 1979.
8. Arneson R.M., Aloyo V.J., Germain G.S. and Chenevey J.E. Lipids 13:383-390:1979.
9. Weiss C., Maker H.S. and Lehrer G.M. Analyt. Biochem. 106:512-516:1980.
10. Germain G.S. and Arneson R.M. Enzyme 24:337-341:1979.
11. Bottenstein J. in: Cell culture. Methods in enzymology. Jakoby W.B. and Pastan
    I.H. eds. 58:97-98:1979.
12. Westermark B. in: Growth control of normal and neoplastic human glialike cells
    in culture. Thesis, University of Uppsala, Sweden: 1973.
13. Castor L.N. Exptl. Cell. Res. 68:17-24:1971.

ACKNOWLEDGEMENTS

This work was supported by grants from the National Swedish Board for Technical Development (Grant no 81-5009). Thanks are due to Ms I Varnbo and Ms Ann-Charlotta Eriks-
son for careful technical assistance.

Primary Rat Astroglial Culture in Serum-Free Supplemented Media and Effect of a Bovine Brain Factor

M. Weibel, B. Pettmann, G. Daune, G. Labourdette, and M. Sensenbrenner

Centre de Neurochimie du CNRS and INSERM U44, 5, rue Blaise Pascal,
F-67084 Strasbourg Cedex, France

ABSTRACT

A serum-free supplemented medium has been developed that supports growth of astroglial cells in primary culture from newborn rat brain hemispheres. This medium consists of a basal medium (Waymouth MD 705/1) supplemented with insulin (I), transferrin (T) and fatty-acid-free bovine serum albumin (BSA). In basal medium without serum only a few cells survived after 15 days. In the presence of I and T the number of cells increased. The same results was observed with the addition of a purified fraction from bovine brain extract (astroglial growth factor : AGF). Addition of AGF to the IT medium stimulated the proliferation of the cells and elicited an increase of the level of S-100 protein and of the activity of glutamine synthetase. The complete defined medium (with I, T and BSA) supported the growth of astroglial cells. After 14 days nearly all cells express glial fibrillary acidic (GFA) protein. These cells could be maintained in the defined medium over a period of 4 weeks.

1. Introduction

Astroglial cells from rat brains have been extensively cultured in basal media supplemented with serum from various sources. In these conditions the effects of brain extracts and of factors partially purified from these extracts on the morphological and biochemical maturation of the astroglial cells have been investigated (1). Serum is a complex mixture containing many components of undefined nature. These compounds may interfere with the effect mediated by growth factors when cells are cultured in a serum-supplemented medium. Therefore, a serum-free environment would be more appropriate to study the effects and mechanism of action of factors on the proliferation and maturation of astroglial cells.

Recently, astroglial cells have been subcultured and maintained in secondary culture in defined media (2, 3, 4). These media contained one or two growth factor(s), like fibroblast growth factor (FGF), epidermal growth factor (EGF) or an undefined mixture (Gimmel factor).

We have developed a defined medium, free of growth factors, for rat astroglial cells in primary culture which supports growth of these cells over a period of four weeks.

2. Materials and Methods

Cells dissociated from cerebral hemispheres of newborn rats were seeded in Falcon plastic Petri dishes and maintained for 4-5 days in a serum-supplemented medium (SSM), then they were switched to a serum-free medium (SFM). These media consist of a basal medium, Dulbecco's modified Eagle medium (DMEM), Ham's F12 medium (F12), Waymouth's MD 705/1 medium (WM) or a combination of DMEM and F12 supplemented either with 10 % fetal calf serum (SSM) or with various components (SFM) (see Results). The medium was changed twice a week. In some experiments an active brain factor (AGF) purified from bovine brain extract was added to the cultures.

DNA was determined by the fluorometric method of Hinegardner (5). S100 protein was determined by radioimmunoassay (6) and glutamine synthetase activity by the method of Miller et al. (7). GFA protein was localized in the astroglial cells by the indirect immunoperoxidase reaction using anti-GFA rabbit serum (1:100 dilution).

3. Results and Discussion

In WM alone, without serum and without additional supplements only a few astroglial cells survived after 15 days. In the presence of I (10 µg/ml) and T (10 µg/ml) the number of cells was higher. The same result was observed with the addition of AGF (1 µg/ml). In the presence of I, T and AGF a 10-fold increase of the cell was observed. In this condition, at 20 days in culture, the level of S-100 protein and of the activity of glutamine synthetase were about 2 and 3.5 times as high as in control cultures containing only I and T (8).

These results show that a bovine brain factor is able to stimulate growth and maturation of cells grown in a defined medium containing only insulin and transferrin.

The IT medium does not allow an intense proliferation of astroglial cells. Therefore, we have developed a more complete defined medium which sustains growth of these cells. When putrescine and hormones (progesterone, β-estradiol, hydrocortisone, dexamethasone and triiodothyronine) were added individually or in different combination to a 1:1 mixture of DMEM/F12 containing I (5 µg/ml) and T (10 µg/ml), a small or no effect was observed on cell proliferation. In contrast, the addition of selenium, vitamins (vitamin A and vitamin E), BSA alone or with linoleic acid enhanced the proliferation of the glial cells. In the presence of selenium or vitamin E beside the flat shaped astroglial cells, small round oligodendroglial cells developed. Therefore, these compounds were not anymore used as supplements in the defined medium for astroglial cell cultures. In basal medium supplemented with I (5 µg/ml), T (10 µg/ml), BSA (1 mg/ml) and linoleic acid (5 µg/ml) a marked response of cell proliferation was obtained, a 7-fold increase over control containing only I and T.

We tested various basal media alone or in mixtures to which I (5 µg/ml), T (10 µg/ml), BSA (1 mg/ml) and linoleic acid (5 µg/ml) were added. The optimal growth response, after 2 weeks in culture, was obtained when astroglial cells were cultured in supplemented DMEM alone or in supplemented 3:1 and 1:1 mixture of DMEM/F12. However, in these media the cells could not be grown over a period of 3 weeks. When cells were cultured in WM, F12 or in different WM/F12 ratios with the supplements the proliferation was less intense. But in supplemented WM alone the astroglial cells could be grown over a period of 4 weeks. Most of these cells were positive for GFA protein (Figure 1).

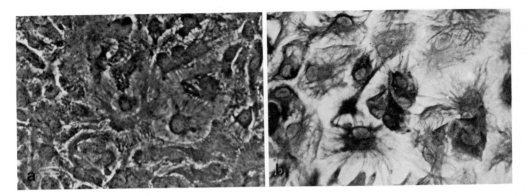

Fig. 1. Astroglial cultures grown in defined medium for 28 days. Phase-contrast (a) and immunoperoxidase for GFA protein (b). X 200.

Recently, we observed that deletion of linoleic acid from the supplement mixture added to WM did not affect the number of cells and the morphology of the astroglial cells in long-term culture. The defined medium for these cells was therefore modified ; it consist of MW with I (5 µg/ml), T (10 µg/ml) and BSA (1 mg/ml). This medium supports growth of astroglial cells and allows their maintenance over a period of 4 weeks. This serum-free medium will facilitate studies on the effects of AGF on proliferation and maturation of astroglial cells.

REFERENCES

1. Pettmann, B., Sensenbrenner, M. and Labourdette, G. (1980) FEBS Letters 118, 195.
2. Brunner, G., Lang, K., Wolfe, R.A., Mc Clure, D.B. and Sato, G.H. (1981) Develop. Brain Res., 2, 563.
3. Morrison, R.S. and De Vellis, J. (1981) Proc. Natl. Acad. Sci. U.S.A., 78, 7205.
4. Fischer, G., Lentz, A. and Schachner, M. (1982) Neurosci. Letters, 29, 297.
5. Hinegardner, R.T. (1971) Anal. Biochem. 39, 197.
6. Labourdette, G. and Marks, A. (1975) Eur. J. Biochem., 8, 73.
7. Miller, R.E., Hackenberg, R. and Gershman, H. (1978) Proc. Natl. Acad. Sci. U.S.A., 75, 1418.
8. Pettmann, B., Weibel, M., Daune, G., Sensenbrenner, M. and Labourdette, G., J. Neurosci. Res. (in press).

This work was supported by a grant from the DGRST (82 V 0012).

Endocrine and Exocrine Cells

Hormone Inducible Specific Gene Expression in an Isolated Whole Mammary Organ in Serum-Free Culture

Mihir R. Banerjee, Prabir K. Majumder, Michael Antoniou, and Jay Joshi

Tumor Biology Laboratory, School of Life Sciences, University of Nebraska, Lincoln, NB 68588-0342, USA

Selective gene expression is believed to play a critical role in cellular differentiation associated with developmental processes (1). Functional differentiation (lactogenesis) of the mammary epithelial cells is accompanied by hormone-inducible expression of several specific gene products including the major milk-proteins, the casein (2). In the murine mammary gland, a glucocorticoid (cortisol or corticosterone) and prolactin are the principal steroid and polypeptide hormones required for lactogenesis including the synthesis of the caseins, a phosphoprotein complex (3,4). Progesterone is also involved in this process and is known to act as a suppressor of lactogenesis (5). This chapter includes a brief discussion of our recent findings on the mode of action of the different steroid and polypeptide hormones involved in the regulation of the expression of the casein genes in an isolated whole mammary organ in vitro. Earlier studies on milk-protein gene expression in the mammary gland in vivo and in vitro have been reviewed in recent years (6-10).

ORGAN CULTURE OF THE WHOLE MAMMARY GLAND

Since the initial report by Ichinose and Nandi (11) the culture procedure of the whole mammary organ of the mouse has been extensively described (12-14). Briefly, as a prerequisite of the culture procedure 3-4 week old BALB/c female mice (used in our studies) are primed by daily injections of a mixture of estradiol-17β and progesterone for 9 days. The whole second thoracic mammary glands from these animals are then excised on a sterile dacron raft. The isolated whole mammary organ resting on the raft is then transferred into a plastic petri dish containing serum-free Waymouth's medium (MB/751), supplemented with combinations of appropriate steroid and polypeptide hormones. The glands are then incubated at 37°C in a humidified atmosphere of 95% oxygen and 5% carbon dioxide. As illustrated in figure 1, incubation of the gland first in a mammogenic hormone containing medium induces the morphogenetic differentiation with resultant development of the lobuloalveolar (secretory) structures within 5-6 days. The parenchyma containing the lobuloalveolar structures during subsequent culture in medium with the lactogenic hormone mixture elicits abundant milk-like secretory material, which includes the caseins (2). Later, culture of the lobuloalveolar glands in a prolactin-free medium containing insulin,

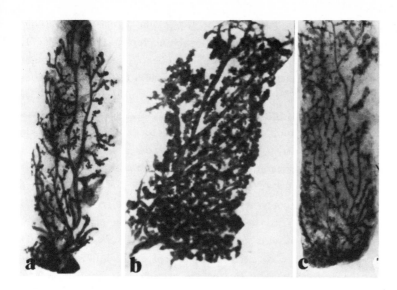

FIGURE 1. Whole mount of second thoracic mammary gland after organ culture. (a) Ductal morphology of the gland after estrogen, progesterone priming of the animal for 9 days. (b) The gland after 6 days of incubation in the medium containing the mammogenic hormone mixture; note the development of extensive lobuloalveolar structures. (c) A gland showing regression of the lobuloalveolar structures after 15 days of incubation in the hormone deficient medium containing insulin, and aldosterone (reference 14).

and aldosterone causes complete regression of the alveolar structures leaving a ductal parenchyma (2). Continued culture of the ductal parenchyma in medium containing the mammogenic hormones and epidermal growth factor stimulates a second round of alveolar morphogenesis (15). Furthermore, treatment of the glands with carcinogenic chemicals during development in vitro, induces neoplastic transformation of the epithelial cells (7). Details of the combinations of polypeptide and steroid hormones needed to obtain alveolar morphogenesis, lactogenesis and alveolar regression in the mammary glands in vitro have been described (14).

TWO-STEP CULTURE MODEL OF THE ISOLATED WHOLE MAMMARY ORGAN

The conventional short-term (95 h) organ culture of the mammary tissue is generally derived from pieces of mammary glands of pregnant animals (16,17). Mammary epithelium in pregnant animals is rich in glucocorticoid receptors and the tissue is exposed to the elevated levels of circulating glucocorticoid (18,19). Mammary tissue in pregnant mice and rats also contains abundant mRNAcsn and casein 20-23). Consequently, the organ culture derived from pregnancy mammary tissue presents serious technical limitations in studies to determine the role of the individual steroid and polypeptide hormones on induction of the milk protein genes (7,8).

In order to avoid this problem the organ culture of the whole mammary gland described in the preceding section has been modified into a two-step culture model (7). During this procedure the casein genes remain in an uninduced state in the lobulo-alveolar glands prior to exposure to the lactogenic hormone mixture, which includes cortisol, prolactin and insulin. Step I incubation for 6 days in a corticosteroid-free controlled medium containing prolactin, growth hormone, insulin, estrogen and progesterone stimulates development of the lobuloalveolar structures in the glands in vitro. During step II incubation the lobuloalveolar glands are incubated for different time periods in the lactogenic medium.

Translation assays in a heterologous ribosome system fails to show mRNAcsn activity in the total RNA from the lobuloalveolar glands after step I incubation (24). Virtually no casein is detectable in these glands by radioimmunological assay. However, mRNAcsn activity and the caseins become abundant in the glands after 6 days of step II incubation in medium with prolactin, cortisol and insulin. Thus in contrast to the mammary gland in vivo (2), the controlled hormone environment in the two-step culture model of the whole mammary organ, permits separation of the developmental stages of lobuloalveolar morphogenesis and lactogenesis. The two-step culture of the whole mammary gland therefore provides a suitable model for reliable measurement of the role of individual hormones during the multiple hormonal regulation of milk protein gene expression.

QUANTITATIVE MEASUREMENT OF CASEIN GENE EXPRESSION IN THE MAMMARY GLANDS IN VITRO

Results of the translational assays described above do not provide an accurate quantitative measure, and consequently, low levels of the mRNAcsn in the glands in vitro may remain undetected. Therefore, the levels of mRNAcsn in the glands in vitro were measured by the more sensitive molecular hybridization assay using a cDNA probe (cDNAcsn) to 15S casein mRNA (7,25,26). After step I incubation, RNA from the glands hybridizes to the cDNAcsn probe but at a very high eR_ot value and mRNAcsn concentration in these glands remains as low as 0.00067% of the total RNA, representing only 147 molecules of mRNAcsn per epithelial cell (Table 1). This low concentration has been established as the basal level of mRNAcsn in the glands after step I culture (7). Thus the casein genes in the lobuloalveolar glands after step I culture remain uninduced in the glands in vitro. This finding is consistent with the virtual absence of mRNAcsn translational activity in the glands after step I culture. On the other hand, like the results of the translational assays, hybrization of the RNA to the cDNAcsn probe showed a high level of mRNAcsn accumulation in the glands after step II incubation in the presence of the lactogenic hormone mixture. Table 1 shows the mRNAcsn in the glands increases 9 fold over the basal level within 24 hr and then progressively rises 255 fold showing a

Table 1   mRNAcsn concentration in total RNA from the glands at different stages of development in organ culture as measured by hybridization to the cDNAcsn*

Incubation Steps	Hormone Combinations	Incubation Time (days)	$eR_ot_{\frac{1}{2}}$	mRNAcsn (%)	mRNAcsn mol./cell	fold increase
I	IPrlEPGH	6	524.8	0.00067	147	–
II	IPrlF	1	104.7	0.033	1,366	9.3
	IPrlF	3	12.0	0.029	4,826	32.8
	IPrlF	6	5.1	0.068	23,699	161.2
	IPrlF	9	3.9	0.09	37,524	255.2

*cDNAcsn probe provides a measure of total casein mRNA sequences. Abbreviations for hormones: I, insulin; Prl, prolactin; GH, growth hormone; E, estradiol-17β; P, progesterone; F, cortisol (reference 7,26).

concentration of 37,524 molecules per cell after 9 days of incubation. This remarkable rise of hybridizable mRNAcsn concentration is accompanied, also by a similar progressive increase of translational activity of the specific milk-protein mRNA, assayed in a wheat germ ribosome system (26). This indicates that the glucocorticoid-prolactin hormone combination also supports processing of the pre-mRNA to mature mRNA for the milk protein in the mammary glands in medium containing insulin.

The observations described above further suggest that the sustained uninduced state of the casein genes in the lobuloalveolar glands is due to the absence of any glucocorticoid in the step I medium. This possibility has been confirmed by our observation that addition of cortisol in the step I medium promotes a 2-fold increase of mRNAcsn accumulation over the basal level in the glands in vitro after 3 days of incubation (27). In view of above observation it is conceivable that in the pregnant animal expression of the casein genes during lobuloalveolar morphogenesis reflects a stimulatory action of the increased level of circulating glucocorticoid in the presence of prolactin in these animals (28). Moreover, as in the mammary gland during pregnancy, mRNAcsn accumulation can also be stimulated in the glands in vitro simultaneously with the lobuloalveolar morphogenesis when the medium with prolactin, and insulin contains the adrenal steroid hormones (29). This indicates that the isolated whole mammary organ in the serum-free medium can mimic the physiological pattern of expression of the milk-protein genes during gestation when the mammogenic hormone mixture contains cortisol. Thus glucocorticoid appears to play a critical role in milk protein gene expression.

INFLUENCE OF INDIVIDUAL POLYPEPTIDE AND STEROID HORMONE

The two-step culture model was then used in the following experiments to determine whether glucocorticoid or prolactin alone can induce expression of the milk-protein genes in medium containing insulin (30).

In all these experiments step I incubation of the glands was done for 6 days in the corticosteroid-free medium containing the mammogenic hormones to obtain the lobuloalveolar structures. Table 2 shows that mRNAcsn in these glands remained at the basal level after the step I incubation. Since no corticosteroid hormone is present in the step I medium these glands also remain free from any residual gluco-corticoid.

Table 2   mRNAcsn in glands incubated with different combinations of the lactogenic hormones cortisol, prolactin and insulin.

Culture Conditions	$eR_0t_{\frac{1}{2}}$	% mRNAcsn
Step I*		
6 day I, Prl, E, P, GH	417.0	0.0009
Step II: Experiment 1		
3 day I, F	832.0	0.0005
3 day I, F → 3 day I, Prl, F	5.02	0.076
3 day I, Prl	N.M.	N.M.
3 day I, Prl → 3 day I, Prl, F	10.0	0.038
Step II: Experiment 2		
3 day I, Prl → 3 day I, F	316.0	0.0012
3 day I, F → 3 day I, Prl	23.4	0.016

*   In all experiments step I incubation for 6 days was done in the corticosteroid-free mammogenic medium containing the hormones indicated. Subsequently step II incubations were done sequentially in medium containing different combinations of the lactogenic hormones. Abbreviations: I, insulin; Prl, prolactin; GH, growth hormone; F, cortisol (5 µg/ml each); E, estradiol-17β (0.001 µg/ml); P, progesterone (1 µg/ml); N.M., not measurable (reference 30).

In experiment I, step II incubation of the lobuloalveolar glands was done in medium with cortisol or prolactin in the presence of insulin. As measured by the cDNAcsn probe, neither cortisol nor prolactin alone was capable of raising the mRNAcsn concentration above the basal level in the glands in vitro after 3 days of incubation. However, additional 3 days of incubation of the glands in medium containing the complete lactogenic hormone mixture (prolactin, cortisol and insulin) resulted in markedly increased accumulation of the mRNAcsn in the glands (table 2). These results strongly indicate that neither the steroid nor the polypeptide hormone alone can induce expression of the milk-protein genes in the lobuloalveolar glands which are competent to respond to the complete lactogenic hormone mixture.

In experiment II, the lobuloalveolar glands during step II incubation were exposed initially for 3 days to prolactin or cortisol in the presence of insulin. This was followed by an additional 3 days of incubation in medium with cortisol or prolactin in the presence of insulin. The glands preincubated with prolactin showed, an extremely low level of mRNAcsn after subsequent incubation with cortisol (table 2) suggesting that residual prolactin if present in the glands is insufficient to exert a significant synergistic action with cortisol present in the medium. However, the glands preincubated with cortisol showed 18-fold increase of mRNAcsn after an additional 3 days of incubation in medium with prolactin and insulin (table 2). This marked increase cannot be attributed to a stimulatory action of only prolactin in the medium because the results from experiment I described above showed that the combination of prolactin and insulin fails to stimulate mRNAcsn accumulation in the glands in vitro. This then raises the possibility whether the increased mRNAcsn is due to a synergistic action between residual cortisol retained in the gland and prolactin in the medium.

RETENTION OF CORTISOL BY MAMMARY GLAND PREINCUBATED WITH STEROID HORMONE

Mammary cells can retain steroid hormones for an extended period of time (31). Therefore, it is conceivable that the stimulatory response observed in the glands preincubated with cortisol described above reflects a synergistic action of residual cortisol in the tissue and prolactin in the medium. Figure 2 shows that the lobuloalveolar glands preincubated with cortisol can indeed retain the steroid hormone. Depletion of the residual cortisol in the glands during subsequent incubation in cortisol-free medium is accompanied by a corresponding loss of mRNAcsn in the glands in medium containing prolactin and insulin. However, addition of cortisol in the medium at the time when the residual cortisol concentration reached near basal levels on the 6th day, mRNAcsn in the glands increased 20 fold after subsequent 3 days of incubation (30). This demonstrates that a continuous presence of glucocorticoid is essential for casein gene expression in the presence of prolactin. A similar synergistic action of residual cortisol with prolactin has also been observed during stimulation of casein synthesis in rat mammary explants (32). Thus, contrary to the conclusion (33,34) that the casein genes in rat mammary gland are induced by prolactin and the presence of glucocorticoid is not required for this process, the results of the studies in the murine mammary organ in vitro clearly demonstrate that glucocorticoid is an obligatory requirement for the induction of the milk protein genes.

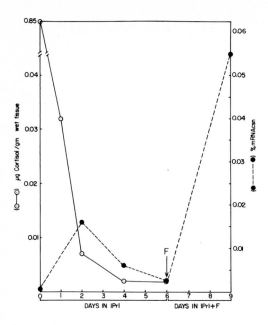

FIGURE 2. Influence of residual cortisol retained by the mammary glands on mRNAcsn accumulation during subsequent incubation in cortisol-free medium (reference 30).

NUCLEAR BINDING OF GLUCOCORTICOID-RECEPTOR COMPLEX AND CASEIN GENE EXPRESSION

Steroid hormone induction of gene expression is believed to require interaction of the hormone-receptor complex with nuclear acceptor sites (35). Pyridoxal-5'-phosphate (PALP), a vitamin B_6 derivative can block the binding of the steroid hormone-receptor complex to the nuclear acceptor site in a specific manner by interacting with the lysine residue(s) of the receptor molecule (36). PALP thus provides a potential physiological modulator of steroid hormonal induction of specific gene expression. Accordingly, PALP has been used in our recent studies to determine whether the stimulatory action of glucocorticoid on the expression of the casein genes is mediated at the level of interaction of the steroid hormone-receptor complex with the nuclear acceptor site in the mammary glands in vitro.

As usual in these studies, the mammary glands from immature female mice were initially incubated in the step I medium containing the corticosteroid-free mammogenic hormone mixture to obtain the lobuloalveolar structures. Step II incubation of the lobuloalveolar glands was then done in medium containing the lactogenic hormone mixture composed of cortisol, prolactin and insulin. The presence of 2 mM or 5 mM PALP in the same medium increased the concentration of PALP in the mammary tissue 4 and 12 fold, respectively, over the basal levels after 3 days of incubation. Table

Table 3   Levels of nuclear binding of ^{3}H-dexamethasone and mRNAcsn concentration at different experimental conditions.

Hormones	^{3}H-DEX Bound f moles/ug DNA	Cell No./gm Tissue	Total RNA Yield/gm Tissue	mRNAcsn	
				$eR_0t_{\frac{1}{2}}$	Percent
IPrlF	0.53	2.9×10^6	777 μg	11.64	0.030
IPrlF + 2 mM PALP	0.25	2.3×10^6	650 μg	83.95	0.0041
IPrlF + 5 mM PALP	0.06	N.M.	525 μg	135.50	0.0026

The glands were initially incubated in the step I medium containing the mammogenic hormones to obtain the lobuloalveolar structures. All determinations were made after 3 days step II incubation of the lobuloalveolar gland. Abbreviations: PALP, pyridoxal-5'-phosphate; DEX, dexamethasone; I, insulin; Prl, prolactin; F, cortisol; N.M., not measured. Epithelial cell number was determined after collagenase dissociation of the glands and RNA was extracted as described (reference 26).

3 shows that corresponding to its increased tissue concentration, PALP at a concentration of 2 mM caused a 52% inhibition of specific ^{3}H-dexamethasone binding (37) in the glands after 3 days of incubation in the step II medium containing the lactogenic hormones. Inhibition of ^{3}H-dexamethasone nuclear binding reached 92% when the level of PALP was increased to 5 mM in the medium containing the same hormones. The nuclear binding of the glucocorticoid-receptor complex measured represented the translocated ligand-receptor complex, because incubation of the glands with 1 mM P-chloromercuric benzoate resulted in total absence of ^{3}H-dexamethasone nuclear binding within 30 minutes. Mercurials are potential inhibitors of steroid hormone interaction with cytoplasmic receptors (38).

    Molecular hybridization analysis shows (table 3) that RNA from the glands not exposed to PALP hybridized to the cDNAcsn probe at $eR_0t_{\frac{1}{2}}$ of 11.64 mols.s.1^{-1} indicating a 0.03% concentration of mRNAcsn sequences in total RNA from the glands incubated for 3 days in the step II medium containing cortisol, prolactin and insulin. The $eR_0t_{\frac{1}{2}}$ value of RNA samples from glands exposed to 2 mM PALP increased to 83.95 mol.s^{-1}.1^{-1} showing an mRNAcsn concentration of 0.0041%. In glands incubated with 5 mM PALP under similar culture conditions, the mRNAcsn concentration was further reduced to 0.0026%. These results clearly show that PALP can cause a dose-dependent inhibition of binding of the glucocorticoid to nuclear acceptor sites in the mammary glands in vitro. The inhibition of nuclear binding of the steroid hormone-receptor complex is accompanied by a corresponding loss of mRNAcsn accumulation in the glands. The inhibitory action of PALP, however, was reversible.

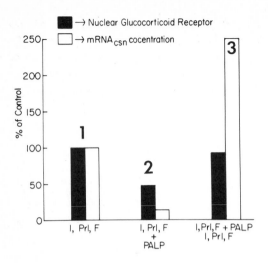

FIGURE 3. Correlation between inhibition of nuclear binding of glucocorticoid-receptor complex and mRNA accumulation at 2 mM concentration of PALP. The histogram also shows that the inhibitory action of PALP is reversible. Column 1 shows the control levels in gland not treated with PALP. Column 2 shows the levels of glands exposed to 2 mM PALP and column 3 shows the levels after withdrawal of PALP (2 mM) from the medium.

Its withdrawal from the medium restored nuclear binding of the steroid–receptor complex and this was accompanied by an increase of mRNAcsn concentration in the glands (figure 3). This demonstrates that the PALP-mediated inhibition of nuclear binding of the glucocorticoid-receptor complex, does not alter the specific hormone responsiveness of the mammary cells in vitro at the concentrations used. It should be mentioned, that while PALP inhibits nuclear binding of the steroid hormone-receptor complex in a specific manner (36,39), it may also act nonspecifically by interacting with the lysine residues of different tissue proteins. However, our estimates of total RNA yield, epithelial cell number from control and PALP treated glands, failed to show any marked differences (table 3). Moreover, the pronounced increase in mRNAcsn accumulated in the glands after withdrawal of PALP from the medium (figure 3) strongly indicates that its nonspecific adverse effect on the mammary tissue if any, remained insignificant at the concentrations used. Thus, the loss of casein gene expression in the glands treated with PALP is very likely a consequence of the specific inhibition of nuclear binding of the glucocorticoid receptor complex. Therefore, the PALP-mediate inhibition of nuclear binding of the glucocorticoid-receptor complex and the corresponding loss of mRNAcsn, strongly indicates that (a) glucocorticoid action is receptor mediated and (b) the adrenal steroid hormone in conjunction with prolactin plays a major modulatory role in the expression of the milk-protein genes in the murine mammary gland.

Since binding of the steroid hormone-receptor complex to nuclear acceptor sites is considered essential for the onset of hormone-inducible gene transcription (40), the loss of mRNAcsn in the mammary glands concurrently with PALP mediated inhibition of nuclear binding of the receptor complex, further indicates that glucocorticoid acts at the transcriptional level of control of the casein genes. This contention is in agreement with our earlier finding on glucocorticoid modulation of transcription of the casein genes in the mammary gland of post-partum mice (7,25). A modulatory influence by glucocorticoid on β-casein gene transcription has also been observed in rabbits. Interestingly, the receptor mediated, dose-dependent inhibitory action of PALP on milk-protein gene expression also suggests that breast tissue concentration of vitamin B_6 may influence the physiology of lactation in nursing mothers. Vitamin B_6 is known to influence nuclear binding of glucocorticoids in rat liver cells (36,39).

PROGESTERONE-GLUCOCORTICOID INTERACTION AND CASEIN GENE EXPRESSION

The role of progesterone as an antagonist to lactogenesis (5) generated the interest concerning its role in milk-protein gene expression. Physiologically, the action of progesterone on lactogenesis should be confined mostly to the mammary gland during gestation. Progesterone is not likely to influence the process of lactogenesis in post-partum animals because the circulating level of this ovarian steroid hormone is reduced to near basal levels at parturition, and progesterone receptors become undetectable in mammary cells of lactating animals (42,43). Nevertheless, progesterone can compete for the glucocorticoid binding sites in the mammary cell cytoplasm. Displacement of glucocorticoid from its receptors caused by progesterone, can inhibit cortisol induction of mammary tumor virus production in murine mammary cells (37). This then raises the possibility whether a similar receptor mediated action of progesterone may also impair glucocorticoid induction of the milk-protein genes. The two-step organ culture model of the mammary gland in the controlled hormone environment in vitro permits a reliable test of this hypothesis.

In these studies (27) step I incubation of the immature glands was done in the corticosteroid-free mammogenic medium to stimulate development of the lobuloalveolar structures. As expected only the basal level of mRNAcsn was detectable in these glands by the cDNAcsn probe. Subsequently, the lobuloalveolar glands were incubated with different concentrations of cortisol in a progesterone-free step I mammogenic medium. In the progesterone-free medium, cortisol at concentrations of 1 and 5 μg/ml stimulated a 19.5 and 17 fold increase of mRNAcsn concentration respectively, over basal levels after 6 days of incubation in the presence of prolactin which is a component of the mammogenic hormone mixture. However, addition of 1 μg/ml progesterone in the medium after an initial 3 days of culture in the progesterone-free medium caused reduction in the rate of mRNAcsn accumulation between the 3rd and 6th days of incubation. This indicates that progesterone suppresses

rather than totally abolishes mRNAcsn accumulation in the glands in vitro. Incubation of the glands with 1 ug/ml each of progesterone and cortisol prompted only a 3
fold increase of mRNAcsn, whereas 5 µg/ml cortisol in presence of 1 µg/ml progesterone evoked a 10 fold increase. These results suggest that although progesterone
acts as an antagonist to mRNAcsn accumulation in the glands, glucocorticoid when
present in excess can limit the suppressive action of the ovarian steroid hormone.
Furthermore, at high concentrations glucocorticoid can progressively reduce the
antagonistic action of progesterone during incubation between the 3rd and 6th day.
This suggests that glucocorticoid when present in excess, can partially overcome the
antagonistic influence of the ovarian steroid hormone.

   This possibility was tested by incubating the glands in different molar concentrations of progesterone (P) and cortisol (F) in the medium. The level of mRNAcsn
progressively declined in the glands with increased P:F molar ratio in the medium.
At equimolar concentrations of progesterone and cortisol (P:F=1) in the medium, the
level of mRNAcsn in the glands was reduced 84% after 3 days of culture. This con-
firms that the antagonistic action of the ovarian hormone in the glands in vitro is
dependent upon the P:F ratio in the medium. At this point a consideration of the
endocrine environment of the pregnant animal, indicates that the P:F ratio used in
the medium mimics a similar relative concentration of the circulating levels of the two
steroid hormones. During pregnancy the level of serum progesterone remains relatively constant, while the circulating glucocorticoid level rises progressively in the
animal (28,45). This then is likely to cause a reduced P:F ratio in the circulating
levels of the two steroid hormones at advanced stages of pregnancy. Consequently,
this should permit an enhancement of glucocorticoid stimulation with resultant limited
expression of the casein gene in the presence of prolactin. Depletion of circulating
progesterone and progesterone receptors in mammary cells at parturition (42,43),
should then account for the maximal response of the mammary cells to the stimulatory
action of the glucocorticoid in the presence of the increased level of prolactin in the
nursing animal.

   The finding that manifestation of progesterone antagonism is related to the
relative concentrations of the two steroid hormones then raises the question whether
action of progesterone on casein gene expression is mediated at the level of its
competitive binding to the glucocorticoid receptor in the mammary cytosol. Accordingly, progesterone interaction with mammary cell glucocorticoid receptor and the
consequences of such an interaction on mRNAcsn accumulation in the glands in vitro,
was determined at different P:F ratios in the medium. Glucocorticoid receptors in
the mammary cytosol were measured by a specific ^{3}H-dexamethasone binding assay as
described (27). The results show that progesterone competition can cause a 60%
inhibition of glucocorticoid binding to its specific cytosol receptor from the glands in
vitro. At increased molar ratios of P:F, both binding of glucocorticoid to its mammary cytosol receptor and mRNAcsn levels in the gland show a corresponding
decrease (figure 4). Our recent observations have further shown that progesterone

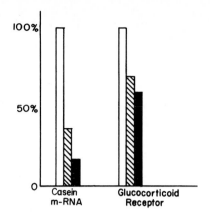

FIGURE 4: The levels of mRNAcsn and glucocorticoid binding to its receptors in mammary glands at different P:F ratios in the medium. [] P:F = 0; ▨ P:F ≠ 0.21; ■ P:F = 1 (reference 24).

competition for the glucocorticoid cytosol receptor can reduce nuclear binding of the glucocorticoid-receptor complex. This receptor mediated inhibition of nuclear binding of the glucocorticoid is accompanied by inhibition of casein synthesis in the glands in vitro (unpublished, Majumder, P., Antoniou, M. and Banerjee, M. R.). These observations strongly indicate that progesterone antagonism on the expression of the milk-protein genes is exerted at the level of its competitive binding to the glucocorticoid receptors in the mammary cytosol. In contrast, earlier it has been postulated that progesterone inhibition of milk-protein gene expression in the rat mammary gland is caused by progesterone mediated blockage of the stimulatory action of prolactin (44). However, in the absence of any information concerning a mechanism of progesterone-prolactin interaction this postulation remains a conjecture at this time. The postulation that progesterone blocks casein gene expression primarily by inhibiting prolactin action may have been prompted by the, apparently, erroneous conclusion that prolactin is the hormone required for the induction of the milk-protein genes and glucocorticoid is not essential in this process (10,33). However, results of several recent studies using controlled hormonal combinations in the culture medium, have demonstrated that glucocorticoid is an obligatory requirement for casein gene expression and α-lactalbumin synthesis in the presence of prolactin (7-9,44,45). A preliminary report has further indicated that glucocorticoid can support α-lactalbumin synthesis in explants of mammary tissue from pregnant mice in the absence of prolactin (46). Some role of insulin in this complex multiple hormone regulatory process has also been proposed (47).

THE HORMONAL REGULATION OF MILK WHEY PROTEIN mRNA ACCUMULATION IN VITRO

Milk contains two major mammary cell specific whey (acid soluble) proteins. These are α-lactalbumin (48) and whey acidic protein, WAP (49,50). Unlike the milk of other species, WAP constitutes the most abundant whey protein in the mouse milk (49,50). WAP and α-lactalbumin have the same molecular weight of 14,100 (48-50) and their mRNAs are also of similar size (51). Using the two-step, whole mammary organ culture model described above, we have performed preliminary experiments which look at the hormonal regulation of the genes for these whey proteins. A cDNA probe was synthesized from an mRNA fraction highly enriched for α-lactalbumin and WAP sequences (see legend to figure 5). This $cDNA_W$ was then used to assay whey protein mRNA sequences in RNA samples extracted from mammary glands cultured in the presence of different hormone combinations. The results are shown in figure 5. WAP and α-lactalbumin mRNA sequences were found to be virtually

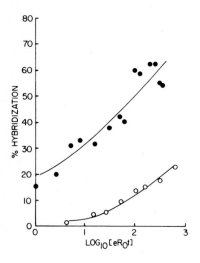

FIGURE 5. An mRNA fraction highly enriched for α-lactalbumin and whey acid protein (WAP) sequences was prepared from total poly(A)-containing RNA from lactating mouse mammary gland. The poly(A)-containing RNA was fractionated according to size by agarose gel electrophoresis in the presence of methylmercury hydroxide as denaturant. An mRNA fraction judged by the immunoprecipition of translation products in a wheat germ cell-free system to contain almost exclusively α-lactalbumin and WAP mRNA sequences, was used as a template for cDNA synthesis (7,25). This $cDNA_W$ was then used as a hybridization probe to measure α-lactalbumin and WAP mRNA sequences in total RNA from mouse mammary gland cultured in the presence of different hormone combinations.

    0, hybridization kinetics with RNA from mammary gland at the end of 6 day step I culture with insulin, prolactin, growth hormone, estrogen and progesterone.

    0, hybridization kinetics with RNA from mammary gland grown for 6 days in step I culture, plus for 3 days in step II culture with insulin, prolactin and cortisol. The $cDNA_W$ probe hybridized with its template to give an $eR_o t_{\frac{1}{2}}$ value of 0.015 mol of nucleotide $s^{-1}.liter^{-1}$.

absent in the glands at the end of the 6 day, step I mammogenic period of culture. This was indicated by a limited protection of the hybridization probe by an eR_0t value of 648 mol of nucleotide $s^{-1}.litre^{-1}$. After 3 days of step II culture with insulin, prolactin and cortisol, α-lactalbumin and WAP mRNA sequences accounted for 0.015% of the total RNA. The RNA from this tissue hybridized with an $eR_0t_{\frac{1}{2}}$ value of 100 mol of nucleotide $s^{-1}.litre^{-1}$. Step II culture with either insulin and prolactin or insulin and cortisol did not induce α-lactalbumin and WAP gene expression above that present at the end of the step I period of morphogenesis (results not shown). Thus, it appears that the accumulation of α-lactalbumin and WAP mRNAs in the murine whole mammary organ in culture is under the same hormonal control as that for the caseins.

In conclusion, our present state of the knowledge on the regulatory mechanisms of milk protein gene expression may be summarized as follows: (a) casein genes are hormone inducible, (b) both glucocorticoid and prolactin are required to induce expression of the casein genes, neither the steroid nor the polypeptide hormone alone can induce this response in murine mammary cells, (c) nuclear binding of the glucocorticoid-receptor complex appears to be required for casein gene expression, and (d) progesterone antagonism to casein gene expression appears to be due to inhibition of glucocorticoid binding to its specific receptors in mammary cytosol, apparently caused by progesterone competition for the same binding site. Studies in murine mammary glands so far have measured cellular accumulation of the mRNAcsn mostly using a cDNA probe to total casein mRNA sequences. Although preliminary evidence indicate that glucocorticoid can influence transcription of the casein gene in mice (25) and rabbits (41) further elucidation of the specific role of the individual steroid and the polypeptide hormones at the levels of transcription, post-transcriptional processing of the pre-mRNA, cytoplasmic migration, and stabilization of the mature mRNA must depend upon future studies. Little is known about the regulatory influence of the hormones on transcription and accumulation of the indivi-dual casein mRNA sequences. Cloned cDNAs for the various milk protein gene sequences from different species including human, are now available for use as molecular hybridization probes and also for sequence analysis (10,51-54). Develop-ment of the unique culture model of the whole mammary organ described in this chapter now makes it feasible to measure hormone responses of the cells in a controlled environment in serum-free medium. These advances now permit future studies for the further elucidation of the role of the individual steroid and poly-peptide hormones during the complex multiple hormonal regulation of expression of the milk-protein genes.

REFERENCES

1. Davidson, E. H. (1976) in: Gene Activity in Early Development. Academic Press, NY.
2. Banerjee, M. R. (1976) Int. Rev. Cytol. 46, 1-97.
3. Nandi, S. (1958) J. Nat. Cancer Inst. 20, 1039-1063.
4. Topper, Y. J. (1970) Rec. Prog. Hormone Res, 26, 287-308.
5. Assairi, L., Delouis, C. Gaye, P., Houdebine, L. M., Olliver-Bousquet, M. and Denamur, R. (1974) Biochem. J. 144, 245-252.
6. Banerjee, M. R., Terry, P. M., Sakai, S., Lin, F. K. and Ganguly, R. (1978) In Vitro 14, 128-139.
7. Banerjee, M. R., Ganguly, N. Mehta, N. M., Iyer, A. P. and Ganguly, R. (1980) in: Cell Biology of Breast Cancer (C. McGrath, M. Brennan and M. Rich, eds) Academic Press, NY, pp 485-516.
8. Banerjee, M. R., Mehta, N. M., Ganguly, R., Majumder, P. K., Ganguly, N. and Joshi, J. (1982) in: Conference on Cell Proliferation (D. A. Sibrasku, G. H. Sato and A. B. Pardee, eds) Cold Spring Harbor Laboratory, NY, vol. 9, pp. 789-805.
9. Topper, Y. J., and Freeman, C. S. (1980) Physiol. Rev. 60, 1049-1106.
10. Rosen, J. M., Matusik, R. Richard, D. A., Gupta, P. and Rodgers, J. R. (1980) Recent Prog. Horm. Res. 36, 157-193.
11. Ichinose, R. R. and Nandi, S. (1966) J. Endocrinol. 35, 331-340.
12. Wood, B. G., Washburn, L. L., Mukherjee, A. S. and Banerjee, M. R. (1975) J. Endocrinol. 65, 1-6.
13. Lin, F. K., Banerjee, M. R. and Crump, L. R. (1976) Cancer Res. 36, 1607-1614.
14. Banerjee, M. R., Wood, B. G., Lin, F. K. and Crump, L. R. (1976) in: Tissue Culture Assoc. Manual (K. K. Sanford, ed) Tissue Culture Assoc., Rockville, MD, vol. 2, pp 457-462.
15. Tonelli, Q. J. and Sorof, S. (1980) Nature 285, 250-252.
16. Elias, J. J. (1957) Science 126, 842-844.
17. Rivera, E. (1971) in: Methods in Mammalian Embryology (J. C. Danial, ed) Freeman, San Francisco, pp 442-471.
18. Wittliff, J. L. (1975) Methods in Cancer Res. 11, 293-354.
19. Gala, R. R. and Westphal, U. (1965) Acta Endocrinologica 55, 47-61.
20. Ganguly, N., Ganguly, R., Mehta, N. M. and Banerjee, M. R. (1982) J. Nat. Cancer Inst. 69, 453-463.
21. Terry, P. M., Ball, E. M. and Banerjee, M. R. (1975) Methods of Immunology 9, 123-124.
22. Rosen, J. M. and Barker, S. (1976) Biochemistry 15, 5272-5280.
23. Benerjee, M. R., Terry, P. M., Sakai, S. and Lin, F. K. (1977) in: Hormone Research III (N. Norvell and T. Shellenberger, eds) Hemisphere Publishing Corp., Washington, DC, pp 281-306.
24. Terry, P. M., Banerjee, M. R. and Lui, R. M. (1977) Proc. Natl. Acad. Sci. U.S.A. 74, 2441-2445.
25. Ganguly, R., Mehta, N. M., Ganguly, N. and Banerjee, M. R. (1979) Proc. Natl. Acad. Sci. U.S.A. 76, 6466-6470.
26. Mehta, N. M., Ganguly, N., Ganguly, R. and Banerjee, M. R. (1980) J. Biol. Chem. 255, 4430-4434.
27. Ganguly, R., Majumder, P. K., Ganguly, N. and Banerjee, M. R. (1982) J. Biol. Chem. 257, 2182-2187.
28. Tucker, H. A. (1974) in: Lactation, a Comprehensive Treatise (B. L. Larson and V. R. Smith, eds) Academic Press, NY, vol. 1, pp 277-326.
29. Ganguly, N., Ganguly, R., Mehta, N. M., Crump, L. R. and Banerjee, M. R. (1981) In Vitro 17, 55-60.
30. Ganguly, R., Ganguly, N., Mehta, N. M. and Banerjee, M. R. (1980) Proc. Natl. Acad. Sci. U.S.A. 77, 6003-6006.
31. Strobl, J. and Lippman, M. (1979) Cancer Res. 39, 3319-3329.
32. Bolander, F. F. Jr., Nicholas, K. R. and Topper, Y. J. (1979) Biochem. Biophys. Res. Comm. 91, 247-252.
33. Guyette, W. A., Matusik, R. J. and Rosen, J. M. (1979) Cell 17, 1013-1023.

34. Hobbs, A., Richards, D. A., Kessler, D. J. and Rosen, J. M. (1982) J. Biol. Chem. 257, 3598-3605.
35. O'Malley, B. W. and Means, A. R. (1974) Science 183, 610-620.
36. Litwack, G. (1979) Trends in Biochemical Sciences, October, 217-220.
37. Shyamala, G. and Dickson, C. (1976) Nature 262, 107-112.
38. Coty, W. A. (1980) J. Biol. Chem. 255, 8035-8037.
39. Disorbo, D. M. and Litwack, G. (1981) Biochem. Biophys. Res. Comm. 99, 1203-1208.
40. Yamamoto, R. and Albert, B. (1976) Ann. Rev. Biochem. 38, 722-746.
41. Teyssot, B. and Houdebine, L. M. (1981) Eur. J. Biochem. 114, 597-608.
42. Tucker, H. A. (1979) in: Seminars in Perinatology (T. K. Oliver and T. H. Kirschbaum, eds) Grun and Stratton, NY, vol. 3, pp 199-223.
43. Haslam, S. Z. and Shyamala, G. (1979) Endocrinology 105, 786-795.
44. Rosen, J. M., O'Neal, D. L., McHugh, J. E. and Comstock, J. P. (1978) Biochemistry 17, 290-297.
45. Ray, D. B., Horst, I. A., Jensen, R. W., Mills, N. C. and Kowal, J. (1981) Endocrinology 108, 584-590.
46. Nicholas, K. R., Sankaran, L. and Topper, Y. J. (1981) Endocrinology 109, 978-980.
47. Bolander, F. F., Jr., Nicholas, K. R., Judson, J. V. W. and Topper, Y. J. (1981) Proc. Natl. Acad. Sci. U.S.A. 78, 5682-5684.
48. Nagamatsu, Y. and Oka, T. (1980) Biochem. J. 185, 227-237.
49. Zamierowski, M. M. and Ebner, K. E. (1980) J. Immun. Methods 36, 211-220.
50. Piletz, J. E. Heinlen, M., Ganschow, R. E. (1981) J. Biol. Chem. 256, 11509-11516.
51. Hennighausen, L. G. and Sippel, A. (1982) Eur. J. Biochem. 125, 125-131.
52. Dandekar, A. M. and Quasba, P. K. (1981) Proc. Natl. Acad. Sci. U.S.A. 78, 4853-4957.
53. Mehta, N. M., El-Gewely, M. R., Joshi, J., Helling, R. B. and Banerjee, M. R. (1981) Gene 15, 285-288.
54. Hall, L., Craig, R. K., Davis, M. S., Ralfs, D. N. L. and Campbell, P. N. (1981) Nature (Lond.) 290, 602-604.

A New Culture Technique: An Approach to the in-Vitro Reconstitution of Endocrine Organs

Elke Lang[1], Klaus Lang[1], Ulrich Krause[2], Kurt Racké[3], Bernd Nitzgen[1], and Gerd Brunner[1]

[1] Institut für Immunologie der Johannes Gutenberg Universität, Obere Zahlbacher Str. 67, D-6500 Mainz, FRG
[2] II. Medizinische Klinik, Abt. Endokrinologie, Langenbeckstr. 1, D-6500 Mainz, FRG
[3] Pharmakologisches Institut der Johannes Gutenberg Universität, Obere Zahlbacher Str. 67, D-6500 Mainz, FRG

ABSTRACT

A new cell culture technique called three-dimensional-rotation culture (3dR-culture) has been developed. Its main characteristics are: (i) cultivation under constant rotation, and (ii) the use of a three-dimensional material that allows the cells to adhere and to grow in a three-dimensional arrangement. Two glassfibre materials and one gelatine-sponge proved suitable for the use in cell culture. The new technique has the advantage to yield in large numbers cells bound on a stable matrix that can easily be handled, e.g. for implantation.

The technique described was used for primary culture of dissociated pituitaries in combination with a serum-free medium. Under these conditions a pituitary "organoid" was reconstituted in-vitro which secreted in average 50 ng ACTH/ml x day into the culture supernatant. The pituitary organoids were implanted subcutaneously into hypophysectomized syngeneic rats. The influence on restoring growth and ACTH blood plasma level was observed. The animals did not increase their body weight, but the ACTH level rose from zero to at least one fifth of normal values.

Hypothalamic organoids, also grown in serum-free medium, secreted vasopressin for up to seven weeks into the culture supernatant.

These experiments show that it may be possible to substitute dysfunctional organs by in-vitro reconstituted organoids, which would open new possibilities for medical therapy and for studying the regulation of endocrine glands.

INTRODUCTION

In most of the reports concerning the cultivation of single cells, the cells are grown in monolayers and are directly attached to the culture dishes. Therefore, interactions between the cell and the artificial substratum are predominant. More physiological conditions can be obtained when the culture dishes are treated with special coats such as collagen, fibronectin, membrane proteins, or lectins (1). Nevertheless,

---

This report is dedicated to Gerd Brunner who died in July 1982 in the Karakorum Mountains, Pakistan since it is based on his last ideas and investigations.

the microenvironment in monolayer cultures is completely different to the in-vivo situation.

To overcome unphysiological culture conditions attempts were made to develop culture techniques that allow specific interactions between cells when they are grown in a three-dimensional arrangement. Several research reports dealing with aggregating cell cultures could show that single cells reestablish specific cell to cell contacts and differentiate similarily in morphology and in biochemistry as they would in vivo (2, 3). In these systems the cells do not need an artificial substratum for attachment.

Another possibility to culture cells in a three-dimensional arrangement was first described by A. Leighton in 1951 (4, 5). His proposal was to cultivate cells in a cellulose sponge. Leighton's technique had the advantages to yield high cell numbers in a small volume, to grow multilayers of cells, and to have cultures that are easy to manipulate.

We have picked up this idea to grow cells on a stable matrix because it seems to be predestinated for attempting an in-vitro organ reconstitution and in this way to transfer cells into an animal by implantation. We have tried to realize an organ reconstitution with pituitary cells. Pituitary substitutions in hypophysectomized animals had been investigated in several ways with more or less success. Ectopic pituitary transplantations had shown to be less effective to substitute the removed gland (6, 7, 8, 9). Only implantations into the hypophyseotrophic area of the brain showed significant effects(10, 11, 12).

The work presented here is concerned with the development of a strategy for the in-vitro reconstitution of endocrine glands, to make a first approach with pituitary substitution and to discuss the possibilities of such a strategy especially in combination with serum-free, celltype-specific culture conditions.

MATERIALS AND METHODS

Cell culture: After preexamination using established cell lines the following three materials were used for the 3dR-cultures: a gelatine sponge "Gelastypt M" (Hoechst, Frankfurt, FRG) of the size 10 x 5 x 1.5 mm, and two glass fibre materials "microlith SM 100/1" and "microlith SAB 0.8" (Schuller, D-698 Wertheim, FRG) of the size 25 x 5 x 0.8 mm. These substrata were washed several times in bidistilled water and sterilized with alcohol. The substrata were placed either unfixed into petridishes for bacteriological purposes or, in the case of hypothalamus cell culture, fixed with silicone glue into Costar six-well plates. 3dR-cultures were kept under constant rotation (60 - 100 rpm) on a rotation plate constructed especially for this purpose.

For primary culture the tissues were disintegrated using a combined mechanical and enzymatic procedure which is described in (13). Pituitaries were taken from two-month-old Wistar-Furth rats; hypothalami were taken from newborn rats. Cells were seeded at a density of 2 x 10^6 cells/dish (pituitary) and 1 - 2 x 10^6 cells/well (hypothalamus).

In one experiment human fetal pituitary cells from therapeutical aborti (20 weeks of gestation) were cultivated in monolayer culture in 3.5 cm Costar dishes at a density of 6 x 10^5 cells/dish. Primary pituitary cells were plated in medium containing 10 % newborn or fetal calf serum (NCS, FCS) for the first day of culture, then the serum-free medium TB (Table I) was used (14). Medium was changed every two days. Hypothalamic cells were kept under serum-free conditions (medium B17, Table I) from the very first day. In these cultures the glass fibre material had been coated with an aqueous brain extract (13). The GH_3 cell line (15, 16) and normal rat fibroblasts were cultured in medium supplemented with 10 % NCS.

All cells were cultivated at 37°C, 5 % CO_2, 95 % humidity in a basal medium of Dulbecco's modified Eagle's medium and Ham's F12 (1:1) with supplements. Culture supernatants were centrifuged at 4°C, 1000 g_{av} x min to remove cells, and stored at -30°C for RIA. Supernatants from pituitary cultures were again centrifuged at 250 000 g_{av} x min, 4°C.

TABLE I.   HORMONE SUPPLEMENTS FOR SERUM-FREE CELL CULTURE

PITUITARY PRIMARY CELLS (TB-MEDIUM)(14)		HYPOTHALAMUS PRIMARY CELLS (B17-MEDIUM, DERIVED FROM N2-MEDIUM(17))	
Insulin	5 µg/ml	Insulin	5 µg/ml
Transferrin	5 µg/ml	Transferrin	100 µg/ml
T_3	5×10^{-10} M	T_3	0.3×10^{-10} M
TRH	1 ng/ml	Thyroglobulin	100 µg/ml
LRH	4 ng/ml	Progesterone	20 µM
Putrescine	2×10^{-4} M	Putrescine	100 µM
Prostaglandin E	100 ng/ml	Hydrocortisone	8 ng/ml
FGF	10 ng/ml	Selenium	3×10^{-8} M
EGF	40 ng/ml		
Selenium	5×10^{-8} M		

Scanning electron microscopy: Cells attached to three-dimensional material were fixed with a 2 % glutaraldehyde solution in PBS (phosphate-buffered saline) for two hours at room temperature, rinsed in PBS, postfixed in 2 % osmium tetroxide in PBS for 30 minutes. Dehydration was carried out in acetone (10, 30, 50, 70, 90, 100,100%, 7 min each step) and after critical point drying they were coated with gold on a rotary platform.

Radioimmuno-assays: The vasopressin content of the hypothalamic cell culture supernatants was determined by a radioimmunological procedure as described in (18), using rabbit antibody to arginine vasopressin (Calbiochem, Behringwerke), ^{125}I-vasopressin (NEN) and synthetic arginine vasopressin (Sigma) as standard. The sensitivity limit of the assay was 0.05 - 0.1 µU vasopressin and the vasopressin in the samples diluted according to standard curves. None of the factors present in the culture medium had any effect on the assay. ACTH in blood plasma and cell culture supernatants was determined by RIA without prior extraction using an antibody induced with $^{1-14}$ACTH in rabbit. Crossreactions of this antibody with β-endorphine, γ-LPH, and β-LPH was negligible (less than 1 %). Crossreaction with β-MSH was 15 %. Synthetic $^{1-39}$ACTH, which had been calibrated with MRC-74/555 was used for calibration. All reagents were from CEA and purchased from IDW, Sprendlingen, FRG.

Animals: Male Wistar-Furth rats were hypophysectomized by the parapharyngeal approach at 1 - 2 months of age. Animals showing less than 5 % increase in body weight during the following two weeks and having no detectable ACTH in the blood plasma were used for further experiments. Hypophysectomized rats (hypox) were kept with 10 % sucrose in the drinking water.

Pituitary organoids were subcutaneously implanted into the neck of syngeneic male rats and were removed later on for further investigations. Blood for the RIA of ACTH was taken from the ventral artery of the tail and gathered in EDTA-coated tubes. 400 KIE Aprotinin/ml blood was added. After centrifugation (10 000 g_{av} x min, 4°C) the plasma was stored at -30°C.

Immunofluorescence analysis: The removed implants were fixed in Bouin's solution and embedded in paraffine. Immunofluorescence of sections was performed with the indirect method, using a rabbit antiserum against ACTH (Ferring GmbH, Kiel, FRG) and a FITS-labelled goat-anti-rabbit antibody (Boehringer, Ingelheim, FRG). For details see (19, 20).

RESULTS

3dR-technique: The three-dimensional-rotation culture technique is characterized by the fact that cells are grown attached to the fibres of a three-dimensional material in high density and compact structure. To achieve this it has to be prevented that the cells attach to the bottom of the culture dish. We have selected untreated culture dishes designated for bacteriological purposes, whereas tissue culture dishes are already treated for better cell attachment. In addition, attachment is prevented by constant rotation of the cultures. As the cells cannot attach to the dish they form cell-to-cell contacts and aggregates or they attach to the fibres of the three-dimensional substrata. Furthermore, aggregates entangle in the fibres, and the outer cells of the aggregates form contacts with the fibre's surface or with cells that have already attached to the material. This can be seen in Fig. 1a, b.

In a coculture of GH$_3$-cells and normal rat fibroblasts we observed two totally different behaviours of the two cell types. This is demonstrated in figures 1c and 1d. Cells were cultivated in the gelatine sponge. GH$_3$-cells are distributed between the fibres, while the fibroblasts, which had been added to the culture after seven days, form a capsule around the material by enveloping it very tightly (Fig. 1d).

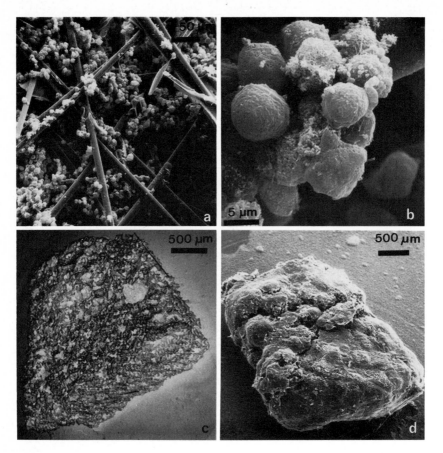

Fig. 1. Micrographs of scanning electron microscopy of 3dR-cultures:
(a,b)   GH$_3$-cells are cultivated on a glass fibre fleece. Single cells or cell aggregates are attached to the fibres.
 (c)   Structure of a gelatine sponge, when GH$_3$-cells are cultivated on this sponge.
 (d)   Coculture of GH$_3$-cells and fibroblasts on a gelatine sponge: fibroblasts form a tight capsule around the sponge.

Besides the possibility that the cells regain contacts to other cells in a three-dimensional self-assembly 3dR-cultures have some other advantages: they can easily be handled, medium changes can easily be performed, and the constant movement of the medium provides homogeneous culture conditions. For the work presented here it was important that cells are attached in high numbers on a stable substratum which can be implanted into an animal and, after a while, be removed again for further studies.

The capacity of cell attachment in a 25 x 5 x 0.8 mm glass-fibre fleece was determined with cells from the pituitary tumour cell line GH$_3$. Such a fleece has an effective surface of 12 cm^2 (comparable to that of a 3.5 cm dish) in which up to 10^7 GH$_3$-cells were found.

Primary hypothalamic cells in 3dR-cultures: Medium B17, used for these cultures, is a serum-free medium which was developed for the cocultivation of neurons and glial cells. Medium B17 is a combination of the N2-medium, which was developed by Bottenstein et al. (17) for the cultivation of neuroblastoma cells and is meanwhile used for the selective cultivation of various types of primary nerve cells, and of the astroglial specific medium B27 (22). In two-dimensional cultures both neurons and astrocytes can be grown simultaneously in medium B17, and the survival of both types of cells is higher than when they are cultivated alone (neurons in N$_2$- and astrocytes in B27 medium) (K. Lang, unpublished observations).

3dR-cultures of hypothalamic cells were compared to self-aggregating cultures with regard to vasopressin production as a function of neuron survival. Fig. 2 shows a typical vasopressin-production curve of these experiments. In all cases vasopressin-production in self-aggregating cultures stopped after about two weeks in vitro, while 3dR-cultures in most cases produced detectable vasopressin for about one month. In one experiment vasopressin was produced over a period of seven weeks. These data show that neuronal survival in 3dR-cultures is higher than in common two-dimensional systems where neurons normally survive no longer than three weeks (13, 23).The reason why 3dR-cultures produce vasopressin so much longer than common aggregating cul-

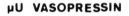

µU VASOPRESSIN

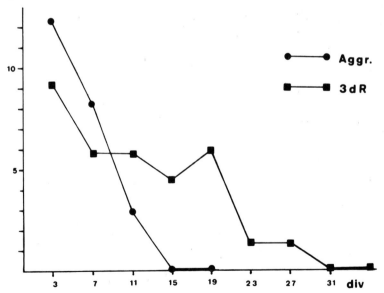

Fig. 2. Vasopressin secretion into the supernatant of hypothalamic cells in serum-free culture.
Comparison between 3dR-culture and cell aggregating culture.

tures may be due to the fact that the cells in the matrix have better access to nutrients and oxygen than cells in the relatively compact aggregates. In these aggregates, which reach a diameter of more than 1000 μm, the inner cells are only supplied by diffusion (24).

Pituitary primary cells: For the primary culture of rat pituitary cells a serum-free, hormone-supplemented medium was developed (TB-medium) (14). This medium is derived from the serum-free medium developed by Hayashi and Sato for the cultivation of the rat pituitary tumour cell line GH_3 (25). Rat pituitary primary cells can be kept under serum-free conditions for up to four months and longer (14).

Using TB-medium we cultivated human fetal pituitary cells in monolayer cultures and we studied the hormone secretion into the culture supernatants by means of radio-immuno-assays (26). Figure 3 shows the amount of secreted pituitary hormones. Prolactin was not detectable, FSH is only secreted during the first days in vitro. ACTH is secreted predominantly under these medium conditions. In the beginning high amounts of ACTH are detectable and a secretion between 50 and 100 pg/ml x day can be observed in vitro until day 25. This indicates that the serum-free culture conditions supply a microenvironment that either selects the survival and growth of ACTH producing cells or stimulates the secretion of ACTH more than that of other hormones.

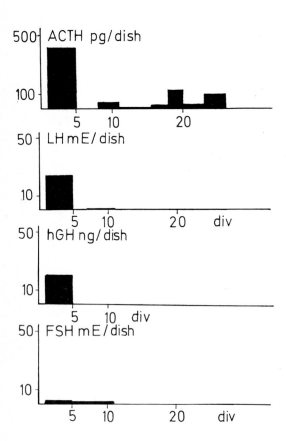

Fig. 3. Secretion of pituitary hormones into the supernatant. Human fetal pituitary cells were cultivated in monolayers under serum-free culture conditions.

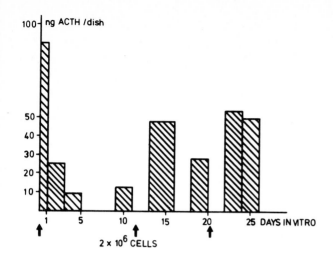

Fig. 4. ACTH-secretion of 3dR-cultured rat pituitary cells under serum-free culture conditions.
Arrows mark the time when cells were added.

In rat pituitary cells cultivated in a glass-fibre fleece we have only measured the ACTH secretion. Like in monolayer cultures the amount of ACTH decreases while the cells are in culture. By adding cells the level of ACTH secretion can be increased. After a third addition of cells a secretion of 50 ng ACTH/ml x day could be maintained in vitro from day 22 on (see Fig. 4).

In contrast to monolayer cultures the amount of secreted ACTH is much higher in 3dR-cultures (10 times as many cells produced 100 times the amount of hormone). This may be due to a better stimulation by the microenvironment of cell-to cell contacts in multilayers.

Pituitary substitution: The 3dR-culture technique offers the possibility of easy implantation of cells into an animal because they are attached to a stable matrix. In vitro the cells retain their special function (ACTH production) and are three-dimensionally organized, similar as in the organ from which they were isolated. For this reason we use the term organ-reconstitution.

In-vitro reconstituted pituitary organoids were tested in vivo by implantation into hypophysectomized rats. After surgical removal of the pituitary juvenile rats stop growing and the ACTH blood plasma level decreases to zero. These two criteria were observed after a reconstituted syngeneic pituitary organoid had been implanted subcutaneously. The results are shown in Table II.

During four weeks control animals (seven weeks of age, not hypophysectomized) gained 37 % in body weight. Hypox-rats did not increase their weight or, in one case, 8 % in four weeks. Also, after implantation, no growth could be observed in hypox-rats. The ectopic implant failed to restore growth.

The normal ACTH blood-plasma level of Wistar-Furth rats ranges between 200 - 400 pg ACTH/ml. Hypox-animals which were used for implantation had no detectable ACTH in the blood. Implantation into non-hypophysectomized control rats did not result in a change of the ACTH level, regardless whether they had received an empty

Table II. Effects of implants of 3dR-cultured pituitary cells (organoids) on growth and ACTH blood plasma level (d = days).

RATS	INTACT CONTROL	INTACT CONTROL		HYPOX	HYPOX
HYPOPHYSECTOMY AT AGE				6.5 WEEKS	8 WEEKS
IMPLANTATION AT AGE	15.5 WEEKS	15.5 WEEKS		15.5 WEEKS	44 WEEKS
IMPLANTATION OF	MATERIAL WITHOUT CELLS	PITUITARY ORGANOID		PITUITARY ORGANOID	PITUITARY ORGANOID
GAIN IN BODY WEIGHT IN 4 WEEKS BEFORE IMPLANTATION	37 %	38 %	GAIN IN BODY WEIGHT IN 4 WEEKS AFTER ECTOMY	8 %	-20 %
GAIN IN BODY WEIGHT IN 4 WEEKS AFTER IMPLANTATION	14 %	12 %		2 %	10 %
DAYS BEFORE IMPLANTATION	63 d	63 d	DAYS AFTER ECTOMY	63 d	256 d
ACTH BLOOD-PLASMA - LEVEL	220 pg/ml	260 pg/ml		0 pg/ml	0 pg/ml
DAYS AFTER IMPLANTATION	28 d	28 d		28 d	26 d
ACTH BLOOD-PLASMA- LEVEL	240 pg/ml	250 pg/ml		240 pg/ml	45 pg/ml

glass-fleece or a pituitary organoid. Nevertheless, a significant change was observed in hypox rats. 28 days after implantation of an organoid in one animal a normal level of ACTH (240 pg/ml) was regained; in another animal the level increased from zero to 45 pg/ml. This clearly indicates that the implanted cells secrete ACTH even when situated in ectopic places. A partial pituitary substitution is possible with 3dR cultivated pituitary cells.

After several weeks the implants were removed from the animals. Four weeks after implantation the material was very well vascularised and surrounded by connective tissue which was already macroscopically obvious and also could be shown in histological sections. No signs of rejection of the graft could be observed, which was not unexpected because we implanted syngeneic cells.

Immunofluorescence studies with ACTH-antiserum were positive in sections of the graft. ACTH-containing cells could be found seven weeks after implantation spread over the whole implant. This fact supports the finding of ACTH-secretion in the animal.

DISCUSSION AND PERSPECTIVES

This paper is a first approach to the idea of an in-vitro organ-reconstitution by means of a new cell culture technique and the application of serum-free, hormone-supplemented culture media, and to the substitution of dysfunctioning organs or parts thereof. The data presented here are not yet sufficient, but they are promising. They indicate that such a strategy may become successful and may become important in medical therapy.

Several groups have reported the advantages of aggregating cultures with regard to cell differentiation (27, 28), cell proliferation (2), and the biochemistry of cells (3). These effects are due to three-dimensional cell interactions. 3dR-cultures offer similar conditions as aggregating cultures with the same advantages as can be seen from our results: we could show that primary pituitary cells in three-dimensional cultures produce much more ACTH than cells in monolayer cultures. This is also true for hypothalamic cells with regard to vasopressin secretion (K. Lang, unpublished results). In the case of hypothalamic cells 3dR-cultures even show a prolonged vasopressin secretion compared to common aggregating cultures, which could be due to a better supply with nutrients and oxygen (24).

Because the cells in our culture system are actively producing hormones and because they are attached to a stable matrix the possibility is opened to try a substitution therapy on an animal which is deficient in the secreted hormone.

Also, in other subjects of cell biology the application of the new technique could be useful; in such cases where it is required to grow high numbers of cells - for instance for virus production - or for the isolation of cell-specific proteins and nucleic acids.

The use of serum-free media for the purpose of organ reconstitution can be valuable since they enable the selective cultivation of distinct cell types (29). Most endocrine glands in mammals are composed of different cell types which, moreover, produce different hormones. Nevertheless, in most endocrine diseases only one cell type is deficient and, therefore, only one hormone is lacking. Selective substitution with cells that produce the deficient hormone could be possible without changing the production level of other hormones in the same gland. As we have shown with the pituitary cell cultures, in TB-medium ACTH-secreting cells are predominantly represented.

3dR-cultivated pituitary cells secrete high amounts of ACTH into the culture supernatant, although the hypothalamic corticotropin releasing factor (CRF) is not present in TB-medium. This fact raises hopes to receive an ACTH-substitution in hypophysectomized rats even with an ectopic implantation of pituitary organoids.

The finding that the substituted hypox-rats did not restore growth may have two reasons: (i) TB-medium may be selective only for ACTH-producing cells - in this case other cells would not survive, or (ii) growth hormone-producing cells do not secrete the hormone without stimulation by hypothalamic factors. The second hypothesis is supported by the findings of other groups (6, 7, 9, 11). In these experiments transplanted pituitaries only restored growth of hypox-rats when they were implanted into hypophyseotrophic areas. Futher experiments will show whether co-implants of hypothalamic and pituitary organoids will overcome this problem.

In our experiments we observed the ACTH-secretion of the grafts into the blood of the treated animals by radioimmunoassays. Significantly higher values were observed in these animals than in hypox rats which had not received an organoid. In one case a normal ACTH level was reached. Other groups have checked ACTH-secretion of their pituitary-transplants via the increase of adrenal weight. In all cases of ectopic implantations adrenals did not increase in weight (6, 7, 8, 9, 30). In two cases (30 pituitaries implanted into muscle (6); one gland implanted into the medial basal hypothalamus (30)) the adrenal weight increased but did not reach the value of intact animals. Therefore, this report is the first one in which an ectopic implant increased the ACTH blood level of hypophysectomized animals.

Our experiments were performed with pituitary cells, but similar experiments are possible with cells from other endocrine tissue. Especially the application of the described technique to pancreatic β-cells may be more successful due to the direct regulation of insulin secretion. This has been shown in experiments by transplantation of pancreas or by implantation of pancreatic islets (31, 32).

The implantation of in-vitro reconstituted organoids has two advantages over common organ transplantations:

(i)   specific cell types may be selected by serum-free culture conditions or other methods, e.g. cell sorting or density centrifugation, then cultivated until organoids are formed, and afterwards implanted to cure special diseases.

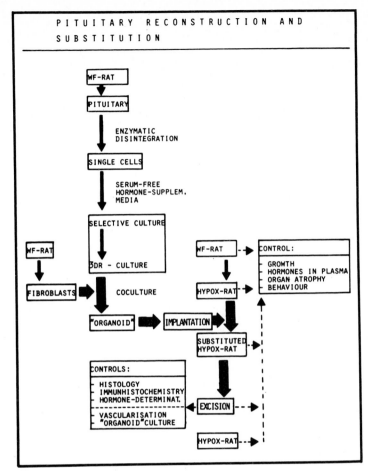

Fig. 5. Strategy of an in-vitro organ reconstitution and organ-substitution.

(ii)   the rejection of allogeneic grafts can be reduced by a pre-incubation in-vitro, as was reported recently by two groups (32, 33, 34). The reduction of graft rejection may be due to the fact that Ia antigen-bearing leuco-cytes leave the tissue during the incubation period. This could be en-forced by the use of selective media.

By following this strategy (demonstrated in Fig. 5) further investigations on the in-vitro reconstitution of endocrine organs may lead towards new methods for medical therapy and research.

Acknowledgements

We are grateful to Hoechst AG, Frankfurt, FRG for their generous gift of Gelas-typt M-materials and to Glaswerk Schuller, Wertheim, FRG, for supplying us with the glass fibre fleeces.

REFERENCES

1) Brunner, G., Nitzgen, B., Wieser, R., Speth, V. 1982. Importance of the contact environment on the behavior of mammalian cells. In: Growth of Cells in Hormonally Defined Media (G. Sato, D. Sirbasku, A. Pardee, eds.) Cold Spring Harbor Laboratory, New York, No. 9, 179 - 201.

2) Moscona, A.A. 1974. Surface specification of embryonic cells: lectin receptors, cell recognition and specific cell ligands. In: The Cell Surface Development (A.A. Moscona, ed.) J. Wiley, New York, 67 - 99.

3) Seeds, N.W. 1971. Biochemical differentiation in reaggregating brain cell culture. Proc. Natl. Acad. Sci. USA 68, 1858 - 1861.

4) Paul, J. 1975. Cell and Tissue Culture. Fifth Edition, Churchill Livingstone, Edinburgh, London, New York, p. 186 - 188.

5) Leighton, J. 1973. Collagen-coated cellulose sponge. In: Tissue Culture - Methods and Applications (P. Kruse, M.K. Patterson, eds.).Academic Press, 378 - 383.

6) Gittes, R.F., Kastin, J. 1966. Effects of increasing numbers of pituitary transplants on hypophysectomized rats. Endocrinology 78, 1023-1031.

7) Goldberg, R.C., Knobil, E. 1957. Structure and function of intraoccular hypophyseal grafts in the hypophysectomized male rat. Endocrinology 61, 742 - 752.

8) Hertz, R. 1959. Growth in the hypophysectomized rat sustained by pituitary grafts. Endocrinology 65, 926 - 931.

9) Meites, J., Kragt, C.L. 1965. Effects of a pituitary homotransplant and thyroxine on body and mammary growth in immature hypophysectomized rats. Endocrinology 75, 565 - 570.

10) Knigge, K. 1980. Relationship of intracerebral pituitary grafts to central neuropeptide system. J. Anatomy 158, 549 - 563.

11) Hymer, W.C., Harkness, J., Bartke, A., Wilbur, D., Hatfield, J.M., Page, R., Hibbard, E. 1981. Pituitary hollow fiber units in vivo and in vitro. Neuroendocrinology 32, 339 - 349.

12) Weiss, S., Bergland, R., Page, R., Turban, C., Hymer, W.C. 1978. Pituitary cell transplants to the cerebral ventricles promote growth of hypophysectomized rats. Proc. Soc. Exp. Biol. Med. 159, 409 - 413.

13) Brunner, G., Lang, K., Wolfe, R., McClure, D.B., Sato, G. 1981. Selective cell culture of brain cells by serum-free, hormone-supplemented media. A comparative morphological study. Develop. Brain Res. 2, 563 - 575.

14) Brunner, G. 1980. Importance of attachment factors for long term primary culture in serum-free, hormone-supplemented media. Hoppe Seyler's Z. Physiol. Chem. 361, 1272.

15) Sonnenschein, C., Richardson, U.J., Tashijan, A.H. 1970. Chromosomal analysis, organ-specific function and appearance of six clonal strains of rat pituitary tumor cells. Exp. Cell Res. 61, 121 - 128.

16) Tashijan, A.H., Brancraft, P.C., Levine, L. 1970. Production of both prolactin and growth hormone by clonal strains of rat pituitary tumor cells. J. Cell Biol. 47, 61 - 70.

17) Bottenstein, J.E., Sato, G.H. 1979. Growth of a rat neuroblastoma cell line in serum-free supplemented medium. Proc. Natl. Acad. Sci. USA 76, 514 - 517.

18) Rackê, K., Ritzel, H., Trapp, B., Muscholl, E. 1982. Dopaminergic modulation of evoked vasopressin release from the isolated neurohypophysis of the rat. Naunyn Schmiedeberg's Arch. Pharmacol. 319, 56 - 65.

19) Choy, V.J., Watkins, W.B. 1977. Maturation of hypothalamo-neurohypophysical systems. I. Localization of neurophysin, oxytocin and vasopressin in the hypothalamus and neural lobe of the developing rat brain. Cell Tiss. Res. 197, 325 - 336.

20) Watkins, W.B. 1981. Differential immunostaining of adenohypophyseal cells with antisera to ACTH and β-endorphin. Regulatory Peptides 1, 375 - 385.

21) Yuhas, J.M., Li, A.P., Martinez, A., Ladman, A. 1977. A simplified method for production and growth of multicellular tumor spheroids. Cancer Res. 37, 3639 - 3643.

22) Lang, K., Brunner, G. 1983. Tracing the astroglial cell lineage in vitro by modification of the microenvironmental conditions. See this volume

23) Romijn, H.J., van Huizen, F., Wolters, P.S., Habets, A.M.M.C. 1982. Further attempts to obtain a serum-free medium for long term cerebral cortex cultures. Biol. of the Cell 45, 34.

24) Folkman, J., Hochberg, M., Knighton, D. 1974. Self-regulation of growth in three dimensions. In: Control of Proliferation in Animal Cells (Clarkson, B., Baserga, R., eds.) Cold Spring Harbor Laboratory, 833 - 842.

25) Hayashi, I., Sato, G.H. 1976. Replacement of serum by hormones permits growth of cells in a defined medium. Nature 259, 132 - 134.

26) Lang, E., Krause, U., Brunner, G. 1982. Hormone production of human fetal pituitary cells under serum-free, hormone-supplemented culture conditions. Biol. of the Cell 45, 197.

27) Garber, B., Huttenlocher, P.R., Larramendi, L.H.M. 1980. Self assembly of cortical plate cells in vitro within embryonic mouse cerebral aggregates. Golgi and electron microscopical analysis. Brain Res. 201, 255 - 278.

28) Trapp, B.D., Honegger, P., Richelson, E., Webster, H.D. 1979. Morphological differentiation of mechanically dissociated fetal rat brain in aggregating cell cultures. Brain Res. 160, 117 - 130.

29) Barnes, D., Sato, G.H. 1980. Methods for growth of cultured cells in serum-free medium. Analytical Biochem. 102, 255 - 270.

30) Halasz, B., Pupp, L., Uhlarik, S., Tima, L. 1965. Further studies on the hormone secretion of the anterior pituitary transplanted into the hypophyseotrophic area of the rat hypothalamus. Endocrinology 77, 343 - 355.

31) Usadel, K.H., Schwedes, U., Bastert, G., Steinau, U., Klempa, I., Fassbinder, W., Schöffling, K. 1981. Transplantation of human fetal pancreas - experience in thymusaplastic mice and rats and in a diabetic patient. Diabetes 29, 74 - 79.

32) Bowen, K.M., Lafferty, K.J. 1980. Reversal of diabetes by allogeneic islets transplantation without immunosuppression. Australian J. Exp. Biol. Med. Sci. 58, 441 - 447.

33) Parr, E.L., Lafferty, K.J., Bowen, K.M., McKenzie, I.F.C. 1980. H-2 complex and Ia antigens on cells dissociated from mouse thyroid glands and islets of Langerhans. Transplantation 30, 142 - 148.

34) Simeonovic, C.J., Bowen, K.M., Kotlarski, J., Lafferty, K.J. 1980. Modulation of tissue immunogenicity by organ culture. Transplantation 30, 174 - 179.

Hormonal Regulation of Growth and Function of Insulin-Producing Cells in Culture

J. Høiriis Nielsen

Hagedorn Research Laboratory, DK-2820 Gentofte, Denmark

The endocrine pancreas in mammals is organized in numerous small clusters of cells, the islets of Langerhans, consisting of 1000-3000 cells of which the insulin-producing beta-cells amount to about 60-70%. The islets represent only 1-2% of the total pancreas, and it was not before the introduction of the collagenase digestion technique (Moskalewski, 1965) that larger quantities of isolated pancreatic islets could be obtained for biochemical studies (for a review, see Nielsen and Lernmark, 1983).

Although maintenance of islets in organ culture was already described by Moskalewski (1965),studies on the long-term effect of glucose and other secretagogues were performed in the culture system described by Andersson and Hellerström (1972). The culture conditions were further improved by employing culture medium RPMI 1640 and free floating islets (Andersson, 1978). It was noted that replacement of the commonly used calf serum with human serum resulted in an augmented production of insulin (Nielsen et al. 1979). Under these conditions human islets could be maintained for up to 2 years with continuous insulin production (Nielsen, 1981).

The mitotic activity in the islets decreases rapidly with age both _in vivo_ (Logothetopoulos, 1972) and _in vitro_ (Swenne and Hellerström, 1982). However, in islets from newborn rats a certain mitotic activity can be detected allowing studies on its regulation by hormones and growth factors (Nielsen, 1982, Rabinovitch et al., 1982).

The aim of the present study is briefly to review and extend the results obtained with supplement and/or replacement of serum with hydrocortisone and growth hormone on the insulin release and DNA-synthesis in isolated rodent islets reported previously (Brunstedt and Nielsen, 1981, Nielsen, 1982).

Materials and methods

Islet isolation: Pancreata from male NMRI-mice weighing 20-22 g, male
Wistar rats weighing 125-150 g, or 5-day old Wistar rats of both sex-
es were excised and treated with crude collagenase (Worthington type
II or Sigma type I), 1.5 mg/ml in Hank's balanced salt solution (Flow
Laboratories) with 25 mM HEPES, 100 IU/ml penicillin and 100 μg/ml
streptomycin, pH 7.4 (HBSS). After 15 min of vigorous shaking at 37°C,
the liberated islets were isolated under a dissecting microscope directly or after gradient centrifugation on Percoll (Pharmacia)(Brunstedt, 1980).

Culture methods: Islet cultures were established as described previously (Nielsen, 1982): The islets were placed in Petri dishes for bacteriological use (Nunc), not allowing attachment of the islets to the
bottom. The culture medium was RPMI 1640 (Flow Laboratories) supplemented with 100 IU/ml penicillin and 100 μg/ml streptomycin pH 7.2.

The standard glucose concentration was 11 mM and specially prepared
RPMI 1640 without glucose was employed for experiments at lower glucose
concentrations.

Serum proteins and hormones

Newborn calf serum (NCS) (Gibco) or normal human serum (HS) from the
blood bank was employed. In some experiments serum was replaced with
human serum albumin (HSA) (reinst, Behringwerke). Hydrocortisone (HC)
was added as the water soluble hydrocortisone 21-sodium succinate (So-
lu-Cortef, Upjohn). Human growth hormone (hGH) with a potency of 2.2
U/mg (clinical grade) or 2.9 U/mg (highly purified, prepared by Dr. K.
Heinæs) was obtained from Nordisk Gentofte (Denmark).

^{3}H-thymidine incorporation

Newborn rat islets were cultured for two days in RPMI 1640 with 10%
newborn calf serum (NCS, Gibco) before addition of the hormones. After
24 hrs $\left[^{3}\text{H-methyl}\right]$-thymidine (Tdr)(The Radiochemical Centre, Amersham)
2 μCi/ml was added and the islets incubated for 3 hrs before the medi-
um was replaced with medium containing 0.15 mM thymidine (Sigma) for
further 3 hrs when more than 90% of the radioactivity was found in a
5% TCA-precipitate. The islets were sonicated and the radioactivity
measured (Nielsen, 1982).

Analytical methods

Insulin release and insulin content of the islets were determined by radioimmunoassay (Heding, 1971). DNA was determined by a fluorometric method (Green and Taylor, 1972). Wilcoxon's test was employed for the statistical evaluation of the results. $2\alpha \leq 0.05$ was considered significant.

Results

When mouse islets were maintained at a low serum concentration e.g. 0.5% HS the rate of insulin release gradually decreased (Fig. 1). However, supplement of either HC or hGH resulted in an almost constant rate of insulin release during a 14-day period (Fig. 1). When the islets were subjected to an acute challenge with glucose, theophylline or adrenaline, the islets cultured with HC released significantly more insulin than the control islets and the islets cultured in the presence of hGH (Fig. 2). The capacity to release insulin in the presence of theophylline was increased markedly both in the HC- and hGH-treated islets while the release was suppressed by adrenaline in all groups (Fig. 2).

Addition of HC to rat islets resulted in a small increase in the insulin release to the culture medium but a marked increase in islet insulin content (Fig. 3). hGH induced a marked increase in both insulin

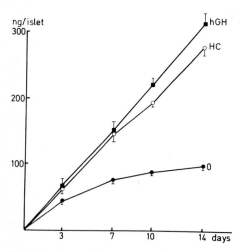

Figure 1. Effect of human growth hormone (hGH) 1 μg/ml and hydrocortisone (HC) 10^{-7} M on cumulative insulin release from mouse islets cultured in medium RPMI 1640 with 11 mM glucose and 0.5% human serum (control medium, 0). Bars indicates SEM (n=6).

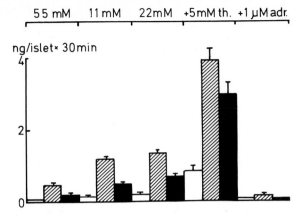

55 mM   11 mM   22mM   +5mM th. +1 μM adr.

ng/islet × 30 min

Figure 2. Acute insulin release from mouse islets collected after 14 days of culture (Fig. 1) in 0.5% human serum (▢), HC (▨) and hGH (▮) in response to glucose 5.5 mM, 11 mM, and 22 mM, and 22 mM glucose with 5 mM theophylline (th) or 1 μM adrenaline (adr.). Results are expressed in ng insulin per islet per 30 min. The HC-groups were significantly different from the control and the hGH groups in all instances, while the hGH groups were significantly different from the controls except for the adrenaline exposure. Bars indicate SEM (n= 6-12).

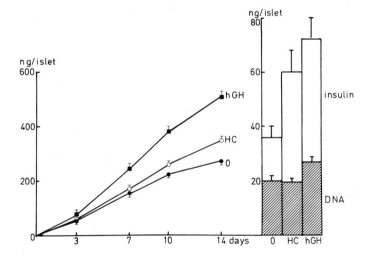

Figure 3. Effect of hGH 1 μg/ml and HC 10^{-7} M on insulin release and insulin and DNA content in adult rat islets cultured in RPMI 1640 with 8.5 mM glucose and 0.5% HS (0). Bars indicate SEM (n=4).

release and insulin content, and in contrast to HC also in the cell number as indicated by the higher DNA content (see below).

The effect was dependent on the glucose concentration in the culture medium since the addition of HC to rat islets cultured at 11 mM glucose resulted in a slight decrease in the insulin release. In contrast, the effect on the insulin content was similar to that found after culture at 8.5 mM glucose, i.e. marked increase at the lowest HC concentrations, while the effect was reversed by increasing the HC concentration to 10^{-5} M (Fig. 4).

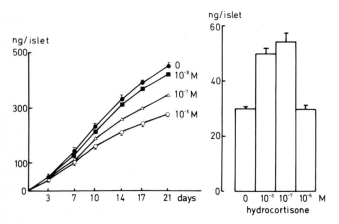

<u>Figure 4.</u> Dose-response effect of HC on insulin release and content of adult rat islets cultured in medium RPMI 1640 with 11 mM glucose and 0.5% human serum (0). Bars indicate SEM (n=4).

When newborn rat islets were exposed to various concentrations of HC for 24 hrs a dose-dependent decrease in the incorporation of ^{3}H-Tdr was found (Fig. 5).

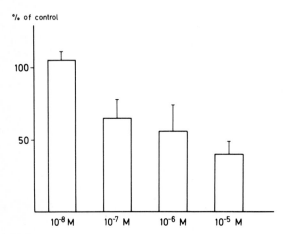

<u>Figure 5.</u> Dose-response effect of HC on ^{3}H-thymidine incorporation into newborn rat islet DNA. The results are expressed as per cent of the incorporation into islets cultured in medium RPMI 1640 with 11 mM glucose and 10% newborn calf serum. Bars indicate SEM (n=6).

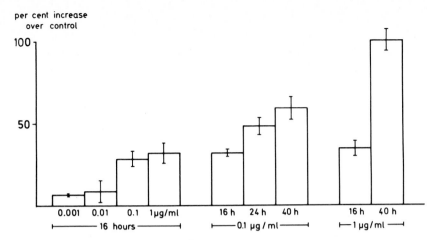

per cent increase
over control

Figure 6. Effect hGH on ^{3}H-thymidine incorporation into newborn rat
islet DNA. The results are expressed as per cent of the incorporation into islets cultured in medium RPMI with 11 mM glucose and 10%
newborn calf serum. The incubation time and the dose of hGH were varied as indicated. Bars indicate SEM (n=4-8).

In contrast islets exposed to hGH showed a marked increase in the
incorporation of ^{3}H-Tdr (Fig. 6). The effect was dose- and time-dependent. Significant stimulation was seen at 100 ng/ml and the effect
was more pronounced after 24 and 40 h exposure to hGH than after 16 h
(Fig. 6).

Discussion

It was previously shown that hydrocortisone exerted a dose-related
bimodal effect on the insulin release of mouse pancreatic islets in
organ culture (Brunstedt and Nielsen, 1981).At near-physiological
concentrations, i.e. 10^{-7}M a marked stimulatory effect was found in
the release (Fig. 1). The subsequent increase in the glucose stimulated insulin release (Fig. 2) suggests an increase in the glucose sensitivity of the beta-cells which we have demonstrated in other experiments (Brunstedt and Nielsen, 1981). There have, however, been
other reports on an inhibitory effect on insulin release from rat
islets (Billaudel and Sutter, 1981). One explanation may be the species difference which is supported by the present experiments. Although a slight stimulation of the release was found in rat islets
maintained in 8.5 mM glucose (Fig. 3) a slight inhibition was seen
at 11 mM glucose (Fig. 4), but under both conditions a marked increase in the islet insulin content was observed in rat islets, but
not in mouse islets (Brunstedt and Nielsen, 1981). This may indicate

that hydrocortisone increases the biosynthesis of insulin and recently it was found that mouse islets treated with HC had a higher content of insulin mRNA than control islets (Brunstedt, 1982). However, HC has been shown to inhibit the intracellular degradation of insulin (Borg, 1982) which may explain the increased insulin content observed in the rat islets (Fig. 3 and 4). Furthermore, the dose of the hormone is critical since slightly higher concentrations, which have been applied in several previous studies, reversed the effect on both insulin release and content in mouse (Brunstedt and Nielsen, 1981) and rat islets (Fig. 4). Maintenance of islets under conditions with no or low serum, may resemble the in vivo condition of adrenalectomy which has been shown to attenuate the glucose response of the pancreatic islets (for references, see Brunstedt and Nielsen, 1981, Borelli et al. 1982). Thus the effect of HC may be explained as a relative reconstitution of the normal physiological milieu of the islets.

Growth hormone seems to have a stimulating effect similar to HC on the insulin release during culture of both mouse (Fig. 1) and rat islets (Fig. 3). However, the response of the islets to secretagogues after removal of the hormones seems to be lower than after exposure to HC (Fig. 2). This indicates a different mechanism of action. GH seems to have to be present in order to stimulate the insulin release, and the subsequent increased response to glucose may be due to the increased insulin production in the islets (Nielsen, 1982) as reflected in an increased mRNA level (Brunstedt, 1982). At least in the rat islets the increased insulin content may be explained by an increase in the number of beta cells since the DNA content was higher in the GH-treated islets (Fig. 3). Again the control condition with GH-deficient medium may resemble the in vivo condition of hypophysectomy where islets have a reduced insulin release and biosynthesis (for references, see Nielsen 1982, Pierluissi et al. 1982). Therefore replacement with GH may also represent another factor important in reconstituting the normal physiological milieu.

Thus, maintenance of normal beta cell function in vitro appears to be accomplished by the presence of a small amount of serum or albumin (Fig. 1 and 3) supplied with a physiological concentration of corticosteroid hormone and an elevated level of growth hormone. The latter may be of importance for the proliferation or regeneration of islet cells (Fig. 6). Growth hormone and the related hormones, prolactin and placental lactogen, have been shown to stimulate cell proliferation of whole islets in organ culture (Nielsen, 1982) and in monolayer cultures of newborn rat islet cells (Nielsen and Brunstedt, 1982) and in beta cells in particular in monolayer cultures of newborn rat pancreatic cells (Rabinovitch et al., 1983) as well as in a rat islet tumor cell line grown in monolayer culture (Fong et al. 1981). This effect is in accordance with *in vivo* observations in rats treated with growth hormone or growth hormone producing tumor transplants (for references, see Nielsen 1982). The inhibitory effect of hydrocortisone on the DNA synthesis (Fig. 5) is in accordance with findings in isolated mouse islets (Andersson, 1975) and monolayer cultures of newborn rat pancreatic cells (Chick, 1973), but in contrast to the increased beta cell replication found *in vivo* in corticosteroid-treated guinea pigs (Hellerström 1963, Kern and Logothetopoulos 1970). However, this phenomenon may be explained by the hyperglycemic effect of the hormones since glucose is reported to induce beta cell replication *in vitro* (Andersson 1975, King and Chick 1976, Swenne et al. 1980, Rabinovitch et al. 1980). In addition, hormone interaction may be responsible for the apparent discrepancy between the *in vivo* and the *in vitro* observations. In preliminary experiments, simultaneous addition of progesterone and placental lactogen resulted in prevention of the decreased islet insulin content induced by progesterone alone and the two hormones counteracted each other on the DNA synthesis (Nielsen et al. 1981). Thus the concomitant beta cell hyperplasia and increased glucose induced insulin release seen in late pregnancy may represent a subtle balance between the hormones. The islet cultures offer possibilities for evaluating adverse effect of disturbed hormone interactions which may result in impairment of the beta cell growth and function similar to that found in diabetes.

Acknowledgement

Mrs. Kirsten Brunstedt, Ragna Jørgensen, and Dagny Jensen are thanked for their expert technical assistance.

References

Andersson A (1975) Synthesis of DNA in isolated pancreatic islets maintained in tissue culture. Endocrinology 96: 1051-1054.

Andersson A (1978) Isolated mouse pancreatic islets in culture: Effects of serum and different culture media on the insulin production of the islets. Diabetologia 14: 397-404.

Andersson A, Hellerström C (1972) Metabolic characteristics of isolated pancreatic islets in tissue culture. Diabetes 21 (suppl. 2): 546-554.

Billaudel B, Sutter BCJ (1981) Modulation of the direct effect of corticosterone upon glucose-induced insulin secretion of rat isolated islets of Langerhans. Diab. Metab. 7: 91-96.

Borelli MI, Garcia ME, Durum CLG, Gagliardino JJ (1982) Glucocorticoid-induced changes in insulin secretion related to the metabolism and ultrastructure of pancreatic islets. Horm. Metab. Res. 14: 287-292.

Borg LAH (1982) Effects of steroid hormones on intracellular insulin degradation in isolated islets of Langerhans of the mouse. Diabetologia 23: 157.

Brunstedt J (1980) Rapid isolation of functionally intact pancreatic islets from mice and rats by Percoll ^{TM}gradient centrifugation. Diab. Metab. 6: 87-89.

Brunstedt J (1982) Expression of the insulin gene: Regulation by glucose, hydrocortisone, and growth hormone. Special FEBS Meeting on Cell Function and Differentiation, April 25-29, 1982 Athens, Greece, Abstracts p. 149.

Brunstedt J, Nielsen JH (1981) Direct long-term effect of hydrocortisone on insulin and glucagon release from mouse pancreatic islets in tissue culture. Acta Endocr. (Cph) 96: 498-504.

Chick WL (1973) Beta cell replication in rat pancreatic monolayer cultures. Effects of glucose, tolbutamide, glucocorticoid, growth hormone and glucagon. Diabetes 22: 687-693.

Fong HKW, Chick WL, Sato G (1981) Hormones and factors that stimulate growth of a rat islet tumor cell line in serum-free medium. Diabetes 30: 1022-1028.

Green IC, Taylor KW (1972) Effects of pregnancy in the rat on the size and insulin secretory response of the islets of Langerhans. J. Endocrinol. 54: 317-325.

Heding L (1971) Radioimmunological determination of pancreatic and gut glucagon in plasma. Diabetologia 7: 10-19.

Hellerström C (1963) Effects of steroid diabetes on the pancreatic islets of guinea pigs with special reference to the A_1 cells. Acta Soc. Med. Upsal. 68: 1-16.

Kern H, Logothetopoulos J (1970) Steroid diabetes in the guinea pig. Diabetes 19: 145-154.

King DL, Chick WL (1976) Pancreatic beta cell replication: Effects of hexose sugars. Endocrinology 99: 1003-1009.

Logothetopoulos J (1972) Islet cell regeneration and neogenesis. In: Steiner DF, Freinkel H (eds.) Handbook of Physiology, Sect. 7, vol. 1. American Physiological Society, Washington DC, pp. 67-76.

Moskalewski S (1965) Isolation and culture of the islets of Langerhans of the guinea pig. Gen. Comp. Endocr. 5: 342-353.

Nielsen JH (1981) Beta cell function in isolated human pancreatic islets in long-term tissue culture. Acta Biol. Med. Germ. 40: 55-60.

Nielsen JH (1982) Effects of growth hormone, prolactin, and placental lactogen on insulin content and release and deoxyribonucleic acid synthesis in cultured pancreatic islets. Endocrinology 110: 600-606.

Nielsen JH, Brunstedt K (1982) Growth hormone as a growth factor for normal pancreatic islet cells in primary culture. In: Sirbasku DA, Sato G (eds.): Growth of cells in hormonally defined media. Cold Spring Habor Conference on ·Cell Proliferation vol. 9 (in press).

Nielsen JH, Lernmark Å (1983) Purification of islets and cells from islets. In: Pretlow TG and Pretlow T (eds.) Cell Separation: Methods and selected applications. Academic Press, New York, vol. 2 (in press).

Nielsen JH, Brunstedt J, Andersson A, Frimodt-Møller C (1979) Preservation of beta cell function in adult human pancreatic islets for several months in vitro. Diabetologia 16: 97-100.

Nielsen JH, Jørgensen R, Jensen D, Brunstedt K (1981) Direct effect of pregnancy hormones on growth and function of pancreatic islets in tissue culture. Diabetologia 21: 308-309.

Pierluissi J, Pierluissi R, Ashcroft SJH (1982) Effects of hypophysectomy and growth hormone on cultured islets of Langerhans of the rat. Diabetologia 22: 134-137.

Rabinovitch A, Blondel B, Murray T, Mintz DH (1980) Cyclic adenosine-3',5'-monophosphate stimulates islet B cell replication in neonatal pancreatic monolayer cultures. J. Clin. Invest. 66: 1065-1071.

Rabinovitch A, Quigley C, Russell T, Patel Y, Mintz DH (1982) Insulin and multiplication stimulating activity (an insulin-like growth factor) stimulate islet β-cell replication in neonatal rat pancreatic monolayer cultures. Diabetes 31: 160-164.

Rabinovitch A, Quigley C, Rechler MM (1983) Growth hormone stimulates B-cell replication in neonatal rat pancreatic monolayer cultures. Diabetes (in press).

Swenne I, Hellerström C (1982) Pancreatic B cell regeneration in rats of various ages. Diabetologia 23: 203.

Swenne I, Bone AJ, Howell SL, Hellerström C (1980) Effects of glucose and amino acids on the biosynthesis of DNA and insulin in fetal rat islets maintained in tissue culture. Diabetes 29: 686-692.

Studies on Regulation of Ovarian Steroidogenesis in Vitro: The Need for a Serum-Free Medium

Joseph Orly, Patricia Weinberger-Ohana, and Yigal Farkash
Department of Biological Chemistry, Institute of Life Sciences, The Hebrew University of Jerusalem, Jerusalem 91904, Israel

SUMMARY

Granulosa cells from rat ovary can be readily grown in serum-free medium. The defined medium consists of a basal nutrient mixture of DMEM and Ham's F-12 media, supplemented by insulin, transferrin, hydrocortisone and fibronectin (4F medium). In 4F medium the granulosa cells expressed all their known differentiated functions: in response to gonadotropic hormone such as follitropin (FSH), the cells produced progestins and estrogen as well as expressed new receptors to lutropin (LH). In contrast to the cells' responsiveness in 4F medium, the presence of serum in the culture medium clearly suppressed the expression of all three hormonally-induced functions. As low as 0.2% serum was sufficient to block 90% of the progestin production in response to FSH.

Since cyclic AMP is now accepted to be the intracellular mediator of all the gonadotropin-induced functions, we tested whether serum impairs the accumulation of cAMP triggered in the granulosa cells by FSH. It was evident that cells grown in the presence of serum accumulated 17 times less cAMP compared with cells exposed to FSH in 4F medium. However, addition of a phosphodiesterase inhibitor (IBMX) to the serum-containing medium, practically abolished the serum inhibition of cAMP accumulation. These results ruled out the possibility that serum suppresses FSH-induced functions merely by inhibition of FSH binding to its receptor or by impairing, by as yet an unknown mechanism, the FSH induced activation of adenylate cyclase. Alternatively, these findings suggest that serum diminishes the rising intracellular cAMP pool by apparently activating a phosphodiesterase enzyme which rapidly degrades the freshly generated cyclic nucleotide. Although there is still room for further study of phosphodiesterase effect in both intact granulosa cells and cell-free lysates, the concept seems attractive regarding the possibility that serum can modulate the cultured cell responsiveness to hormones by activating the cyclic nucleotide catabolizing enzyme, rather than directly inhibiting the cAMP generating system, namely, adenylate cyclase.

INTRODUCTION

Many *in vitro* studies using various cultured cell types have suggested that the expression of the cell's differentiated phenotype was markedly influenced by the culture's environmental conditions, mainly by the presence or absence of serum in the culture medium. Thus, chick cartilage cells did not produce cartilage *in vitro*, unless serum and embryo extracts were removed from the medium (1); serum enhanced the growth of neuroblastoma cells, but only removal of serum from the culture medium resulted in axonal outgrowth (2, 3). In addition, Darmon and collaborators have recently shown that neural differentiation of embryonal carcinoma cells *in vitro* was exclusively induced after serum deprivation and growth of the cells in serum-free medium (4, 5); serum exerted inhibitory effects also on the differentiation process of a myogenic cell line which fused to create muscle cell fibers only upon lowering the serum concentration in the culture medium (6).

Similarly, the present report demonstrates the absolute necessity for serum-free medium also for the study of ovarian physiology *in vitro*. We were preferentially interested in the follicular granulosa cells because of their major physiological role throughout the entire maturation process of the gonade follicle, leading eventually to ovulation. Moreover, the granulosa cells surrounding the oocyte are practically suitable for tissue culture studies as they can be readily expressed from the follicle as a pure population freed from contaminating cells of other types. Taken from immature rats, these cells provide an attractive model for studying their hormone-controlled cytodifferentiation. However, studies of others and ours with the isolated granulosa cells have encountered difficulties in demonstrating the hormonally induced functions when the cells were cultured in media containing serum. We thus formulated a serum-free defined medium to support both the growth and the function of long-term primary cultures of rat granulosa cells.

METHODS

Culture media, expression of granulosa cells, cell counts, steroid measurments, and other standard procedures were as previously described (7).

Preparation of fibronectin-coated dish: The tissue culture dishes (35 mm) or multi-well plates (24 wells, 16 mm diameter) were coated with fibronectin at least 30 minutes *prior* to inoculation of the cells. Human plasma fibronectin was purified on gelatin-Sepharose affinity column, as previously described by Ruoslahti *et al.*(8). It is important to point out that all manipulations with fibronectin should be carried out using only polypropylene labware (tubes, micro-pipettes, etc.). The purified fibronectin eluted from the gelatin-Sepharose column in 8 M urea should be dialysed against phosphate buffered saline (PBS) containing 1 M urea at pH 7.4. The final concentration of fibronectin stock solution should *not* exceed 0.8 mg/ml. In our experience, the presence of up to 30 mM urea in the final culture medium does not harm the cell monolayers. Fibronectin should be added into the dish *already containing* the suitable amount of medium and immediately mixed to create a homogeneous solution. Within 15-30 minutes of incubation at 37°C, most of the fibronectin should by adsorbed to the dish substratum. Hormones and factors are added *after* the cells have been inoculated into the dish.

276

RESULTS AND DISCUSSION

Serum-free medium for growth of primary rat granulosa cells in culture

We have previously described a defined-medium formula for maintenance and growth of primary rat granulosa cells in culture (7). This serum-free medium consisted of a 1:1, v/v, mixture of Dulbecco-Voigt's modified Eagle medium (DMEM) and Ham's F-12 nutrient mixture, supplemented with insulin (2 µg/ml), transferrin (5 µg/ml), hydrocortisone (40 ng/ml), and fibronectin (1.5 µg/cm²). Fig. 1 clearly demonstrates the need for the four supplemented factors (4F medium) to maintain the granulosa cells cultured in the absence of serum. In DMEM:F-12 medium alone, 99% of the cells died within 5 days (Fig. 1A), while insulin and fibronectin were the most needed components to prevent such cell death. However, the plating efficiency of the cells cultured into medium containing 5% serum was still better than that obtained in 4F medium. Nevertheless, the growth profile (Fig. 1A) and the morphology of the cells in 4F medium (Fig. 2) were comparable to that observed in serum containing medium, thus allowing us to maintain healthy granulosa cells in culture for weeks.

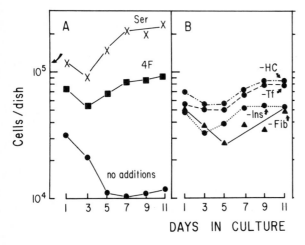

Fig. 1. Effect of various factors on growth of cultured granulosa cells in serum-free medium. Rat granulosa cells were expressed by puncturing ovaries of immature rats treated with diethylstilbesterol (DES) (7). Cells (1.12 x 10⁵, arrow on ordinate) were cultured in medium containing 5% serum (horse serum:fetal calf serum 2:1, respectively) (x — x) or in DMEM:F-12 medium (● — ●) supplemented with the following factors: insulin, transferrin, hydrocortisone and fibronectin (4F, ■ — ■); 4F without fibronectin (-Fib); 4F without insulin (-Ins); 4F without transferrin (-Tf); and 4F without hydrocortisone (-HC).

Granulosa cell functioning in serum-free and serum-containing media

Having long-term cultures of granulosa cells in defined medium, we were now able to study the expression of the cells' specific differentiated functions *in vitro*. Other groups have previously encountered difficulties in demonstrating follitropin (FSH) induced functions in isolated rat granulosa cells cultured in medium con-

277

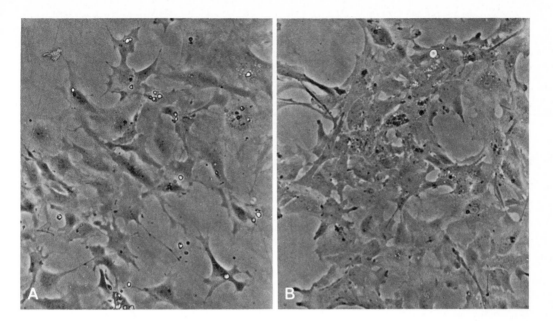

Fig. 2. Phase-contrast micrographs of 4 day granulosa cells cultured in 4F medium (A) or medium containing 5% serum (B)

taining serum (9-11). We therefore assayed three major responses to FSH in cells grown either in the presence of serum or, alternatively, grown in serum-free 4F medium:

(a) Progestin production: The primary response of the granulosa cells to FSH is expressed in progestin production. Progesterone and progesterone-reduce metabolites (mainly dihydroprogesterone, 20α-OH-P) are secreted into the culture medium and can be readily determined by specific radioimmunoassay (RIA). Serum remarkably inhibited (92%) the FSH induced progestin production as compared with cell responsiveness in 4F medium (Fig. 3). Addition of the four factors to the serum-containing medium did not restore the FSH stimulation of the steroid formation. However, the factors were an absolute requirement for the cells' responsiveness in serum-free medium. Examination of the importance of each individual factor revealed that transferrin had no effect on steroidogenesis, whereas omission of insulin and particularly hydrocortisone resulted in significant inhibition (70%) of FSH-induced progestin production.

A more detailed study of serum inhibitory effect on progestin production revealed that as low as 0.2% of serum in the culture medium was sufficient to block 90% of 20α-OH-P production induced by FSH (Fig. 4). As decreasing the serum concentration in the medium below 0.5% severely reduced the plating efficiency of the inoculated granulosa cells (Fig. 4), we conducted a control experiment in which the cells were inoculated also onto plastic substratum that had been pretreated with

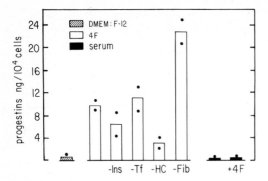

Fig. 3. Effect of serum and 4F medium on FSH induced progestin production. Cells (9.3 x 10^4) were cultured with FSH (50 ng/ml) in DMEM:F-12 medium alone, 4F medium (4F) or serum (5%) as indicated. Factors were added or deleted from the media as indicated. After a 2 day incubation, the progestin content in the medium was measured by RIA. Cells incubated in 4F medium *without FSH* did not secrete detectable amounts of progestin.

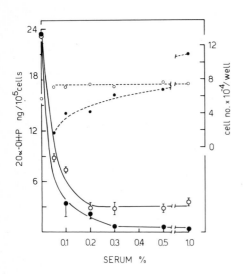

Fig. 4. Dose-dependent inhibition of serum on FSH induced steroidogenesis. Cells (7 x 10^4) were inoculated into DMEM:F-12 medium containing graded doses of serum (horse serum:fetal calf serum, 2:1 respectively). A similar inoculation was performed also into wells (d = 1.6 cm, 24 wells/plate) which had been precoated (7) with 3 μg human fibronectin. After 48 hours of incubation with FSH (100 ng/ml), the culture media were collected for steroid RIA (●-● and o-o symbols represent naked or fibronectin-coated substrate, respectively) and cell number was determined (7) after trypsinization (●---● and ó---o symbols represent with or without fibronectin, respectively).

fibronectin. On such a fibronectin 'carpet' the cells exhibited improved growth properties and high cell counts uniformly independent of the serum concentration. Nevertheless, the presence of fibronectin clearly did not alter the inhibitory effect of serum on the cell function, thus ruling out the possibility that the weak responsiveness of the cells at low serum concentrations results from physiologically incompatible growth conditions.

(b) FSH-induced estrogen formation: An advanced step during the course of the differentiation process in granulosa cells involves the FSH induction of estrogen production. Although it is well established that FSH induces aromatase activity in granulosa cells cultured in serum-free medium (12, 13), the effect of serum on the induction of this enzyme complex has not been examined. Figure 5 (1) shows that after priming the cells for two days in 4F medium containing FSH, the cells converted substantial amounts of exogenously added androgen into estrogen. In contrast, when cells were primed with FSH in the presence of serum, little, if any, of the estrogen was produced during the subsequent incubation of the cells with androgen (Fig. 5C).

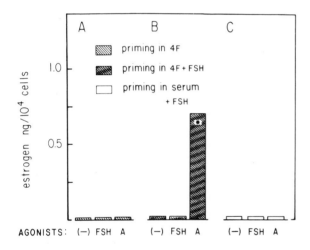

Fig. 5. Effect of serum on the FSH induction of aromatase activity. Cells (1.3 x 10⁵) were primed for two days under the following conditions: (A) 4F medium only; (B) 4F medium containing FSH; (C) serum containing medium with FSH. At the end of the incubation period all the cultures were washed and further incubated in 4F medium containing the indicated additions: no additions (-); FSH (FSH); androstenedione, 10^{-6} M (A). After 48 hours of incubation, the media were collected and 17β-estradiol was determined by RIA. The need for addition of exogenous androgen (androstenedione) as aromatase substrate is due to the inability of the rat granulosa cells to produce androgens from progesterone.

(c) Serum inhibits FSH induction of LH receptors: Previous studies have shown that in response to an *in vivo* administration of FSH, the granulosa cells developed receptors for lutropin (14, 15). As a result of the FSH induction of LH receptors, the granulosa cells acquire competence to undergo their last step of differentiation in response to the pre-ovulatory surge of LH. However, attempts to mimic FSH induction of LH receptors in isolated granulosa cells failed, apparently due to the presence of serum in the culture medium (9, 10).

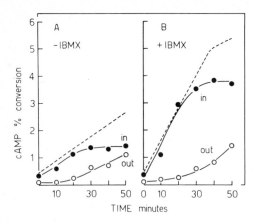

Fig. 6. Time dependent accumulation of cAMP in response to FSH. One day old granulosa cell monolayers (8 x 10^4 cells/well) were incubated in 0.2 ml of 4F medium containing 2 μCi of [^{3}H]adenine. After 2 hours of incubation, the monolayers were washed and further incubated in 4F medium containing FSH (100 ng/ml) with (A) or without (B) 0.5 mM IBMX. At the indicated time points, the culture media were removed from duplicate wells and the cells were lysed by addition of 0.3 ml ethanol solution (70%) and 0.2 ml 'stop solution' (16). The [^{3}H]cAMP content released from the lysed cells (in) and the cyclic nucleotide that spontaneously leaked into the culture medium during the incubation periods (out) were determined using sequential chromatography on Dowex AG 50W-X4 and aluminum oxide columns, as previously described (16). The counts corresponding to purified [^{3}H]cAMP were normalized when expressed as percentage of conversion of total intracellular tritium cpm to [^{3}H]cAMP (% conversion).

As both FSH and LH are accepted to trigger steroidogenesis via cAMP as a second messenger, we chose to demonstrate the serum inhibitory effect on the induction of LH receptors by measuring the ability of newly appeared LH receptors to activate the adenylate cyclase in the intact cells. By doing so, we studied functioning and hence physiologically relevant receptors, rather than estimating number of LH receptors by direct [^{125}I]hCG binding assay. For study of adenylate cyclase in intact cells, we incubated the cell monolayers with [^{3}H]adenine which was rapidly incorporated into intracellular [^{3}H]ATP (16, 17). Consequently, in the presence of adenylate cyclase agonist, the cellular [^{3}H]ATP was readily converted into [^{3}H]cAMP, the content of which was assessed as described under the legend to Fig. 6. This method was found more accurate, highly sensitive, inexpensive, and much less tedious than the one using RIA for cAMP determinations. Fig. 6 demonstrates a time-dependent accumulation of cAMP in granulosa cells responding to FSH. Maximal cAMP production is obviously monitored in the presence of a phosphodiesterase (PDE) inhibitor, 3-isobutyl-1-methyl xanthine (IBMX). This experiment also indicates that within the first 30-40 minutes of incubation, the majority of the generated cAMP stays inside the cell and does not leak out.

We now studied the inhibitory effect of serum on the formation of functional LH receptors. For that purpose we primed the cells for two days with (or without) FSH, prior to adenylate cyclase assay itself, which was carried out in 4F medium and in

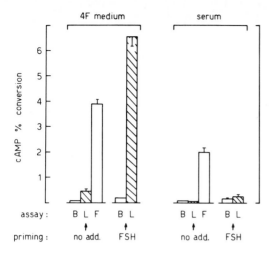

Fig. 7. Failure of FSH to induce LH receptors in the presence of serum. One day old granulosa cells (8 x 10^4 well) were primed for two days in either 4F medium or medium containing 5% serum (horse:fetal calf sera, 2:1, respectively) in the absence (no add.) or the presence of FSH (FSH). Prior to adenylate cyclase assay, the cells were labeled with [^{3}H]adenine (see legend to Fig. 6). After thorough washings, all the cells were further incubated in 4F medium without additions (B = basal) or in the presence of 100 ng/ml LH (L) or 100 ng/ml FSH (F). After 40 minutes of incubation at 37°C, 0.2 ml of ethanol solution and 0.3 ml of 'stop solution' were added to each dish, and the total (inside + outside the cells) content of [^{3}H]cAMP was assessed and expressed as percentage of conversion, as described in the legend to Fig. 6.

the presence of IBMX to reflect maximal adenylate cyclase capacity. Fig. 7 shows that in 4F medium, little but significant amount of cAMP was generated in the presence of LH (four-fold over basal), even without priming with FSH. However, after two days of priming with FSH in 4F medium, LH caused a drmatic 32-fold increase in intracellular cAMP levels accumulated during 40 minutes of incubation with the gonadotropin. In striking contrast, when the priming period with FSH was conducted in the presence of serum, LH totally failed to cause any significant rise in cAMP formation, thus reflecting the severe serum impairment of the hormonally induced expression of LH receptors. In summary, these results are in agreement with previous studies of Erickson *et al.* showing successful induction of LH and prolactin receptors when the granulosa cells were primed with FSH in McCoy's 5a culture medium without serum (11, 18).

Serum inhibition of hormonal response: Search for mechanism of action

In recent years, a large body of evidence was presented to support the general concept that cAMP regulates the entire differentiation process of ovarian granulosa cells. Thus, it has been shown that progestin production (19), induction of LH receptors (20, 21), and expression of aromatase activity (22), are all FSH-induced responses mediated by cAMP. Therefore, it seemed reasonable to test whether serum impairs the accumulation of intracellular cAMP triggered by FSH. Table 1 summarizes a typical experiment in which two groups of granulosa cells were grown for 36 hours

282

Table 1. EFFECT OF SERUM ON FSH-INDUCED cAMP ACCUMULATION

Growth period[1]	Culture medium with FSH[2]	PDE inhibitor[3]	Purified [3H]cAMP[4] cpm per dish	Relative accumulation
4F medium	4F medium	-IBMX	4500	17
		+IBMX	8100	
	5% serum	-IBMX	1100	
		+ IBMX	3400	
5% serum	4F medium	-IBMX	700	
		+IBMX	4000	
	5% serum	-IBMX	270	1
		+IBMX	2500	9

1 Cells (2 x 10⁵/35 mm dish) were grown for 36 hours in either 4F medium or medium containing 5% serum, prior to labeling with [3H]adenine, as described in the legend to Fig. 6.

2 After washing, the cells were incubated for 45 minutes at 37°C with 100 ng/ml FSH in either 4F medium or serum-containing medium.

3 IBMX (0.5 mM) was included or omitted from the culture medium.

4 [3H]cAMP was recovered from the lysed cells and its content assessed, as described in the legend to Fig. 7. Each experimental variation represents the mean of duplicate dishes.

in the presence or absence of serum. After labeling with [3H]-adenine, the cells were challenged with FSH while bathing in either 4F medium or serum-containing medium, in the presence or absence of IBMX. It is evident that in the absence of IBMX, cells grown and challenged with FSH in 4F medium accumulated 17-fold higher levels of cAMP when compared with cells maintained in serum containing medium. However, addition of IBMX to these very cells held in serum, remarkably caused a 9-fold increment in the cyclic nucleotide levels produced in response to FSH. This clearly ruled out the possibility that serum severely alters the gonadotropin interaction with its receptors or that it impairs the hormone induced activation of the adenylate cyclase. Alternatively, these findings suggest that the serum apparently *activates a phosphodiesterase* enzyme which rapidly degrades the intracellular pool of cAMP.

An additional clue for the possible involvement of phosphodiesterase in the regulation of the granulosa cell function originated from studies we recently carried out in trial to correlate the responsiveness of the granulosa cells in steroid production with their ability to accumulate cAMP during growth in culture. Fig. 8 represents a time-dependent responsiveness of granulosa cells to FSH in both ste-

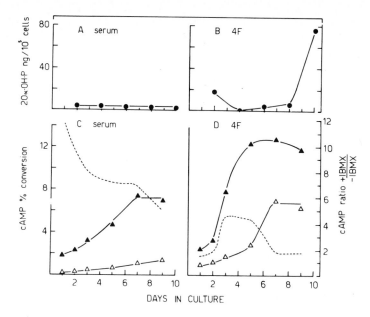

<u>Fig. 8</u>. Hormonal responsiveness of granulosa cells in steroid formation. Cells
(8 x 10⁴/well) were cultured for up to 10 days in either serum containing medium
(A, C) or 4F medium (B, D). *Steroidogenesis*: The cells were exposed to 100 ng/ml
FSH for 48 hour periods. For example, time point on day 6 means that the FSH was added to duplicate wells on day 4. After 48 hours of incubation, the steroid content in
the medium was assayed by RIA (●-●) and the cells were trypsinized and counted.
Cyclic AMP accumulation: At the days indicated, duplicate wells were preincubated
with [³H]adenine and the FSH-induced cAMP accumulation was measured after 45 minutes
(37°C) of incubation with (▲-▲) or without (Δ-Δ) 0.5 mM IBMX. The [³H]cAMP content
was assayed as described in the legend to Fig. 7. The calculated ratio of cAMP content accumulated in the presence of IBMX and in the absence of the PDE inhibitor is
illustrated by the dashed lines (---).

roidogenesis (panels A and B) and cAMP accumulation (panels C and D). Steroid
measurements indicate that serum completely inhibited the steroid production
throughout the 10 day period in culture. In contrast, the cells responded to FSH
in 4F medium but, surprisingly enough, temporarily lost their responsiveness during
days 4-8 *in vitro* (23). However, after 10 days or more, the cells regained their
ability to produce large amounts of dihydroprogesterone.

When cAMP formation in the intact cells was monitored throughout 10 days in
culture, it was evident that much less cAMP accumulated in the cells cultured in
serum (panel C) as compared with the nucleotide content in cells grown in 4F medium
(panel D). Again, this remarkable difference was much diminished if a PDE inhibitor
was included in the assay medium. A calculated ratio between cAMP content accumulated in the presence of IBMX and in the absence of the inhibitor, provided us with
an indirect measure of the phosphodiesterase activity in the cells grown under the
two culture conditions. Thus, while the cells inoculated into 4F medium responded
satisfactorily in steroidogenesis during the first two days in culture and respec-

tively exhibited 'low' PDE activity (ratio of 2), those grown in serum containing medium showed a 'high' phosphodiesterase activity (ratio of 12, panel C), which may explain the cells' failure to accumulate cAMP and, consequently, to trigger steroido-genesis.

We are currently seeking a direct assay of phosphodiesterase activity in intact cells as well as in cell-free lysates which, hopefully, will help us to assess the possible role of PDE in the regulation of the ovarian cell responsiveness to hormones.

ACKNOWLEDGMENT

We thank Dr. F. Kohen from The Weizmann Institute of Science, Rehovot, Israel, for generously providing us with the 20α-OH-P antiserum. We are also grateful to Ms. Edith Dicker for her excellent editorial and secretarial assistance.

This work was supported by the United States-Israel Binational Science Foundation Grant # 2656/71, and by the Bat-Sheva Fund for the Encouragement of Science and Technology.

REFERENCES

1. Coon, H.G. (1966) Proc. Natl. Acad. Sci. USA 55, 66-73.
2. Seeds, N., Gilman, A., Amano, J. and Nirenberg, M. (1970) Proc. Natl. Acad. Sci. USA 66, 160-167.
3. Bottenstein, J.E. and Sato, G.H. (1979) Proc. Natl. Acad. Sci. USA 76, 514-517.
4. Darmon, M., Bottenstein, J. and Sato, G. (1981) Develop. Biol. 85, 463-473.
5. Darmon, M., Stallcup, W. and Pittman, Q. (1982) Exp. Cell Res. 138, 73-78.
6. Yaffe, D. and Saxel, O. (1977) Differentiation 7, 159-166.
7. Orly, J., Sato, G.H. and Erickson, G.F. (1980) Cell 20, 817-827.
8. Ruoslahti, E., Vuento, M. and Engvall, E. (1970) Biochim. Biophys. Acta 534, 210-218.
9. Nimrod, A., Tsafriri, A. and Lindner, H.R. (1977) Nature 267, 632-633.
10. Hiller, S.G., Zeleznik, A.J. and Ross, G.T. (1978) Endocrinology 102, 937-946.
11. Erickson, G.F., Wang, C. and Hsueh, A.J. (1979) Nature 279, 336-338.
12. Dorrington, J.H., Moon, Y.S. and Armstrong, D.J. (1975) Endocrinology 97, 1328--1331.
13. Erickson, G.F. and Hsueh, A.J.W. (1978) Endocrinology 102, 1275-1282.
14. Zeleznik, A.J., Midgley, A.R., Jr. and Reichert, L.E., Jr. (1974) Endocrinology 95, 818-826.
15. Richards, J.S., Ireland, J.T., Rao, M.C., Bernath, G.A., Midgley, A.R., Jr. and Reichert, L.E., Jr. (1976) Endocrinology 99, 1562-1570.
16. Schulster, D., Orly, J., Seidel, G. and Schramm, M. (1978) J. Biol. Chem. 253, 1201-1206.
17. Humes, J.L., Rounbehler, M. and Kuehl, F. (1969) Anal. Biochem. 32, 210-217.
18. Wang, C., Hsueh, A.J.W. and Erickson, G.F. (1979) J. Biol. Chem. 254, 11330--11336.
19. Channing, C.P. and Seymour, J.F. (1970) Endocrinology 87, 165-169.
20. Nimrod, A. (1981) FEBS Lett. 131, 31-33.
21. Knecht, M., Amsterdam, A. and Catt, K. (1981) J. Biol. Chem. 256, 10628-10633.
22. Hsueh, A.J.W., Wang, C. and Erickson, G.F. (1980) Endocrinology 106, 1697-1705.
23. Orly, J., Farkash, Y., Hershkovits, N., Mizrahi, L. and Weinberger, P. (1982) In Vitro, in press.

Control of Normal Phenotype and of Thyroid Differentiated Functions in the Epithelial Cell Strain FRTL

D. Tramontano, R. Picone, and F. S. Ambesi-Impiombato
C. E. O. S., c/o Istituto di Patologia Generale, Via S. Pansini, 5; I-80131 Napoli, Italy

The thyroid gland and its functional unit, the thyroid follicle plays a very important and central role in the endocrine system. Controlled by the pituitary gland via the hormone thyrotropin (TSH), the thyroid then controls virtually every cell in the body via the production and secretion of the thyroid hormones T_3 and T_4 (1).

Apart form the calcitonin, produced by the interstitial or 'C' cells, all the differentiated functions of the gland depend from the specialized activity of one single epithelial cell type, the thyroid follicular cell. Both morphologically and functionally very differentiated, this cell posesses several unique characteristics, such as thyroglobulin (Tg) synthesis and I^- trapping, not expressed by any other cell of the organism.

The availability of such cell type adapted to continuous growth in vitro while maintaining its normal and differentiated characteristics has been made possible by the approach here described. It consists of substituting - totally or partially - the animal serum added to culture media with a mixture of several hormones and growth factors. The animal serum was considered until a few years ago a supplement necessary to all synthetic media which were designed to support survival and growth of isolated cells. Its usefulness obviously meant that some important components - other than the minerals, salts, vitamins, essential and non-essential aminoacids which were provided - were still missing from media formulations, even the most rich and complex ones.

The assumption was made that hormones could be the most important missing components in tissue culture media (2). Hormonal requirements were at least partially fulfilled by the addition of serum to cell cultures, but specific cell types could need different hormones. At the light of these considerations, the fact that only mesenchimal (less differentiated) or transformed cells were adapted to grow in vitro could be easily explained. A rapid survey of the cell lines or strains grown in long-term culture to date (3) easily indicate that even presently almost all those cultures are of either mesenchimal or tumor origins, or both. Alternatively, several cultured cells have been transformed in vitro by chemical, viral or - in the case of the so-called 'spontaneous transformants'- by unknown agents or mutational events, and thus adapted to long-term culture as permanent cell lines.

The approach here described, i.e. to define in vitro the hormonal requirements for the very specialized thyroid cell, lead to the establishment of the strain of epithelial, differentiated follicular cells from adult rat thyroids, named FRTL (Fischer Rat Thyroid, Low-serum cells)(4). This strain may be cultured, whenever necessary, even in the absence of serum (chemically defined medium). Thyroid-specific functions such as TSH-dependence, synthesis and membranes-interactions of thyroglobulin, and iodide metabolism are now studied in vitro.

DEVELOPMENT OF THE SYSTEM

Thyroid primary cultures were started from 5-6 weeks old Fischer rats. The choice of the animal species and strain was motivated from our previous work, recently described (5) on the culture of experimental, transplantable rat thyroid tumors (FR-A, 1-5G).

Enzymatic dissociation of the glands was performed with a mixture of Collagenase, Trypsin, Chicken serum (CTC) (6) as already described (4). Primary cultures, when observed in phase-contrast microscopy, consisted of almost pure populations of epithelial cells (follicular cells) typically estimated >90% of the total cells within the first 2-3 days of culture. Later, the use of serum-free or low-serum (0.5% or less) media was critical in preventing fibroblasts from overgrowing the epithelial cells. In higher (5-10%) serum concentrations this would inevitably occur within 4-7 days of culture in higher (5-10%) serum concentrations.

Epithelial cell growth on the other hand, was only obtained - irrespective of the absence or the presence of serum (at any concentration) - when certain hormones and growth factors were added. The best conditions were found to be a combination of a low concentration of serum (0.5%) and 6 hormones and growth factors (6H)(4).In this hormonally defined medium, specific growth of follicular rat thyroid cells could be readily observed in virtually every epithelial colony and cells can be passed, apparently indefinitely. A cell strain (FRTL) has been continuously cultured for more than 5 years at the time of writing, without any apparent 'crysis' period or 'aging' in vitro.It was soon found that not all the hormones were equally important within the 6H mixture, but while some were essential, some were only required in diluite (cloning) conditions (Table I). The low concentration of serum has been routinely used thereafter to increase plating efficiency, but did not affect cell growth significantly. For this reason, serum could be withdrawn during some critical experiments (4) and cells could be grown in its absence.

FRTL cells are characterized by a very slow growth rate, when compared to other cultured cells. Their population doubling time is between 4 and 6 days, in the best conditions. Even at this rate, however, we can estimate that FRTL cells have undergone at least 300 cell generations in culture. This number is of course well beyond the 50 generations limit which has been indicated by Hayflick (7) as the limit for normal cells in culture. The Hayflick limit however has been shown mainly on human skin fibroblasts, and it is our opinion that more long-term cultures of normal and differentiated cell types will be necessary to further define this point. In particular, the limited growth potential of cultured normal cells could be very well due to scarcity of some nutrient supplied with the medium. In the meanwhile, growth beyond the 50 generation limit should not be considered a criterion sufficient by itself to classify those cells as abnormal.

TABLE   I

REQUIREMENTS FOR HORMONES AND GROWTH FACTORS OF FRTL/FRTL5 STRAINS

Hormones	Essential	Less essential*
Thyrotropin	+	
Insulin	+	
Transferrin	+	
Hydrocortisone		+
Somatostatin		+
Glycyl-L-histidyl-L-lysine		+

* Less essential hormones are necessary expecially when cells are plated very diluted.

The possibility existed that FRTL cells continued to behave like normal and differentiated cells after years of continuous culture because of their peculiar slow growth rate. This possibility could be ruled out when a substrain of fast-growing cells (FRTL-5) has been obtained by adapting FRTL cells to grow in a higher (5%) serum concentration (8).FRTL-5 cells can be considered equal to FRTL cells in all their normal and differentiated characteristics, only their population doubling time is 31 hrs, i.e. approximately 4 times less than that of FRTL cells. As a consequence, it can be easily calculated that FRTL-5 cells undergo at least 250 duplications per year.

CHARACTERIZATION OF THE SYSTEM

During the long-term cultures of FRTL and FRTL-5 cells, several parameters have been checked periodically to monitor both the absence of malignancy and the maintenance of thyroid differentiation in the cell populations.

Chriteria of normality

Both FRTL and FRTL-5 cells have a normal chromosomes complement. The chromosome number is periodically checked and occasionally subclones (spontaneous transformants?) have been spotted and eliminated. It is conceivable that, particularly in a fast-growing cell population in vitro, DNA duplication or mitotic errors could occasionally give rise to faster-growing variant clones, with quantitative and/or quantitative chromosomes abnormalities. Those - among these variants - possessing a strong selective advantage could easily overgrow and take over normal population within a few passages. In vivo, the immunological surveillance theory would predict that such variants would be, in the vast majority of the cases, immediately spotted and rejected by the organism because of their novel antigenic determinants.

To maintain cells normal in long-term cultures in vitro we use the strategy of keeping parallel cultures of different sub-strains, periodically (i.e. once a year) checking the kariotype of each subclone. If any abnormality is found in a subclone, this can be easily eliminated. We found this strategy more practical than other methods, widely used in cell cultures, such as periodically cloning the cell population, or keeping frozen stocks of well-characterized cells in liquid nitrogen - both unpractical with slow-growing cells which require some time for cloning or thawing.

Besides chromosomes characterization, other parameters are occasionally checked to determine the normal phenotype of FRTL-FRTL5 cells. These include clonal growth in agarose, growth after injection in syngeneic animals, and of course microscopic scanning for morphological and growth abnormalities - all absent in the cell populations.

Effects of TSH

TSH effects on the thyroid cell in vivo have been difficult to specify at a biochemical level. Isolated, in vitro cultured cells could provide a clean experimental system to address this question. A direct mitogenic action on follicular cells has been questioned, and denied by some Authors (9) using primary cultures derived from human adenomas. In our rat system, derived from normal thyroids, FRTL/FRTL5 cells require continuous presence of TSH for growth. This is also in agreement with results recently obtained by other Authors on primary rat thyroid

follicles grown in suspension cultures, where pure preparations of TSH are clearly
mytogenic(10). In our cell strains several hormone preparations, with different
purity, gave identical results. Preparations provided from the National Pituitary
and Hormones Agency (NPA,NIH) with a high degree of purity (21 I.U./mg) have been
used routinely. Even FRTL-5 cells, despite the higher concentration of serum in the
culture medium, still show absolute requirement for the hormones, particularly TSH.
Cells survive for several days, or even weeks without TSH but never divide except
when TSH is readded (Fig.1) Specific aspects of the mechanisms of hormones action at
a subcellular and molecular level have been investigated. These include receptor
clustering and TSH internalization (11), the role of cyclic-AMP in modulating both
TSH receptor clustering and intracellular hormone response (12). Also the
morphological changes occurring during TSH withdrawal (Fig.1) have been found to be
due to rearrangements in the cell cytoskeleton, namely in the microfilament
component (13).

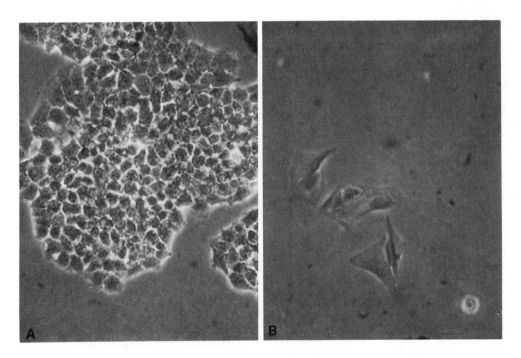

Fig 1. Phase-contrast microphotographs of FRTL5 cells: A - In complete
medium; B - After 10 days in medium plus 5H (lacking TSH) at the same
enlargement.

Synthesis of thyroglobulin

Thyroglobulin (Tg), the unique glycoprotein produced by the thyroid follicular
cell, is a very large protein (660.000 Daltons) synthetized apparently in subunits

of 330.000 Daltons. Although not being a hormone itself, Tg represents the precursor and the storage of the real thyroid hormones, T_3 and T_4 (1). These are synthetized and iodinated on its primary structure. Both FRTL and FRTL5 cells synthetize and secrete Tg in the medium.

This has been first demonstrated by radioimmunoassay for rat Tg on the culture medium from FRTL cells (4). In addition, after labeling with ^{35}S-methionine a radioactive protein band of approx. 330.000 Daltons can be seen in both cell extract and medium, in SDS-polyacrylamide gel electrophoresis under denaturing and reducing conditions. This protein band is immunoprecipitated by purified anti-rat Tg antibodies and displaced by an excess of cold rat Tg (Fig.2).

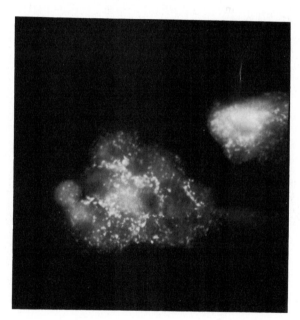

Fig. 2

Fig. 3

Fig. 2. Fluorography of SDS-polyacrilamide (6.5%) gel electrophoresis of FRTL5 culture medium after a 24 hrs labeling with ^{35}S-methionine to evidentiate secreted proteins. Lane 1: Total culture medium; Lane 2: Immunoprecipitation with purified anti-Tg antibodies; Lane 3: Immunoprecipitation with non-specific serum.

Fig. 3. Fluorescence microphotograph of FRTL5 cells treated with purified anti-Tg antibodies and stained with fluoresceine-conjugated goat-anti-rabbit antibodies (sandwich technique). The presence of Tg is clearly evident at the cell surface.

Morphological evidence of the presence of Tg on the surface of the cells can be obtained by immunofluorescence. In a double-antibody assay, fluorescent goat anti-rabbit IgG evidentiate the antigen (Tg) present at the cell surface (Fig.3). Incubations with both first and second antibody were performed on live cells, prior to fixation to evidentiate only surface antigens.

Iodide metabolism

The iodide ion metabolism represents a very specialized function within the thyroid follicle. By active transport, the follicular cell is able to concentrate severalfolds the iodide, a rare ion, from plasma and extracellular fluids. Freshly isolated thyroid cells maintain their iodide trapping ability as demonstrated many years ago by Tong (14). In the intact gland, iodide is organified and the Tg molecule is iodinated at the apical border of the follicular cell, towards and/or - according to some Authors - inside the follicular lumen (15). In monolayer cultures of differentiated cells (FRTL-FRTL5) iodide trapping is very well preserved. After 15 min. of incubation with ^{125}I the C/M ratio (cpm/mg cells vs. cpm/ul medium) reached values between 50 and 100 (i.e. intracellular concentration of I^- between 50 and 100 times higher than the extracellular concentration. Absence of other cell types, connective, vascular tisue, etc. account for these values, even higher than those obtained in vivo. Organification, on the contrary is unefficient, around 2-3%. This is probably due to the absence of the threedimensional follicular structure. It is conceivable that, if Tg is iodinated during or even after its secretion in the lumen in vivo, low iodination should occur in vitro where the newly synthetized Tg is immediately dispersed in the culture medium.

DISCUSSION

Understanding the requirements of differentiated and normal cells dissociated by and kept isolated from the rest of the organism, could be the only means of obtaining in vitro populations of cells stimulated to proliferate but otherwise 'normal' and certainly non-malignant.

This could lead us to find previously unknown cell-cell messages and biochemical signals which could not be evidentiated in the intact animal.

Particularly, the period of primary and early cultures seems extremely critical in obtaining, in the absence of animal serum or unphysiological stimuli, the adaptation of normal and differentiated cells to survival and growth in vitro without fibroblast overgrowth. Once this has been obtained, serum can be additioned to cultures in vitro, even at high concentrations (5% in the case of FRTL5 cells) affecting their proliferation rate but not their normal and differentiated phenotype. At this stage, because all mesenchimal cells have been eliminated by repeated subculturing and/or cloning, overgrowth of contaminant cells is impossible.

FRTL/FRTL5 cells seem capable of indefinite proliferation in vivo, and no signs of senescence have been detected. More cell strains from different organs and animal species are needed to define whether this unlimited growth ability is a peculiarity of rat thyroid cells or this ability is rather shared by other cell types. On the other hand, the limited proliferation in vitro may be due either to intrinsic characteristics of the cell, or to qualitative or quantitative deficiencies in the culture media.

The phenomenon of spontaneous mutational events in a long-term growing cell population must be recognised and taken into account. In the absence of an immune system, our strategy of keeping and periodically checking parallel cultures of separate sublines has proven so far succesful in keeping long-term cultures of normal and fully differentiated thyroid follicular cells.

These results demonstrate that differentiated, normal endocrine cells like FRTL/FRTL5 strains can be used as an effective tool in studying thyroid biology and regulation in vitro, and in understanding structure – function relationships within the thyroid follicle.

AKNOWLEDGMENTS

NIH-bTSH-9 was kindly provided, free of charge, from National Pituitary Agency. We are grateful to Mr. Michele Mastrocinque for skilful technical assistance. This work was partially supported by the NIH Grant 1 RO1 AM21689-03.

REFERENCES

1 - Wollman, S.H. in: Lysosomes in biology and pathology, 2, Dingle, J.T. and Fell, H.B. eds. pp. 483-512. North-Holland Publishing Co., Amsterdam, 1969.

2 - Sato, G.H. in: Biochemical Actions of Hormones, Litwack, G. ed., pp. 391-409, Academic Press, N.Y., 1975.

3 - American Type Culture Collection Catalogue of Strains II, Third Edition, 1981.

4 - Ambesi-Impiombato, F.S.,.Parks, L.A.M., and Coon, H.G.: Proc. Natl. Acad. Sci. USA 77, 3455-3459, 1980.

5 - Ambesi-Impiombato, F.S., Tramontano, D., and Coon, H.G. in: Advances in thyroid neoplasia, pp. 83-93, Andreoli, M. ed., Raven Press, N.Y., 1981.

6 - Coon, H.G.: Proc. Natl. Acad. Sci. USA 55, 66-73, 1966.

7 - Hayflick, L., and Moorehead, P.S.: Exp. Cell Res., 25, 585, 1961.

8 - Ambesi-Impiombato, F.S., Picone, R., and Tramontano, D. in: Growth of cells in hormonally defined media. CSH Conferences on Cell Proliferation 9, Sirbasku, D.A. et al. eds. CSH Press, N.Y., 1982 in press.

9 - Westermark, B., Karlsson, F.A. and Walinder, O.: Proc. Natl. Acad. Sci. USA 76, 2022-2026, 1979.

10 - Nitsch, L., and Wollman, S.H.: Proc. Natl. Acad. Sci. USA 77, 2743-2747, 1980

11 - Avivi, A., Tramontano, D., Ambesi-Impiombato, F.S. and Schlessinger, J.: Molec. Cell. Endocrinol. 25, 55-71, 1982.

12 - Avivi, A., Tramontano, D., Ambesi-Impiombato, F.S., and Schlessinger, J.: Science 214, 1237-1239, 1981.

13 - Tramontano, D., Avivi, A., Ambesi-Impiombato, F.S., Barak, L., Geiger, B., and Schlessinger, J.: Exp. Cell Res. 137, 269-275, 1982.

14 - Tong, W.: in Methods Enzymol. 32, 745-758, 1974.

15 - Ekholm, R., and Wollman, S.H.: Endocrinology 97, pp. 1432-1444, 1975.

Butyrate-Induced Growth Arrest of GH₃-Cells is not Linked to a Distinct Morphological Phenotype

Georg Tschank and Gerd Brunner

Institut für Immunologie der Johannes Gutenberg Universität, Obere Zahlbacher Str. 67, D-6500 Mainz, FRG

N-butyric acid is known to be a potent proliferation-inhibitor of a great number of cell types, both normal and neoplastic (1). In many cases growth arrest is accompanied by striking changes in morphology, e.g. formation of cell processes or increased spreading (1). These changes can be traced back to altered glycolipide and glycoprotein patterns of the plasma membrane and to a reorganization of the cytoskeleton (2, 3).

The aim of the work presented here was to look whether there is any correlation between cell morphology and growth inhibition. As a model system we chose the GH₃-cell line, a tumor cell line of rat pituitary origin (4). The cells were grown in F12/DMEM as basal medium that was supplemented either with 8 % newborn calf serum or with a mixture of insulin (5 g/ml), transferrin (5 g/ml), T₃ (100 pM), TRF (1 ng/ml), FGF (10 ng/ml), MSA (1 ng/ml). All factors were obtained from Sigma, except FGF and MSA (both from Collaborative Research). During all experiments plating density was

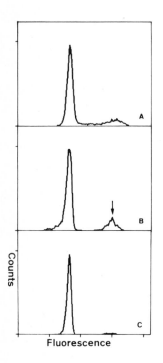

Fig. 1. FCM-analysis of cell cycle distribution of GH₃-cells cultivated in the presence of 0.75 mM n-butyrate.
A - exponential culture
B - 48 hrs after addition of blocker
C - 65 hrs after addition of butyrate
Arrow in B indicates G₂/M compartment.

1×10^5 cells per cm^2 on 35 mm tissue culture dishes (Costar). Proliferation in the above serum-free medium was about 60 % of the serum control, as measured by counting the cells after six days in culture. If the cells were incubated with n-butyrate (0.75 mM) for 65 hours -regardless whether they were grown in serum-containing or in factor-supplemented medium - they accumulated in the G_1-compartment of the cell cycle (90 %), whereby a transient increase in the percentage of cells in G_2/M occurred (Fig. 1B, see arrow). Autoradiographic and cytofluorometric measurements showed that the cells had identical accumulation kinetics under both culture conditions (5). G_1-arrested cells could be restimulated by washing them in fresh medium and replating in butyrate-free medium (data not shown). Cell cycle kinetics are independent of the culture conditions, whereas the morphological behaviour is not. In serum-supplemented medium GH_3-cells grow adherent to the substratum (80%) or are freely suspended as small aggregates in the medium (20 %) (Fig. 2A.

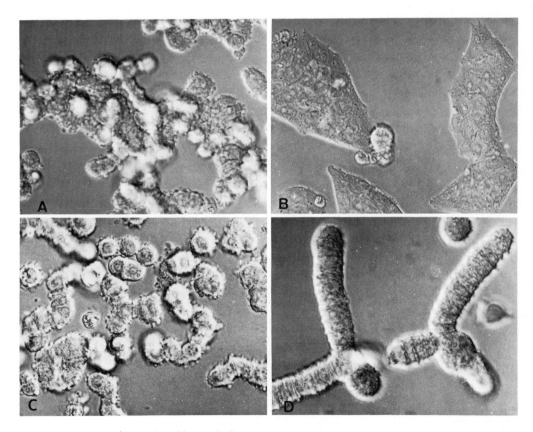

Fig. 2. Butyrate-induced cell morphology

A: GH$_3$-cells grown for 65 h in F12/DMEM, containing 8 % newborn calf serum

B: same as in A, but in the presence of 0.75 mM n-butyrate

C: GH$_3$-cells grown for 65 h in serum-free medium (see text)

D: same as in C, but in the presence of 0.75 mM n-butyrate

This growth pattern is not yet well understood. Possible explanations may be the shedding of mitotic cells, followed by aggregation and growth of these cells and/ or by the existence of subpopulations differing in their attachment behaviour.

In serum-free medium the cells are only loosely attached to the culture dish and the number of floating aggregates is greatly increased as compared with cultures grow: in the presence of serum (Fig. 2C). In the presence of n-butyrate (0.75 mM) GH₃-cells undergo remarkable morphological changes depending on the supplementation of the basal medium. Butyrate-induced cells grown in F12/DMEM containing 8 % serum cease to grow into the "third dimension" - no aggregates. This is not caused by selective death of floating cells (data not shown). The cells are well spread and form typical clusters (Fig. 2B). The number of surface protuberances is greatly decreased. In serum-free medium no spreading is induced. The cells remain loosely attached but tend to form yeast-like cell rods (Fig. 2D). The number of blebs is unaltered compared to controls (Fig. 2C).

This shift in morphology increases with time and is completed after 48 hours. It can be reversed when the blocker is withdrawn. In a preliminary study SDS-polyacryl-amide gel patterns of ^{35}S-labeled proteins from GH₃-cells, grown in serum-supplemented medium in the presence of butyrate, were compared with the patterns of untreated cultures (Fig. 3). Differences were found in both the nuclear and cytoplasmic compartmen especially in the 50 - 30 kD region of the gels. It is not yet clear whether these differences are due to induction by butyrate or are caused by the synchronization of the cells in G_1 (G_1-specific proteins).

In summary, the data presented here show that the morphology of butyrate-synchro ized GH₃-cells is under control of the microenvironment (factor(s) present in newborn

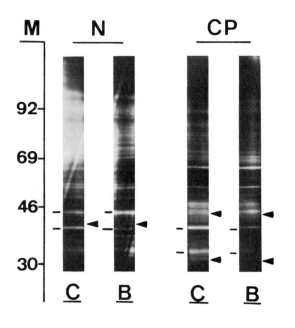

Fig. 3. SDS-PAGE of ^{35}S-labeled GH₃-proteins

C - proteins from control cultures (8 % newborn calf serum)

B - proteins from butyrate-treated cells (65 h, 0.75 mM)

N - nuclear proteins (nuclei were prepared by detergent-mediated lysis of cells)

CP- cytoplasmic proteins

For better identification of protein bands a negative image of the auto-radiograph is presented.

Bars point out quantitative differ-ences and arrows depict qualitative differences of protein patterns.

calf serum) which indicates that the changed cell shape is not the cause of growth arrest. Furthermore, it is shown that the phenotype of cells accumulated in G_1 is rather plastic and can only be described in relation to the special culture conditions.

This work was carried out in partial fulfillment of the requirements for a doctoral thesis at the University of Innsbruck, Austria (G.T.). It was supported by the Deutsche Forschungsgemeinschaft.

References

1) Prasad, K.N., Sinha, P.K. 1976. Effect of sodium butyrate on mammalian cells in culture. A review. In Vitro 12, 125 - 132.

2) Henneberry, R.C., Fishman, P.H. 1976. Morphological and biochemical differentiation in HeLa cells. Exp. Cell Res. 103, 55 - 62.

3) Hormia, M. et al. 1982. Vimentin filaments in cultured endothelial cells form butyrate-sensitive juxtanuclear masses after repeated subculture. Exp. Cell Res. 138, 159 - 166.

4) Hayashi, I., Larner, J., Sato, G. 1978. Growth control of cells in culture. In Vitro 14, 23 - 30.

5) Tschank, G., Stöhr, M., Brunner, G., in preparation.

Hemopoietic and Immune System

Human B Cell Function in 20 μl Hanging-Drop Microcultures Under Serum-Free Conditions

John Farrant[1], Christine A. Newton[1], Christine Weyman[2], Margaret North[1], and Malcolm K. Brenner[1]

[1] Division of Immunological Medicine, Clinical Research Centre, Harrow, U. K.
[2] Courtauld Institute of Biochemisty, The Middlesex Hospital Medical School, London, U. K.

Introduction

The function of human B cells in vitro has been studied by measuring the production of immunoglobulin in response to Pokeweed mitogen and the production of IgG specific antibody to tetanus toxoid in vaccinated donors.

Initial problems were threefold. The majority of vaccinated donors were non-responders for antibody production, serum introduced variability and high background levels and conventional cultures required large numbers of cells. Our approach to overcome these difficulties was as follows. A pokeweed mitogen induced factor increased the proportion of responding donors. The serum-free medium developed for mouse cell culture by Iscove and Melchers (1978) has been adapted for human B cells and finally a hanging-drop microculture system allowed many variables to be studied with small numbers of cells.

Methods

Media

The culture medium used was essentially that devised by Iscove and Melchers (1978) containing transferrin, delipidated albumin and soybean lipid. Iscove's modified Dulbecco's medium (IMDM) was prepared from powder (1 litre pack, Gibco, Cat. No. 430-2200), which was dissolved in water for injection (Antigen Ltd) in the dark and sodium bicarbonate (3.024g Analar) added. The additives transferrin (T), albumin (A) and soybean lipid (S) were prepared as previously described (Iscove and Melchers, 1978; Iscove et al, 1980),
Preparation of culture medium.

Immediately before use, penicillin/streptomycin (a final 100 I.U./ml) and L-glutamine (an extra 2mM/ml) were added to the medium now designated IMDM(U). For the completely supplemented medium IMDM(TAS), the following were added to 20ml of IMDM(U): transferrin (90mg/ml,1/3 saturated with iron, 5ul), delipidated BSA (5%, 400ul) and sonicated soybean lipid (400ul). The final concentration of transferrin was 22.5ug/ml, of BSA 2 mg/ml and of lipid 20 ug/ml, unless otherwise stated.

Cells and cultures

Mononuclear cells were obtained from defibrinated peripheral blood of exercised normal human volunteers who had been immunized with Adsorbed Tetanus Toxoid (Wellcome). The cells were prepared using Leibovitz L-15 Medium (Flow), and Ficoll-paque. Adherent cells were depleted by a 90 min incubation in a 5 cm diameter Petri dish (Nunc). T and non-T cells were obtained by a single rosetting with neuraminidase-treated sheep red blood cells (n-SRBC). After another Ficoll-paque separation the cells at the interface were removed, resuspended in IMDM(TAS) and used as the non-T preparation. T cells were prepared by lysis of the red cells in the

rosettes. When appropriate the T cells were irradiated (2000 rads). Aliquots (10ul) of twice the final required concentration of non-T cells were dispensed into Terasaki plates using a repeating Hamilton syringe . Similar aliquots of T cells were added. Finally, the stimulant was added in a 1ul aliquot,to give a final well volume of 21 ul. The cells were cultured by inverting the Terasaki plates and placing them in humidified boxes in a 5% CO_2 incubator as previously described (O'Brien et al, 1979; Farrant et al, 1980).
Stimulants
Tetanus Toxoid (TT,Wellcome) and Pokeweed mitogen (Sigma) were used. One set of grids of Terasaki wells was used for assaying production of immunoglobulin and for the measurement of specific antibody; others were used for DNA synthesis.
Assays
Immunoglobulin production was measured by a double antibody inhibition microradioimmunoassay (Newton et al, 1981). DNA synthesis was measured by the uptake of 3H-thymidine (2h pulse, 2Ci/mMole, 0.1ug total thymidine/ml) (Farrant et al, 1980). The procedure and controls for the assay for the specific antibody have been described (Brenner and Munro, 1981).
Factor Preparation.
This has been described in detail (North and Brenner, 1982). Irradiated T cells were cultured in IMDM(TAS) with autologous B cells at a ratio of 2:1 in the presence of PWM 4ug/ml. After 36hrs the cells were washed in fresh Iscove's medium, and recultured for a further 72hrs. At the end of this period the supernatants were harvested and called conditioned medium (CM).

RESULTS

Hanging Drop microcultures respond to low doses of mitogen.
On measuring DNA synthesis by the uptake of 3H-Tdr, the response of non-T cells was greatest at a PWM dose of 50 ng/ml.
Immunoglobulin production by B cells requires lipid.
When T cells are stimulated with PHA, the addition of lipid has only a small effect on DNA synthesis. When the non-T population was stimulated with PWM, and irradiated T cells used as the source of help, then thymidine incorporation was greatly reduced when soybean lipid was left out of the medium. This requirement for lipid was equally marked when mitogen induced IgG and IgM production was examined
Total Immunoglobulin production is T cell dependent.
The data also shows the T-cell dependence of IgG and IgM synthesis by PWM stimulated non-T cells. Also, unirradiated T cells can provide help, but in this system, the maximal level of Ig induced is lower, and inhibition at high T cell numbers is more marked, if the T cells are unirradiated.
Serum-free Medium supports antigen dependent IgG antibody Production.
We have previously described a system for the production of anti-tetanus antibody from human T and B cells grown in serum containing medium (Brenner and Munro,1981). The antibody produced by these cultures is almost exclusively IgG. Our data illustrates that serum free medium is also able to support specific antibody production. In the absence of T cell help no antibody was produced. As the number of irradiated T cells

added was increased, the initial help for antibody production was reversed. The data also shows that the dose of antigen affects the response, and the higher level of antibody is detected with the lower of the two antigen doses (0.005iu/ml). TT induces little change in total IgG in the same cultures, indicating that TT is not acting as a polyclonal activator of Ig production.

Antibody Production is enhanced by the addition of conditioned medium (CM).

When CM and TT are both present there is a fourfold increase in antibody levels detected with TT alone. Even in the presence of CM, the production of anti-TT antibody remains strictly T dependent. The ability to make in vitro antibody after TT stimulation, for a prolonged period (4-24 months) after immunisation, is normally shown by only 15% of donors (Brenner et al 1981). The addition of conditioned medium raises this proportion to nearly 60% (8 out of 14).

DISCUSSION

In this paper we have established reliable serum-free culture conditions for antibody production from human B cells, in the manner described for mice (Iscove and Melchers,1978). The absence of serum permits a clearer interpretation of the responses to the added stimuli of antigen or lymphokine. This serum-free medium can be used in a microculture technique (20 ul hanging drops), which allows sufficient numbers of wells within each experiment to study the interactions between variables, such as cell concentration and antigen dose. A recent paper by Tanno et al.(1982) has shown that mitogen stimulated human B cells are capable of producing immunoglobulin under serum free conditions. The serum-free medium they described included fibronectin and insulin. We have found that a medium adapted from that of Iscoves and Melchers is fully effective without either substance.

REFERENCES

Brenner. M.K., Bright., S., Munro A.J. (1981) The MHC and cell interactions in man. Trans. Proc. 13 1527

Brenner M. K., Munro A.J. 1981. T cell help in human in vitro antibody producing systems: role of inhibitory T cells in masking allogeneic help. Cell. Immunol. 57 280

Farrant,J., J.C.Clark, H.Lee, S.C.Knight and J.O'Brien. 1980. Conditions for measuring DNA synthesis in PHA stimulated human lymphocytes in 20 ul hanging drops with various cell concentrations and periods of culture. J. immunol. Meth. 33:301.

Iscove,N.N., L.J.Guilbert and C.Weyman. 1980. Complete replacement of serum in primary cultures of erythropoietin-dependent red cell precursors (CFU-E) by albumin, transferrin, iron, unsaturated fatty acid, lecithin and cholesterol. Exp. Cell Res. 126:121.

Iscove,N.N., and F.Melchers. 1978. Complete replacement of serum by albumin, transferrin and soybean lipid in cultures of lipopolysaccharide-reactive B lymphocytes. J. exp. Med. 147:923.

Newton,C.A., R.S.Pereira and J.Farrant. 1981. Simple hanging drop (20ul) double antibody radioimmunoassay of human IgM, IgG, IgA, IgD and IgE. J. immunol. Meth. 45:41.

North. M.E., Brenner. M.K. (1982) Induction of immunoglobulin and antigen dependent antibody synthesis in human lymphocytes using supernatants from mitogen stimulated cultures. Immunology (in press)

O'Brien,J., S.Knight, N.A.Quick, E.H.Moore and A.S.Platt. 1979. A simple technique for harvesting lymphocytes cultured in Terasaki plates. J. immunol. Meth. 27:219.

Tanno. Y., Arai. S., Takishima. T., (1982) Induction of immunoglobulin producing human peripheral blood lymphocytes in serum free medium. J.Imm. Methods 52. 255.

Adipose Conversion of Murine Bone Marrow-Derived Macrophages in Serum-Free Medium

Inge Flesch, Uwe-Peter Ketelsen, and Ernst Ferber

Max-Panck-Institut für Immunbiologie, Stübeweg 51, D-7800 Freiburg, FRG

Abstract

A serum-free culture medium to obtain macrophages from the murine bone marrow was established. The medium includes sodium pyruvate, sodium selenite, insuline, transferrin, either linoleic or oleic acid, bovine serum albumin and L-cell supernatant. In the case of oleic acid macrophage colonies are obtained. If linoleic acid is added, macrophages are developing which convert into fat cells. Obviously linoleic acid has adipogenic activity.

1. Introduction

In long-term cultures of murine bone marrow cells supplemented with 20% horse serum but without any addition of colony stimulating factors, an adherent layer is obtained which provides an in vitro equivalent of the haemopoietic microenvironment (1,2). One element of the adherent cell population is the large fat cell which seems to be important for stem cell maintenance and haemopoietic differentiation. In the serum-supplemented culture system according to Dexter et al. (2,3) the maturation of adipocytes from a nonfat precursor cell is dependent upon a factor present in horse serum (4). We established a serum-free culture system which induces bone marrow derived macrophages to convert into fat cells after addition of linoleic acid.

2. Experimental

Cells are flushed from the femora of 6-8 week-old C57BL/6 female mice. 2×10^5 cells/ml are incubated without any medium change in uncoated Greiner dishes.

The high glucose formulation of Dulbecco's modified Eagle's medium is used as basal medium, enriched with sodium pyruvate (1mM), sodium selenite (10nM), sodium hydrogen carbonate (3.7 mg/ml), insulin (5 µg/ml), transferrin (5 µg/ml), either linoleic or oleic acid (5 µg/ml), 0.1% of fatty acid free bovine serum albumin and 30% of serum-free L-cell supernatant.

Adipose conversion

Without any addition of long-chain fatty acids only poor macrophage development is observed. If oleic acid bound to bovine serum albumin is added to the culture medium large macrophage colonies are obtained within eight days (Fig. 1). The macrophages adhere to the culture dish, are able to phagocytose zymosan, and bear Fc-receptors.

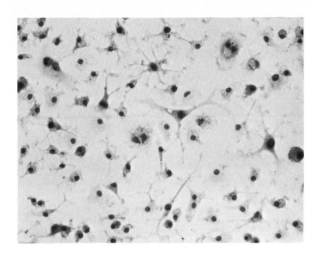

Fig. 1 Macrophages (day 10) obtained in serum-free culture medium conditioned with oleic acid (x 224). Oil Red O staining

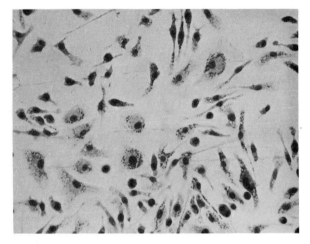

Fig. 2 Macrophages after conversion into large fat cells (x 224). Oil Red O staining

If oleic acid is replaced by linoleic acid macrophages are obtained which change morphology and start accumulating lipid droplets after eight days (Fig. 2). After three weeks some confluence of lipid droplets is evident.

Fc-receptors

The number of Fc-receptor bearing cells was determined as described in (5). During the adipogenic conversion the macrophages retain their Fc-receptors but they lose their ability to phagocytose zymosan (Tab. 1).

Tracing of long-chain fatty acids

Bone marrow cells were cultivated in the presence of 14-C-labelled oleic or linoleic acid. After ten days lipids were extracted and analyzed as described in (6). Linoleic acid but not oleic acid is stored in form of neutral lipids (Tab. 2).

Tab. 1 Fc-receptors of macrophages and large fat cells

	Percentage of rosettes
Fat cells	61
Macrophages grown with oleic acid	74
Macrophages grown in serum-supplemented medium	62

Tab. 2 Incorporation pattern of 14-C-labeled fatty acids into phospholipids of bone marrow cells.
(PC: phosphatidylcholine, PE: phosphatidylethanolamine, FFA free fatty acids, NL: neutral lipids)

	% PC	% PE	% FFA	% NL
Linoleic acid	44.1	17.8	4.3	29.9
Oleic acid	59.1	25.0	2.8	8.7

3.   Discussion

Our results indicate that the monocyte represents a possible precursor cell for fat cell formation in the bone marrow. The adipose conversion of bone marrow-derived macrophages in serum-free medium only depends on the presence of linoleic acid. Lipid analysis of several batches of horse serum revealed a high content of linoleic acid (about 60 mol%), in contrast to fetal calf serum were only trace amounts of linoleic acid were found. Obviously the adipogenic factor of horse serum as described by Dexter et al. (5) is linoleic acid.

References
1.   T.D. Allen & T.M Dexter, Differentiation 6, 191 (1976)
2.   T.M. Dexter, T.D. Allen & L.G. Lajtha, J. Cell. Physiol., 91, 335 (1976)
3.   T.M. Dexter, E. Spooncer, D. Toksoz & L.G. Lajtha, J. Supramol. Struc., 13, 513 (1980)
4.   M. Lanotte, D. Scott, T.M. Dexter, T.D. Allen, J. Cell. Physiol., 111, 177 (1982)
5.   R. van Furth, J.A. Raeburn & T.L. van Zwet, Blood, Vol 54, No. 2, 485 (1979)
6.   J. Trotter, I. Flesch, B. Schmidt & E. Ferber, J. Biol. Chem. 257, 1816 (1982)

Supported by the Max-Planck-Gesellschaft.

Analysis of the Mitogenic Effect of Fibrinogen

Jacques A. Hatzfeld and Antoinette Hatzfeld

Institut de Pathologie Cellulaire, Hôpital de Bicêtre, F-94270 Kremlin Bicêtre, France

Fibrinogen is absent in serum but is a major component of plasma, where its concentration is about 3 mg/ml. Blood clotting results from the polymerisation of fibrinogen into fibrin (1). Here we present evidence that fibrinogen may play another role by stimulating the proliferation of certain human hemopoietic cells. A strong proliferative response of certain cell lines resulted from the synergism elicited by the addition of fibrinogen (3-30 nM) to transferrin in defined medium. Fibrinogen was also found to increase the plating efficiency and colony size when human bone marrow cells were cultured in semi-solid media containing serum. Purified fibrinogen fragment D possessed a stimulating activity similar to that of the intact fibrinogen molecule. This fragment cannot form fibrin thus eliminating fibrin as a source of the mitogenic effect.

MATERIAL AND METHODS

Reagents, fibrinogen purification, cell lines and growth assays have been detailed elsewhere (2,3). Fibrinogen was more than 99% pure and the aα, bβ and γ chains were not damaged by the purification procedure. Removing fibronectin contaminant of fibrinogen on a gelatin agarose column did not change the mitogenic effect. No contaminant growth factors have been found in fibrin exsudate after clotting of purified fibrinogen preparation.

RESULTS

EFFECT OF FIBRINOGEN ON GROWTH IN MINIMAL MEDIA

A minimal medium is composed of defined factors which are all necessary in a particular combination for the growth of a particular cell type: removal of each factor individually prevents growth. These media facilitate the study of each growth requirement and its effects.

a) JM cell line

This cell line was derived from a human T lymphoma. When JM cells grown in medium containing 10% FCS were washed twice and resuspended in IMDM at a concentration of 2×10^5 cells/ml, no residual growth was observed. However, when transferrin was added and cell concentration was carefully maintained between 2×10^5 and 10^6 cells/ml, a doubling time of 31 hours was observed for at least 30 days. By adding 1-10 μg/ml (3-30 nM) pure fibrinogen, growth was strongly stimulated and a doubling time of 18 hours was obtained.

When cells were seeded in IMDM supplemented with transferrin at low density (i.e. 2×10^3 instead of 2×10^5 cells/ml), no growth occured. However, if 10 μg/ml fibrinogen was added, all of the single cells started to grow and formed clones which could be isolated and expanded for continuous growth in this medium. Therefore IMDM supplemented with transferrin and fibrinogen constitutes a minimal medium for growth of the JM cell line at low cell density. In low cell density cultures no stimulating cell contacts occur and diffusible factors, such as TCGF, produced by the cells are diluted. Such conditions have been used to study the proliferative dose response to fibrinogen of JM cells. A maximal effect was obtained with 10 μg/ml fibrinogen, a concentration 300 times lower than that normally found in plasma.

The mitogenic effect of fibrinogen was tested in a situation where fibrin could not be formed. Plasmin treatment progressively degrades the fibrinogen molecule producing two D fragments and one fragment E per molecule. Fragment D, not only cannot form fibrin, but even inhibits its formation. Purified fragment D had a proliferative effect similar to that of the intact fibrinogen molecule. An optimal response was obtained for 10 μg/ml fragment D (0.1 μM). These results suggest that fibrin formation is not a prerequisite for the proliferative effect of fibrinogen.

b) Other cell lines

A strong positive proliferative response at high and low cell density has also been obtained with the pre B cell line Raji (3). A positive response is observed only for residual growth at low cell density with HL-60 and U-937 cells. With K-562 no response has been observed in all experimental conditions tested (3).

EFFECT OF FIBRINOGEN ON THE PROLIFERATION OF HUMAN BONE MARROW COLONY-FORMING CELLS

a) Colony assay

The effect of fibrinogen on normal human bone marrow colony-forming cells grown in a medium with serum and methyl-cellulose was studied. Cultures seeded at 5×10^4 and 2×10^5 cells/ml with or without fibrinogen were compared. After 3 days, regardless of the starting cell density, clones with 2, 4 and 8 cells were more numerous in cultures supplemented with fibrinogen. Eleven days later, cultures seeded at 5×10^4 cells/ml were dead. On the other hand, in cultures seeded at the higher concentrations, addition of fibrinogen increased the number of 20-50 cell colonies by a factor of 4 and the number of colonies with more than 50 cells by a factor of 20. In the presence of erythropoietin, fibrinogen was also found to increase the number and size of erythroid colonies. In the absence of a reliable serum free colony assay to analyse specific physiological parameters, results may be highly fluctuant from one donor to the other.

b) Long-term bone marrow cultures

The addition of fibrinogen to a long-term serum containing culture greatly reduced the time-associated decrease in the production of colony-forming cells. After 6 weeks, cultures with fibrinogen produced 50 CFU-GM/10^5 cells, while control cultures without fibrinogen no longer produced any.

DISCUSSION

Further analysis are in progress in order to determine whether fibrinogen binds specifically to certain cells as has been reported for activated platelets (4). Fibrinogen could also have a binding site for a growth factor. These molecules, present in serum or produced by certain cells, could be active only after binding to fibrinogen or its fragment D which would serve as a carrier protein.

ACKNOWLEDGEMENTS. We are greatly indebted to Dr. G.H.Sato and his laboratory for an enriching apprenticeship. This work was supported by grants from INSERM (CRL n°812031), UER Kremlin Bicêtre and Ministère de la Recherche et de la Technologie (n°82V0011).

BIBLIOGRAPHY

1. Doolittle, R.F. (1973) in Adv. Prot. Chem., eds. Anfinsen, C.B., Edsall, J.T. & Richards, F.M. (Academic Press) 27, 2-109.
2. Hatzfeld, J.A., Hatzfeld, A., Maigné, J., Sasportes, M., Willis, R. & Mc Clure, D.B. (1982) in Growth of cells in Hormonally Defined Media, eds. Sirbasku, D.A., Sato, G.H. & Pardee, A.B. (Cold Spring Harbor Laboratory Press, Cold Spring Harbor, New-York) 9, 703-710.
3. Hatzfeld, J.A., Hatzfeld, A. & Maigne J. (1982) Proc. Natl. Acad. Sci. USA 79,
4. Marguerie, G.A., Plow, E.F. & Edgington, T.S. (1979) J. Biol. Chem. 254, 5357-5363.

Hybridoma Formation in Serum-Free Medium

Tomoyuki Kawamoto, J. Denry Sato[1], Anh Le, Don B. McClure, and Gordon H. Sato

Cancer Center, Q-058, University of California, San Diego, La Jolla, CA 92093, USA
[1] Present address: Molecular Genetics Department, City of Hope Research Institute, 1450 E. Duarte Road, Duarte, CA 91010, USA

INTRODUCTION

The production of Ig-secreting hybridomas from fusions between mouse myeloma cells and mouse immunized spleen cells in serum-free medium has several practical advantages in monoclonal antibody research in terms of simplification of the process of preliminary screening for biological activities of the monoclonal antibodies as well as their purifications from the culture supernatants (1-3). Several attempts in applying serum-free media which have been developed specifically for the growth of established NS-1 myeloma derived hybridomas (4,5) in the isolation of nascent NS-1 meyloma-derived hybridomas have been unsuccessful (Kawamoto et al, in preparation). This failure leads us to focus our attentions on the conditions which would support the growth of the parent myeloma cell lines, NS-1, which as we anticipated, would also promote the formation and the outgrowth of their derived hybridomas.

Pursuing this strategy, we succeeded in developing a hormone-supplemented lipid-enriched serum-free medium, designated KSLM, which supports the growth of NS-1 myeloma cells as well as does serum containing medium and permits the isolation of antibody-secreting hybridomas at a similar efficiency as with serum-supplemented medium. Likewise, following the same approach, lipid-deficient KSLM, a medium adapted for growth by NS-1-503 myeloma cells (a clonal cell line derived from NS-1 myeloma) which lacks oleic acid and human low density lipoprotein (LDL), allows for the isolation of nascent NS-1-503 myeloma-derived hybridomas at efficiencies equally close to those under serum-supplemented medium or complete KSLM.

MATERIAL AND METHODS

The serum-free medium formulated for the growth of NS-1 myeloma cells consists of a basal nutrient medium (a mixture of RPMI:DME:Ham's F12 at a 2:1:1 ratio) supplemented with insulin (10 µg/ml), human Fe^{+++}-free transferrin (10 µg/ml), 2-aminoethanol (10 µM), 2-mercaptoethanol (10 µM), sodium selenite (1 x 10^{-9} M), human low density lipoprotein (density 1.019-1.063) (1.0-2.0 µg/ml) and oleic acid (4 µg/ml) complexed with fatty acid-free bovine serum albumin (FAF-BSA) in a 2:1 molar ratio as described previously (6). NS-1-503 myeloma is a clonal cell line, isolated from NS-1 myeloma cells which were adapted to growth in lipid-free KSLM (for details, Kawamoto et al, in preparation). Cell fusions were carried out according to the method of Galfré et al (7) with some slight modifications (J. D. Sato et al, in preparation).

RESULTS AND DISCUSSION

Growth of NS-1 myeloma in serum-free medium:

Despite the resemblance in the four common factors; insulin, transferrin, ethanolamine and selenium, which were previously reported by other groups (4,5), KSLM differs remarkably in its inclusion of an exogeneous lipid supplements, provided through oleic acid-free fatty acid bovine serum albumin complex and human low density lipoprotein (LDL). The lipid supplements present in KSLM prove to be essential for serum-free growth of NS-1 myeloma cells (Fig. 1) and support NS-1

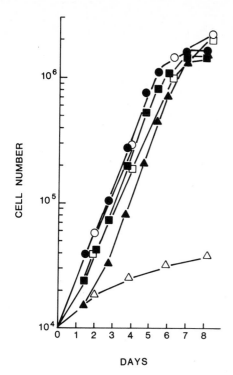

Figure 1. NS-1 myeloma and NS-1-503 myeloma cells were resuspended at 1 x 10^4 cells/ml in either KSLM medium (□), KSLM minus oleic acid and LDL (△), or RDF + 10% FCS (O) and plated into wells of a 24-well dish (Costar). Cell numbers in duplicate wells were determined on the indicated days by counting with a Coulter counter. Open signs are for NS-1 growth and closed signs for NS-1-503 myeloma growth.

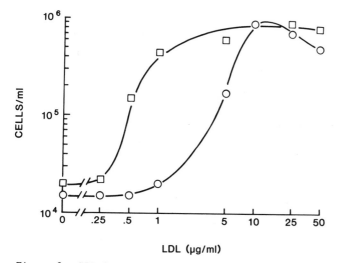

Figure 2. LDL Concentrations. NS-1 myeloma cells (1 x 10^4) were plated on day 0 into 24-well dishes containing 1 ml KSLM medium, either with (□) or without oleic acid (O), and the indicated concentrations of LDL. Cell numbers in duplicate wells were determined on day 6.

myeloma proliferation at a mean generation time closely comparable to that in serum containing medium (~22 hours). The distinction between the role of LDL and fatty acid, particularly oleic acid, becomes clear if we delete LDL from KSLM (Fig. 2) which results in impairment of NS-1 myeloma growth.

LDL as the sole lipid supplement in the medium appears to serve both as an exogeneous fatty acid source via its cholesterol ester and phospholipid components as well as a sterol source through its cholesterol moiety, since at a high concentration, 10 μg/ml, LDL eliminates entirely the oleic acid requirement for NS-1 cell growth. This role contributed by LDL is further confirmed by preliminary experiments (data not shown) which indicate that cholesterol, when added to LDL-free KSLM medium under the appropriate conditions, mimics LDL in promoting NS-1 myeloma cell growth.

NS-1 myeloma X spleen cell fusion in KSLM medium:

The lipid requirement which is stringent for the growth of NS-1 myeloma appears to be more relaxed in the formation and outgrowth of its derived hybridomas. Experiments done by deleting LDL and/or oleic acid from KSLM medium (Table I) indicate no positive contribution of LDL in the success of hybridoma formation.

Table I. Effect of Oleic Acid and LDL on Myeloma X Spleen Cell Fusion in KSLM Medium.

Deletion from KSLM	Positive Wells (%)		A431 Antibody (% positive wells)	
	Parent Myeloma			
	NS-1-503	NS-1	NS-1-503	NS-1
None	50	90	20	70
LDL	70	100	20	90
Oleic acid	10	95	20	50
LDL + Oleic acid	10	100	30	90

See legend of Table II for experiment details. For each medium condition, oleic acid, LDL or both factors were added to HAT containing KSLM medium deleted of oleic acid and LDL.

However, fatty acid, in particular, oleic acid, added in association with FAF-BSA, is essential for the manufacture of NS-1 derived hybridomas in serum-free medium. This fatty acid requirement for hybridoma formation seems to be linked to the use of the cloning technique which is a necessary part of the hybridization protocol if a unique colony derived from a single cell progenitor is desired.

Growth of NS-1-503 in serum-free medium:

Pursuing the same strategy, NS-1 myeloma cells can also be adapted to growth in a serum-free medium and this medium used in conjunction with the adapted NS-1 meyloma is applied directly to the isolation of antibody-secreting hybridomas. In our study, we have adapted NS-1 myeloma cells to growth in a lipid-free (without either oleic acid or LDL) version of KSLM medium and have isolated a clonal cell line, NS-1-503 myeloma, which grows in lipid-deficient KSLM in terms of mean generation time of 18.5 hours, a rate comparably close to that in complete KSLM or serum-supplemented medium (Fig. 1) except for a slightly longer lag phase in the former medium. The stringent exogeneous lipid requirement for growth exposed by NS-1 myeloma is more relaxed for NS-1-503 myeloma cells, presumably due to the fact that this lipid-free KSLM medium adapted myeloma line can de novo synthesize enough cholesterol and fatty acid to satisfy their cellular needs.

NS-1-503 myeloma X spleen cell fusion in serum-free medium:

The efficiency of hybridoma formation in either KSLM medium or serum-supplemented medium was roughly 7.5 fold higher when NS-1-503 myeloma instead of NS-1 myeloma was used as the parent myeloma (~1.5 fold increase in the number of positive wells X ~5 fold increase in hybridoma colonies per well) (Table II).

Table II. Myeloma X Spleen Cell Fusion in KSLM Medium and RDF + 10% FCS

Parent Myeloma	Condition	Positive Wells (%)	Colonies/ well	A431 antibody (% positive wells)
NS-1	KSLM	55	1-2	25
	RDF + 10% FCS	50	1-2	30
NS-1-503	KSLM	85	5-10	60
	RDF + 10% FCS	80	5-10	60

Fusion was carried out by the method of Galfré et al (7) with some modifications (J. D. Sato, in preparation). Fusion products were resuspended in either RDF + 10% FCS + HAT medium or KSLM + HAT medium and finally seeded in 96-well microtiter plates at 50-100 µl per well. Two weeks after fusion, hybridoma colonies were counted and screened for presence of positive, A431 specific immunoglobulin secretion by indirect binding assay (Kawamoto et al, in preparation).

At this point, it is not clear why NS-1-503 meyloma is a more efficient fusion partner, both in serum-free and serum-supplemented medium, than is NS-1.

Following the anticipation that a serum-free medium developed for growth of the parent myeloma will allow for the isolation of its nascent hybridomas, we performed a NS-1-503 X spleen cell fusion in oleic acid, LDL deleted KSLM medium (Table II). Results indicate that lipid-free KSLM medium was capable of supporting hybridoma formation from a NS-1-503 X spleen cell fusion in a similar yield as with serum-supplemented medium (>95% of wells positive for hybridoma colonies). Lipid supplements are not critical for the efficient isolation of NS-1-503 myeloma derived hybridomas, however, from our unshown data, we have evidence that fatty acid, particularly oleic acid-free fatty acid bovine albumin complex contributes to the increase in the number of colonies per well from 2-3 to 5-10.

ACKNOWLEDGEMENTS

This work was supported by USPHS NIH grants CA 33397 and CA19731.

REFERENCES

1. Sato, G. H. (1975) in Biochemical Actions of Hormones, Vol. III, pp. 391-396, (G. Litwack, ed.), Academic Press, New York.
2. Barnes, D., and Sato, G. H. (1980a) Anal. biochem. 102: 255-270.
3. Barnes, D., and Sato, G. H. (1980b) Cell 22: 649-655.
4. Chang, T. H., Steplewski, Z., and Koprowski, H. (1980) J. Immunol. Methods 39: 369-375.
5. Murakami, H., Masui, H., Sato, G. H., Sueoka, N., Chow, T. P. and Kano-Sueoka, T. (1982) Proc. Natl. Acad. Sci. USA 79: 1158-1162.
6. Wolfe, R., Sato, G. H. and McClure, D. B. (1980) J. Cell Biol. 87: 434-441.
7. Galfré, G., Howe, S. C., Molstein, C., Butcher, G. W. and Howard, J. C. (1977) Nature 266: 550-552.

Immune (γ) Interferon Produced by Murine T-Cell Lymphomas

Santo Landolfo[1] and Bernd Arnold[2]

[1] Institute of Microbiology, University of Torino, I-10126 Torino, Italy
[2] Institut für Immunologie und Genetik, Deutsches Krebsforschungszentrum, D-6900 Heidelberg, FRG

ABSTRACT

Various cloned murine T-cell hybridomas and T lymphomas were evaluated for their ability to produce immune (γ) IFN and other lymphokines such as interleukin-2 (IL-2) and macrophage activiating factor (MAF). The 2 T-cell clones, L12-R1 and -R4, dereived from a spontaneously in vitro transformed cell line L12 which was originally established from fetal calf serum (FCS)-primed C57BL/6 spleen cells (Rubin et al., 1980, Scand. J. Immunol. 12:407) were found to produce IFN after mitogen stimulation (1.000 IU) in presence of 2% FCS. By contrast in complete absence of FCS IFN titres decreased to 500 IU. None of the cell lines tested produced IFN either constitutively or upon lipopolysaccharide (LPS) stimulation. The IFN was characterized as immune (γ) IFN by being labile at pH 2 and neutralized by 2 rabbit anti-murine IFN-γ antisera but not by antiserum to murine IFN-α and -ß. L12-R4 IFN-γ chromatography on Sephacryl S-200 and Phenyl Sepharose columns indicates a molecular weight of about 45.000 and a significant apparent hydrophobicity just as other murine IFN-γ. In addition to IFN-γ IL-2 and MAF were also found in the supernatants of the mitogen treated L12-R4 cells. Our data provide further evidence that IFN-γ is a product of T cells of the Lyt-1[+], 23[−] phenotype and establish a system which could be used for the IFN-γ purification as well as for the characterization of the molecular mechanisms involved in T cell differentiation leading to IFN production.

Activation of T lymphocytes by a variety of antigens leads to the release of soluble factors collectively called "lymphokines" (1). Several data indicate that lymphokines are capable to activate and modulate cell populations of the immune system involved in the defense against bacteria, viruses, protozoa and tumors (2). The exact definition of their role, however, has been hampered so far by insufficient amounts of purified material. The conventional system, in fact, employing normal lymphocytes stimulated with mitogens in the presence of foetal calf serum (FCS) require several steps of purification with constant loss of activity. In search for a more convenient system for lymphokine production we screened various T cell hybridomas and lymphomas for their ability to produce IFN-y, interleukin-2 (IL-2), macrophage activating factor (MAF) and macrophage migration inhibition factor (MIF). A T cell clone, L12-R4, derived from a spontaneously in vitro transformed cell line L12, which was originally established from FCS primed C57BL/6 spleen cells (3), was to produce significant amounts of lymphokines (Table 1).

Table 1. Lymphokines produced by L12-R4 stimulated with Phorbol myristate acetate (PMA) (2×10^{-7} M).

Lymphokines tested	Activity found
IFN-y	+
MAF	+
IL-2	+
MIF	−

Using monoclonal antibodies we characterized with the aid of a fluorescence activated cell sorter (FACS) the phenotype of the L12-R4 cells. As shown in Table 2, the lymphokine producing lymphoma displays Lyt-1, found on T helper cells, reinforcing the hypothesis that both helper and cytotoxic T lymphocytes can produce lymphokines such as IFN-y and MAF.

Table 2. Membrane phenotype of L12-R4 cells.

Cells	H-2^b	Thy 1.2	Lyt 1.2	Lyt 2.2	Lyt 3.2	Ig
L12-R4	95%	95%	88%	< 5%	< 5%	< 5%

Having established an in vitro system for lymphokine production we attempted to produce the lymphokine in complete absence of FCS in order to facilitate purification and to characterize biochemically the IFN-y produced. As shown in Table 3, the IFN amount produced in serum-free medium is about half of that produced in the presence of FCS.

Table 3. Comparison of IFN-y production in the presence or absence
of FCS.

| PMA concentration | % FCS | |
	2%	0%
10^{-6} M	243 IU	81 IU
10^{-7} M	>729 IU	243-729 IU
10^{-8} M	243-729 IU	81 IU

As far as the biochemical characterization of IFN-y produced by
L12-R4 cells are concerned, Table 4 shows that this L12-R4 IFN-y is
pH-2 labile, has a molecular weight of 45.000 d., has an elevated
hydrophobicity and affinity for lectines the same as IFN-y produced
by normal T lymphocytes stimulated with mitogens (4).

Table 4. Physico-chemical characteristics of IFN-y produced by L12-R4
cells.

Treatment	Characteristics
pH-2	labile
Sepharyl-S-200	45.000 d
Phenyl-Sepharose	high affinity
Con A - Sepharose	high affinity

Our data establish an experimental system which could be used
for the IFN-y purification as well as for the characterization of the
molecular mechanisms involved in T cell differentiation leading to
lymphokine production.

REFERENCES

1. De Weck, A., F. Kristeenen and M. Landy (eds.)(1980) Biomedical
Characterization of Lymphokines. Academic Press, New York.
2. Cohen, S., E. Pick and J.J. Oppenheim (eds.)(1979) Biology of the
Lymphokines. Academic Press, New York.
3. Rubin, B., M.A. Cooley, C. Le Bourgne deKaouel, R.B. Taylor and
P. Golstein. (1980) Scan. J. Immunol. 12, 401.
4. Baron, S. and F. Bianzani (1982) The Interferon System. Tex. Rep.
Biomed., Galveston, USA.

TCGF-Dependent Growth of Naturally Autoreactive Cells: Regulatory Role of the Thymus

Carlo Riccardi, Graziella Migliorati, and Luigi Frati

Institute of Pharmacology, University of Perugia and Institute of Pathology, University of Rome

ABSTRACT

Culture of non-immune spleen cells in the presence of T-cell-growth-factor (TCGF) generate Natural Killer (NK) cells with autoreactive activity against syngeneic normal non-neoplastic cells. These cells are under thymic control. The possible relevance of these observations is discussed.

INTRODUCTION

NK cells has been shown to play an important role in vivo against neoplastic as well as normal non-neoplastic cells (1-2). In the attempt to better analyze the role and regulation of NK cells, we cultured mouse spleen cells in vitro in the presence of TCGF.

RESULTS

Mouse spleen cells from non-immune animals were cultured in RPMI supplemented with 10% FBS, 1% glutamine, 1% sodium pyruvate, 1% non-essential aminoacids, 10^{-5}M 2-mercaptoethanol and 10 1/2 u TCGF/ml, in 96 well tissue culture treated micro-plates (5×10^{5} cells/well) in the presence of 5×10^{4} feeder cell (3000R irradiated syngeneic spleen cells)/well. At the end of the culture period (8 days) cells were harvested and tested for cytotoxic activity in a 4-hr ^{51}Cr-release assay. As shown in Table I cultured cells showed a significantly higher cytotoxicity than fresh uncultured spleen cells as measured against the NK sensitive YAC-1 cells. These data suggest that the cultured cell population was highly enriched for spontaneously cytotoxic effector cells.

Table I

Natural reactivity of uncultured and cultured CBA/J spleen cells against YAC-1 target

Effector cell	% Cytotoxicity		
	100:1	50:1	25:1[a]
Uncultured cells	35.5	25.0	15.9
Cultured cells	80.8	78.2	75.6

a) Effector: target ratios.

To further analyze such naturally cytotoxic cells we compared their reactivity against the NK-sensitive YAC-1 target with that against the NK-insensitive EL-4 target cells. As reported in Table II these cells were able to lyse YAC-1 cells. Interestingly enough these cells were also able to lyse Concanavallin-A induced syngeneic blasts but less efficient or not lytic at all when tested against different allogeneic blasts, suggesting a "self-preference" of this spontaneous autoreactivity.

Table II

Natural reactivity of cultured BALB/c spleen cells against different target cells.

Target cells	% Cytotoxicity		
	100:1	50:1	25:1[a]
YAC-1	75.6	75.0	70.1
EL-4	11.0	5.7	4.5
BALB/c blasts	48.0	37.4	28.9
CBA/J blasts	4.0	3.7	1.0
B10.A blasts	2.4	2.4	0.7
SJL/J blasts	3.0	1.9	2.0
C57B1/6 blasts	12.0	7.6	4.1

a) Effector: target ratios.

Using similar culture conditions we have shown that is possible to grow progenitor-NK cells and that such growth and differentiation is under the regulation of "T-helper" as well as "T-suppressor" cells (3). We then examined the possible regulatory role of the thymus by implantation of syngeneic thymus into athymic BALB/c nu/nu mice.

Table III

Frequency of progenitor-NK cells growing in the presence of TCGF.

Donor of cultured spleen cells	Frequency of progenitor-NK cells[a]
BALB/c nu/nu, sham-operated	$1/1 \times 10^6$
BALB/c nu/nu, thymus implanted	$1/3 \times 10^4$

a) As measured against YAC-1 target cells.

Three thymus lobes were implanted s.c. for each mouse and after 20 days the frequency of NK cells growing in the presence of TCGF was estimated by the "limiting dilution assay". As shown in Table III, thymus implant resulted in an actual augmentation of the frequency of cells spontaneously cytotoxic against YAC-1 target cells.

CONCLUSIONS

The above reported data point to an <u>autoreactive</u> role of NK cells confirming our previous observations (2). This autoreactivity shows a self-preference, which is not surprising since in physiological conditions the immune system is involved in syngeneic rather than allogeneic interactions. Alloreactivity can not represent a pressure mechanism which could have been involved in the evolution of the species and of their immune reactivity. Self-reactivity does. We have also shown that such reactivity is under the thymic regulation, which is in line with the important regulatory role of the thymus which is involved in many immunological processes (4). Such kind of observations are made possible by <u>in vitro</u> studies which imply culturing with specific growth factors which can selectively expand and amplify selected cell populations. In our "syngeneic" cultures TCGF is able to expand spontaneously autoreactive cells which are under thymic control. Such kind of studies could be more informative than studies on allogeneic mixed lymphocyte reaction, on the physiological regulation of the immune system and some important aspects of its homeostatic role (2).

Supported by C.N.R., PFCCN contract n° 82.00395.96.115.9782.

References

1. C. Riccardi, P. Puccetti, A. Santoni and R.B. Herberman., J. Natl. Cancer Inst., 63, 1041, 1979

2. C. Riccardi, A. Santoni, T. Barlozzari and R.B. Herberman., Cellular Immunology, 60, 136, 1981

3. C. Riccardi, B.M. Vose and R.B. Herberman., In "NK Cells and Other Natural Effector Cells" R.B. Herberman (Ed.) Academic Press, N.Y., 909, 1982

4. L.R. Ruben., In "Immune Regulation: Evolutionary and Biological Significance". L.R. Ruben and M.E. Gershwin (Eds.) Marcel Dekker Inc. N.Y., vol. 17, 217, 1982

Serum Replacement in Culture of Human Erythroid and Megakaryocytic Precursors

G. Vinci[1], N. Casadevall[2], C. Lacombe[2], J. Chapman[3], W. Vainchenker[1], B. Varet[2], and J. Breton-Gorius[1]

[1]INSERM, U.91, Hôpital Henri Mondor, F-94010 Creteil, France
[2]INSERM, U.152, Hôpital Cochin, F-75674 Paris, France
[3]INSERM, U.35, Hôpital Henri Mondor, F-94010 Creteil, France

Iscove et al. (1) have recently, succeeded in the complete replacement of serum for cloning of murine CFU-E. In the cultures, serum was replaced by albumin, iron saturated transferrin and lipids prepared as liposomes. Aye et al. (2) could also replace the serum in human cultures. The source of lipids was low density lipoproteins (LDL). In this work, first we have used the method described by Aye et al. (2) to compare the erythropoietin (Epo) sensitivity of normal and polycythemia vera (PV) erythroid progenitors. Indeed, it has been demonstrated that in serum cultures, a part of the PV erythroid progenitors differentiates without Epo addition while their normal counterparts have an absolute Epo requirement (3,4,5). These PV spontaneous colonies can be either Epo independent or exquisitely sensitive to the hormone present in the serum (6). Results of this study have been already published (7). Second, we have preliminary tried to replace the serum in the human megakaryocytic (MK) colony assay. However, this technique was not serum free since the semi solid medium consisted of bovine plasma clot. A part of the results has been published elsewhere (8).

MATERIAL AND METHODS

Bone marrow or blood cells were obtained from normal donors or 6 PV patients. For erythroid progenitors, cultures were grown in 0.8 % methylcellulose in Iscove's medium (9). In this medium, serum albumin (1 mg/ml Cohn fraction 5, Sigma), purified human transferrin (300 µg/ml Sigma), $0.8 \ 10^{-7}$ M $Fecl_3$ and LDL isolated by a density gradient procedure (1.028 – 1.050 g/ml) from human serum (10) were added. The Epo preparation was obtained from Connaught Laboratories (Canada) and was a step III purification (10 IU per mg of protein). 2.10^5 bone marrow light density cells and 5.10^5 blood light density cells were plated. Bone marrow cultures were studied at day 8 while blood cultures were removed at day 14.

For megakaryocytic colonies, the plasma clot technique was used as previously described (8). The α medium was supplemented with sodium selenite (9). A batch of bovine plasma which was unable to sustain MK colonies by itself was choosen. The same ingredients as for erythroid progenitor cultures were employed. PHA-LCM (8) was the stimulating factor. Cultures were studied at day 12 of culture either by cytological procedure or by fluorescent labelling (11).

RESULTS

1. Erythroid progenitors

− Culture of normal erythroid progenitors

On bone marrow cultures, the first CFU-E colonies appeared at on Epo concentration slightly below 0.1 IU/ml. A plateau was usually achieved at about 1.5 IU/ml Epo. The Epo dose response curve for blood BFU-E did not differ markedly from that of marrow CFU-E. Comparison with serum cultures has shown that :
- The number of colonies at the plateau dose of Epo was similar.
- Below 0.5 IU/ml of Epo, the number of colonies was always higher in serum cultures.
- The first colonies were observed at 0.01 IU/ml.

In addition, LDL could not be kept for more than 2 weeks without loss of their biological activities.

− PV Cultures

In these conditions of culture, no Epo independent colony was observed in PV cultures either from marrow or blood cells while spontaneous colonies were grown in serum cultures. In four cases, the Epo dose response curve was studied. The first colonies appeared at an Epo concentration of 0.01 IU/ml while a plateau was typically observed at 1.5 IU/ml Epo concentration (Table I).

322

TABLE I

COMPARISON OF Epo DOSE RESPONSE OF PV CFU-E IN SERUM FREE
CULTURES AND OF THE SPONTANEOUS COLONIES IN SERUM CULTURES

			PATIENTS			
			1	2	3	4
SERUM FREE CULTURES	Added Epo (IU/ml)	0	0	0	0	0
		0.001	0	0	0	0
		0.01	9	6	3	6
		0.1	70	60	6	17
		0.2	91	84	11	24
		0.5	100	96	40	46
		1	100	100	89	85
		2	100	100	100	100
SERUM CULTURES	Spontaneous culture		80	50	11	39

Results are expressed as % of the number of colonies obtained at
the plateau-dose of Epo (1.5 IU/ 2 IU/ml) in serum free cultures.

2. MK Cultures

- Serum cultures

In the human MK colony assay, MK colonies can be grown in the absence of a stimulating factor, but PHA-LCM increased 2 to 5 times the number of colonies. Normal human AB serum can inhibit MK colony formation since in all cases the number of MK colonies was higher (130 % - 300 %) at a 5 % serum concentration than at 20 %. The maximum number of colonies was observed at a serum concentration from 2.5 % to 5 %. A similar results was observed for spontaneous or PHA-LCM stimulated colonies. In addition the size of the MK colonies was reduced by 20 % serum (average MK value per colony 5.5 MKs at 5 %, 3.3 MKs at 20 %).

- Replacement of serum

When serum was replaced as above, similar results to that described at 5 % serum concentration were obtained. "Spontaneous" colonies were still present. Addition of LDL to a volume equivalent to 20 % human serum did not elicit an inhibition of MK colony formation. LDL could also be replaced by HDL_2 (density 1.063 - 1.125 g/ml) or HDL_3 (density 1.125 - 1.121 g/ml) but not by VLDL. However, the volume of HDL necessary to sustain MK colony formation was higher than for LDL and was equivalent to at least a concentration of 15 % human serum.

CONCLUSION

Serum free cultures for the growth of erythroid progenitors could be obtained. However, these cultures were not entirely equivalent to their homologous with serum. In PV, no erythroid colonies were observed in the absence of Epo, but the PV erythroid progenitors were 10 times more sensitive to Epo than their normal counterparts. However, further studies are required to investigate the Epo dose response with a totally purified Epo and with serum free cultures containing only synthetic lipids since it has been described that some lipoproteins could inhibit cellular proliferation (12). In the MK colony formation, serum could also be replaced, but this substitutin was incomplete since the semi solid medium is a bovine plasma. However, it could be demonstrated that human serum may inhibit MK colony formation. This result has to be compared to recent data (13, 14) which demonstrate that human plasma permits a superior MK growth to human serum. Further studies are required to demonstrate whether this phenomenon is linked to trivial culture conditions or to the presence of platelet factors regulating megakaryopoiesis in the serum.

REFERENCES

1. Iscove NN, Guilbert LJ, Weyman C, Exp. Cell Res. 126:121, 1980
2. Aye MT, Seguin JA, Mc Burney JP, J. Cell Phys. 99:233, 1979
3. Prchal JF, Axelrad AA, N. Engl. J. Med. 290:1392, 1974
4. Eaves CJ, Eaves AC, Blood 52:1196, 1978
5. Lacombe C, Casadevall N, Varet B, Brit. J. Haematol. 44:189, 1980
6. Zanjani ED, Lutton JD, Hoffmann R et al. J. Clin. Invest. 59:841, 1977
7. Casadevall N, Vainchenker W, Lacombe C et al. Blood 59:447, 1982
8. Vainchenker W, Chapman J, Deschamps JF et al. Exp. Hemat. 650, 1982
9. Guilbert LJ, Iscove NN, Nature 263:594, 1976
10. Chapman J, Goldstein S, Lagrange D et al. Lipid Res. 22:339, 1981
11. Vainchenker W, Deschamps JF, Bastin JM et al.Blood 59:514, 1982
12. Zucker S, Lysik RM, Chikkappa G et al. Exp. Hemat. 8:895, 1980
13. Messner HA, Jamal N, Izaguirre J Cell Phys. (suppl. 1) 45, 1982
14. Kanz L, Straub G, Bross KG et al. Blut, 45:267, 1982

Participation of Pterins and of a Pteridine Binding Variant of Alpha₁-Acid Glycoprotein in the Control of Lymphocyte Transformation and of Lymphoblast Proliferation

I. Ziegler, U. Hamm, and J. Berndt

Institut für Toxikologie und Biochemie der Gesellschaft für Strahlen- und Umweltforschung, Abteilung Zellchemie, Arcisstr. 16, D-8000 München 2, FRG

1. Introduction

Dihydroneopterin triphosphate is the first product of pterin synthesis from guanosine triphosphate. It is further metabolized to tetrahydrobiopterin via sepiapterin and dihydrobiopterin (1). The anabolic biopterin derivatives have been found to accumulate in blood cells during hemopoietic cell proliferation in Beagle dogs (2) and especially, to be a marker of increased proliferation during leukemias; in blasts high concentrations of biopterin were found (3) and neopterin has been identified in the medium of alloantigen-induced lymphocytes (4). – Furthermore from blood of patients with malignant diseases a pteridine binding variant of alpha₁-acid glycoprotein (AGP$_M$) has been characterized (5). The glycoprotein moiety differs from normal AGP in its secondary structure; the pteridine chromophore is bound by the sialic acid antennae, resulting in a decreased negative charge as compared to normal AGP (6). Blood biopterin and AGP$_M$ levels followed during clinical cases (7) also suggest a participation of the pterin system in (hemopoietic) cell proliferation. These observations prompted us to screen the major intermediates of pterin metabolism to determine whether they are not only lymphocyte products but also whether they have an effect on lymphocyte transformation and lymphoblast proliferation.

2. Materials and methods

Mouse spleen lymphocytes and a lymphoblastoid cell line (LS-2 from a patient with acute lymphatic leukemia) were processed in RPMI 1640 tissue culture medium with 5% inactivated fetal calf serum at 5% CO_2 and 37°. Cell growth was determined by the Microtiter assay system using ³H-thymidine incorporation as an indicator.

3. Results and discussion

A screening of the major intermediates pf pteridine metabolism showed that only a few exert an effect on Con A mediated lymphocyte activation. The activity is highly dependent on the structural and optical isomers (table 1). Three anabolites are promoting, two of the catabolites are inhibitory.

Xanthopterin, but not dihydroxanthopterin causes half maximal inhibition at 1.5 x 10^{-5}M (fig.1). Its inhibitory action on prestimulated lymphocytes and on the growth of LS-2 shows that it interferes with lymphoblast proliferation rather than with lymphocyte transformation. Isoxanthopterin inhibition only takes place if FCS is reduced or if it omitted (fig.2), since isoxanthopterin but not xanthopterin is trapped

Table 1. Effect of pteridines (1.1×10^{-6} to 1.4×10^{-4}M) on Con A ($0.4 - 4.0$ ug/ml) induced lymphocyte stimulation. The activation was read after 72 h of simultaneous Con A + pteridine incubation. All effective pteridines are des‑ cribed below in more detail.

DESIGNATION OF THE COMPOUND AND THE RING SYSTEM	SUBSTITUTION		EFFECT ON LYMPHOCYTE ACTIVATION
	R	R'	
PTERIN	–	–	NONE
6-METHYLPTERIN	CH₃	–	NONE
6-HYDROXYMETHYLPTERIN	CH₃	–	NONE
D-NEOPTERIN	CHOH – CHOH – CH₂OH (D-ERYTHRO)	–	NONE
7,8-DIHYDRO-D-NEOPTERIN	CHOH – CHOH – CH₂OH (D-ERYTHRO)	–	NONE
L-BIOPTERIN	CHOH · CHOH – CH₂OH (L-ERYTHRO)	–	NONE
7,8-DIHYDRO-L-BIOPTERIN	CHOH – CHOH – CH₃ (L-ERYTHRO)	–	PROMOTING
5,6,7,8-TETRAHYDRO-L-BIOPTERIN	CHOH – CHOH – CH₃ (L-ERYTHRO)	–	PROMOTING
7,8-DIHYDRO-6-LACTOYLPTERIN = SEPIAPTERIN	CO – CHOH – CH₃	–	PROMOTING
LEUCOPTERIN	OH	OH	NONE
XANTHOPTERIN	OH	–	INHIBITING
ISOXANTHOPTERIN	–	OH	INHIBITING
7,8-DIHYDROXANTHOPTERIN	OH	–	NONE
LUMAZINE	–	–	NONE
6-HYDROXYLUMAZINE	OH	–	NONE

PTERIDINE

PTERIN

LUMAZINE

by the AGP of the serum (7). The reduced inhibitory action which was found even in serum free medium (as compared to xanthopterin) may be due to the trapping of isoxan‑ thopterin at the cell membrane by AGP since this glycoprotein is produced as an ex‑ ternally located integral membrane protein by proliferating lymphocytes (8).

Sepiapterin, dihydrobiopterin and tetrahydrobiopterin promote Con A induced lym‑ phocyte activation, especially at suboptimal and supraoptimal Con A concentrations (fig.3). The promoting effect follows an optimum curve; e.g. with sepiapterin maximum stimulation occurs with 3×10^{-5}M. Neither resting lymphocytes nor prestimulated ones show an effect of statistical significance.

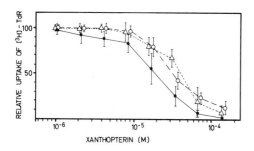

Fig.1 Inhibition of ³H-TdR incorporation into proliferating cells with xan‑ thopterin. ●——● Con A stimulation in the presence of xanthopterin; o- - -o lymphocytes prestimulated with Con A; △·····△ LS-2 cells

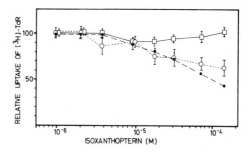

Fig.2 Inhibition of LS-2 with isoxan‑ thopterin. □———□ 5% FCS; o····o 1% FCS; ●- - -● serum free medium (assays in tripli‑ cate which showed virtually no variation)

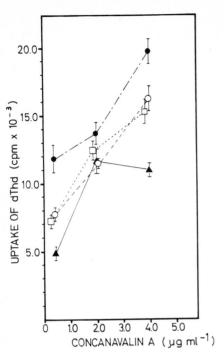

Fig. 3 Promoting effect of reduced biopterin in and of sepiapterin (1.4 x 10⁻⁵M) on lymphocyte activation at different Con A concentrations.

▲——▲ controls
○– –○ sepiapterin
□···□ dihydrobiopterin
●·–·● tetrahydrobiopterin

AGP_M alone induces lymphocyte activation; normal AGP is largely inactive. In serum free medium significantly less AGP_M is needed for optimum stimulation as compared to the level required in medium containing 5% FCS (fig.4).

Our experiments show that pterins are not only synthesized during hemopoietic cell proliferation but also act on this process in specific ways. Thus they fulfill the criteria for a control system which is governed by the equilibria present between the various anabolic and catabolic steps. The production of AGP_M during malignant diseases adds another component of activating ability to this equilibrium. Although

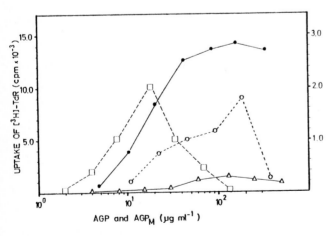

Fig. 4 Activation of lympho-cytes by AGP_M. ●——● AGP_M from a case with metastatic tera-toma of testicle(partial re-mission) in 5% FCS; ○– –○ AGP_M from a case with acute myelomonocytic leukemia, in 5% FCS; □– –□ same in serum free medium; △——△ normal AGP, 5% FCS. 5% FCS: left scale; serum free medium; right scale

the pterins are similar to lymphokines their classification must await further investigation. Moreover it is necessary to determine whether they exert a direct effect or whether they only provide the tetrahydrobiopterin cofactor for cleavage of glycerylethers, yielding fatty acids and fatty alcohols (9), known to control hemopoiesis (see ref.10).

4. References

1. Fukushima,K., Eto,I., Mayumi,I., Richter,W., Goodson,S., Shiota,T. in: Pfleiderer,W.(Ed.), Chemistry and Biology of Pteridines.Walter de Gruyter,Berlin 1975

2. Ziegler,I., Kolb,H.J., Bodenberger,U., Wilmanns,W.: Blut 44, 261 (1962)

3. Ziegler,I., Fink,M., Wilmanns,W.: Blut 44, 231 (1982)

4. Fuchs,D., Hausen,A., Huber,C., Margreiter,R., Reibnegger,G., Spielberger,M., Wachter,H.: Hoppe Seiler's Zeitschr.f.Physiol.Chemie 363, 661 (1982)

5. Ziegler,I., Maier,K., Fink,M.: Cancer Res.42, 1567 (1982)

6. Ziegler,I., Armarego, W.L.F., Fink,M. in: Blair J.A. (Ed.). Chemistry and Biology of Pteridines. Walter de Gruyter (in press)

7. Fink,M., Ziegler,I., Maier,K., Wilmanns,W.: Cancer Res.42, 1574 - 1578 (1982)

8. Gahmberg, C.G., Andersson, L.C.: J.Exp.Med. 148, 507 (1978)

9. Tietz,A., Linberg,M., Kennedy,E.P.: J.Biol.Chem. 239, 4081 (1964)

10. Morton,R.A.: Biochemical Spectroscopy.Adam Hilger,London 1975, Vol.1,pp.112-115

Liver- and Kidney-Derived Cells

Conversion of Heterogeneous Liver Parenchyma Cells into a Homogeneous Cell Population During Cell Culture with Respect to PEPCK

B. Andersen and K. Jungermann

Institut für Biochemie, Humboldtallee 7, D-3400 Göttingen, FRG

ABSTRACT

Hepatocytes from the periportal zone of the liver parenchyma mediate predominantly gluconeogenesis. Glycolysis is preferentially catalyzed by perivenous hepatocytes. Using indirect immunofluorescence microscopy it could be shown that shortly after isolation hepatocytes contained different amounts of phosphoenolpyruvate carboxykinase (PEPCK). Also after 1 h of culture the hepatocytes were still heterogeneous. Hepatocytes cultured for 24 h in the presence of 1 nM insulin and 10 nM dexamethasone showed a very weak fluorescence staining of PEPCK. Not all cells fluoresced to the same extent. Hepatocytes cultured for 20 h as described above and then applied to inducing conditions (10 nM glucagon for 4 h) possessed essentially equal amounts of PEPCK. Thus, it appears that the original heterogeneous population of hepatocytes can be converted in cell culture into a homogeneous population if appropriate conditions are used.

1. Introduction

The model of metabolic zonation proposes that in the liver e.g. gluconeogenesis is predominantly mediated by periportal hepatocytes and that glycolysis is preferentially catalyzed by perivenous cells (1). Using indirect immunofluorescence microscopy it could be shown (2, fig. 1) that phosphoenolpyruvate carboxykinase (PEPCK), a key enzyme of gluconeogenesis, was heterogeneously distributed over the liver parenchyma as the periportal marker enzyme succinate dehydrogenase (SDH). In agreement with the model of metabolic zonation periportal hepatocytes contained more PEPCK than perivenous cells.

Freshly isolated hepatocytes and hepatocytes maintained in primary culture are widely used for metabolic studies often with the implicit assumption of cellular homogeneity. The purpose of this study was to investigate whether isolated and cultured hepatocytes each contained different amounts of PEPCK.

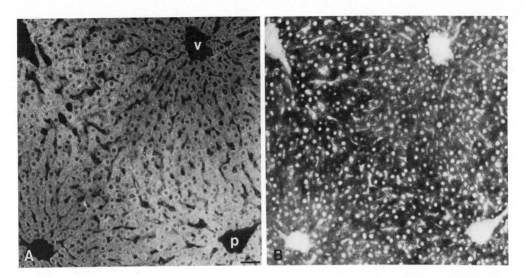

Fig. 1. Parallel liver sections (8 μm) of an 24 h fasted animal were
stained for PEPCK (A) or SDH (B). - p Terminal portal vein. - v Terminal hepatic vein. - Bar 50 μm.

2.   Methods

Rat liver parenchymal cells were isolated by recirculating collagenase perfusion (3) and inoculated onto collagen-coated coverslips in
Medium 199 (Earle's salts) containing 4% foetal calf serum, 10 nM
dexamethasone and 1 nM insulin. After 3 h medium was changed and foetal serum then omitted. Incubation was carried out at $37^{O}C$, 5% CO_2,
13% O_2, 82% N_2.

For details of immunofluorescence microscopy see (2).

3.   Results

1. Isolated hepatocytes in suspension and after 1 h of culture
contained different amounts of PEPCK (fig. 2).

2. Hepatocytes cultured for 24 h in the presence of 10 nM dexamethasone and 1 nM insulin showed a weak fluorescence. The heterogeneity with respect to PEPCK was not totally lost (fig. 3a).

3. Hepatocytes cultured for 20 h as under 2. and then treated
with 10 nM glucagon for 4 h possessed essentially the same amounts of
PEPCK (fig. 3b).

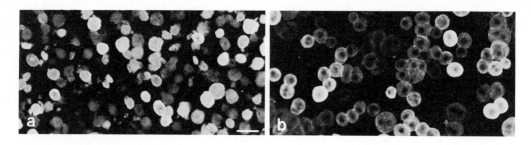

Fig. 2. Hepatocyte suspension (a) and 1 h cultured hepatocytes (b) were stained for PEPCK. - Bar 50 μm

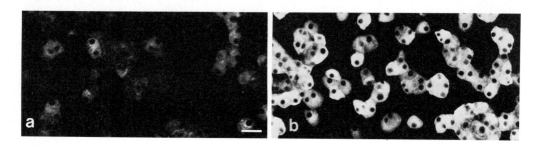

Fig. 3. Hepatocytes cultured for 24 h in the presence of 10 nM dexamethasone, 1 nM insulin (a), and for the last 4 h 10 nM glucagon was added (b): staining for PEPCK. - Bar 50 μm

4. Conclusion

    Under inducing conditions with glucagon heterogeneous liver parenchymal cells can be converted into a homogeneous cell population with respect to PEPCK.

5. References

(1) Jungermann, K. and N. Katz (1982). Hepatology 2, 385-395.
(2) Andersen, B., A. Nath and K. Jungermann (1982). Eur. J. Cell Biol. 28, 47-53.
(3) Katz, N., M. Nauck and P. Wilson (1979). Biochem. Biophys. Res. Commun. 88, 23-29.

Preservation of the Adult Functionality of Hepatocytes in Serum-Free Cultures

J. V. Castell, M. J. Gómez-Lechón, J. Coloma, and P. Lopez

Centro de Investigacion, Hospital La Fe, Ministerio de Sanidad Avda, de Campanar 21, Valencia-9, Spain

ABSTRACT

We have studied the effects of hormone supplementation of culture medium on the maintenance of adult biochemical functions of serum-free cultured hepatocytes. The results suggest a role for glucocorticoids in the control of differentiated state of cultured adult liver cells.

1. INTRODUCTION

Cultured hepatocytes initially retain the morphology and the expression of differentiated biochemical cell functions when maintained in primary cultures, but on adaptation to culture conditions cells lose many adult capabilities and show fetal characteristics. This is the case when cells are cultured in chemically defined serum-free media. Our effort has been directed to maintain in this culture conditions highly differentiated adult liver cells and to investigate the role played by Insulin and Glucocorticoids.

2. MATERIAL AND METHODS

Hepatocytes were obtained by liver perfusion with collagenase in presence of protease inhibitors (1). Plastic culture dishes were previously coated with Fibronectin (2). Hepatocytes were seeded in Ham's F-12 medium supplemented with 0.2% bovine albumin, 10^{-8}M Insulin, 10^{-6}M Glucagon (2), and antibiotics. Cells were shifted to protein-free medium 24 h later. Dexamethasone (DEX) 10^{-8}M and Insulin 10^{-8}M were daily added to the cultures when medium was renewed. Tyrosine aminotransferase (TAT) was measured as described (3). Gamma glutamyl transpeptidase (GGT) was assayed after isozyme separation (4) as reported (5). Glycogen distribution in cultures was estimated citophotometrically after PAS staining.

3. RESULTS AND DISCUSSION

One of the most characteristic function of liver cells is the synthesis and metabolism of glycogen. Short after cell attachment hepatocytes showed in presence of 10mM glucose and 10nM Insulin an average glycogen content of 600 nmol glucose/mg protein, that gradually decreased during the following hours. By 24 h culture cells had an average con-

334

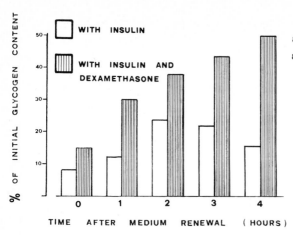

Fig.1. Glycogen synthesis after stimulation with Insulin (10^{-7}M) and/or DEX (10^{-7}M).

tent of 50 nmol glucose/mg prot. then undergoing daily periods of maxi mal glycogen accumulation 4 h after medium renewal (140 nmol gluc./mg prot.). DEX added to cultures increased glycogen storage up to 300 nmol gluc./mg prot., probably as result of glycogen synthase activation (6) Fig.1. Cells cultured in absence of Insulin gradually lost the ability to deposit glycogen when later stimulated by a higher dosis of Insulin (10^{-7}M), Fig.2. Cells in culture were not homogeneously influenced by Insulin. While the glycogen loss rate was gradual in all cells but more pronounced in the high glycogen content group, the synthesis and storage upon Insulin stimulation was almost due to a cell subpoblation ($\sim$30%) reaching up to 80% of initial glycogen content.

TAT induction by hormones is a well accepted marker of a differentia ted liver cell. Glucocorticoids (10^{-7}M) induced a maximum of activity 18 h after stimulation (lag:0-4 h). Glucagon (10^{-6}M) showed no lag period and maximal activity was found 9 h after incorporation to the cul ture. When both hormones were simultaneously present the TAT activity

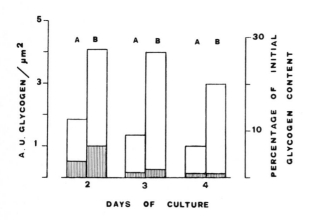

Fig.2. Response to Insulin by hepatocytes cultured in presence of Insulin (clean) versus control (shadowed). A: time 0 h. B: 4 h.

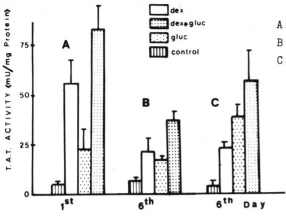

Fig.3. TAT induction by hormones
A: control, freshly isolated cells
B: non supplemented culture
C: 10^{-7}M DEX supplemented culture

closely resembled the activity induced by each hormone separately. We
did not find a clear potentiation effect. In non supplemented cultures
TAT activity induced by Glucagon or DEX decreased along a week of culture (25 to 15 and 60 to 20 mU/mg prot. respectively), however when DEX
was continously present cells still maintained a fasely good ability
to induce TAT upon adition of hormones after a week of culture (Fig.3).

In continous presence of DEX the synthesis and excretion of adult plas
ma proteins was maintained in a greater extend than in controls (14 ver
sus 10 µg/mg prot.hour). Pre-albumin, albumin, transferrin, fibrinogen
α_2Macroglobulin and other plasma proteins were found in one week cultu
res supernatant as evidentiated by SDS-PAGE and inmunoelectrophoresis.

The integrity of the cell membrane was evaluated on the basis of enzymatic leakage to the medium. GPT activity increased from 28±4 to
50±9 in controls while in presence of DEX, 13±1.5 to 8.5±0.1 mU/mg prot.
from day 1 to 5th. During the same period GOT increased in controls from
26±6 up to 420±50 while in DEX supplemented cultures only 14±4 to 31±5.
DEX also slowed the rapid decrease of cit.P-450 microsomal enzymes. Bi-
liverdin reductase was 50% the 2nd day. If DEX was absent only 5%.

DEX also blocked the expression of proteins like αFetoprotein and GGT
which are assigned to fetal behaviour of cells. Cultures show a progre
sive rise of GGT activity along the days of culture reaching a value
100× greater by the 8th culture day (7). At the same time there is a
progresive displacement by the fetal isozyme. As shown in Fig.4 DEX
selectively blocked the expression of the fetal isozyme. We had previously shown (8) that the isozyme pattern of two key metabolic enzymes Pyruvate Kinase and Aldolase shifted to a fetal type along the days
of culture. The presence of DEX prevented this displacement by inhibiting the expression of the fetal isozyme. Those findings suggest a role for glucocorticoids in the control of differentiated state of cultu
red adult liver parenchymal cells.

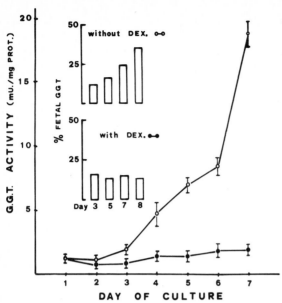

Fig.4. GGT activity in cultures

4. REFERENCES

1) Coloma J. et al. *Proc. of the II Congress FESBE* Madrid 1981, nr.595
2) see paper by Gomez-L. M.J., and Castell J.V. this volume
3) Granner D.K., Tomkins G.M. *Methods in Enzymology* 17-A, 633 (1970)
4) Coloma J., Castell J.V. *Biol. Cell.* 45, 71 (1982)
5) Sirica A.E., Richards W.C. et al. *P.N.A.S.* 76, 283 (1979)
6) De Wulf H., Hers H.G., *Eur.J. Biochem.* 244, 1701 (1969)
7) Coloma J., Gomez-L. M.J., et al. *Experientia* 37, 941 (1981)
8) Feliu J.E., Coloma J., et al. *Mol. Cel. Biochem.* 45, 73 (1982)

Isolation and Characterization of MDCK-Subcultures

E. M. Giesen, C. Welsch, M. Schmidt, J. L. Imbs, A. Steffan*, and J. Schwartz

Institut de Pharmacologie and *Institut de Virologie, Faculté de Médecine, F-67000 Strasbourg, France

ABSTRACT

In order to obtain uniform populations derived from the MDCK cell line, the technique of centrifugal elutriation has been used. Seven cell types, which differ from each other by their size have been sub-cultured and characterized with regards to their morphology and stimulation of adenylate cyclase. The latter is inducible by isoproterenol in a rapid and dose dependent way. The smallest cells are the most sensitive to isoproterenol; the increase of enzyme activity brought about by these cells is higher than that of the original cell line.

1. Introduction

The MDCK cells are derived from the whole kidney of a normal dog and form confluent epithelial monolayers on a glass or plastic culture dish. In culture, these cells retain a differentiated morphology (apical brush border, apical tight junctions and lateral spaces (1) as well as certain physiological and enzymatic properties of the distal and collecting tubules such as a pattern of adenylate cyclase activity (2, 3,4). They seem cytologically more uniform than the kidney despite a certain diversity of cell size and number of nuclei and nucleoli. A homogeneous population of differentiated cells would therefore be usefull to improve the MDCK cell line as a model of kidney physiology.

2. Methods

Cell culture and adenylate cyclase induction

MDCK cells (70-80 serial passages, Flow Laboratories) were grown in Falcon 75 dishes in Eagle's medium containing 10% calf serum (Flow). Adenylate cyclase induction was performed on 4.10^{-7} trypsinized cells in 250 µl serum-free medium in the presence of papaverine (5.10^{-4}M) and/or isoproterenol as indicated. The incubation time was 5 min. The cAMP content was determined by the method of Brown et al. (5), the protein content according to Lowry et al. (6).

Staining

Cells were fixed in situ and embedded as described elsewhere (7). Toluidine Blue and PAS staining were performed on semi-thin sections.

Centrifugal elutriation

The cells were spun at 1600 rpm in a Beckman JE-6 rotor. The flow rate varied from 30 ml/min to 130 ml/min.

3. Results

Subcultering by elutriation

By the technique of centrifugal elutriation, viable cells are separated according to their rate of sedimentation. This is possible without using a density gradient, by opposing the tendency of the cells to sediment in a centrifugal field to a liquid flowing in the centripetal direction. At a constant rotor speed, the increase of fluid velocity reduces the g forces and cells, with increasing sedimentation rates, will be washed (elutriated) out of the rotor.

Seven fractions of equal-sized cells were obtained. We measured the cell size of all seven fractions : 1) 18μ x 9μ; 2) 25μ x 13μ; 3) 42μ x 31μ; 4) 60μ x 45μ; 5) 92μ x 60μ; 6) 100μ x 65μ; 7) 110μ x 80μ. The smaller cells (1 to 4) proliferated quickly after plating (24h generation time), the big cells seemed unable to divide. After 8 days of culture, however, very small cells (17μ x 10μ) appeared among the cells of fractions 6 and 7. The small cells grew rapidly and soon covered the available surface.

Staining properties

No differences between the subcultures derived from the seven elutriated fractions were observed. When stained with Toluidine Blue, all cells had one or more big central nuclei with one or several nucleoli. Only the smallest cells seem to be mononuclear. No abnormal mitotic figures were observed. Abaza et al. (8) described three types of reaction to PAS : 1) staining of nuclear membranes; 2) uniform staining of the cytoplasm and 3) negative reaction. We distinguished unstained cells and cells containing distinct vacuoles with PAS positive material.

Adenylate cyclase induction

Induction of adenylate cyclase was previously reported in MDCK cells (9), we therefore decided to investigate whether the different fractions have a different enzymatic equipment, using adenylate cyclase as a marker. The response to isoproterenol of unelutriated MDCK cells (Table 1) and of three fractions of elutriated cells (Figure 1) was studied.

A significant induction by papaverine and isoproterenol was obtained with the MDCK cells (p < 0.001, Scheffé's test). The maximum of adenylate cyclase induction appears after 3 to 5 min (data not shown).

The sensitivity to the beta-agonist seems to be typical for each of the three fractions, since the highest induction rate was obtained with the smallest cells while larger cells are much less responsive. This

Table 1. *cAMP content of unelutriated cells*

	cAMP content (%) (m ± SD)		
Papaverine	215	30	(n=4)
Isoproterenol	198	36	(n=4)
Papaverine + Isoproterenol	440	42	(n=4)

The increase of cAMP was expressed as the ratio of cAMP content brought about by papaverine and/ or isoproterenol ($10-6M$) compared to the basal level of cAMP.

Figure 1. *Dose-response curve with isoproterenol*

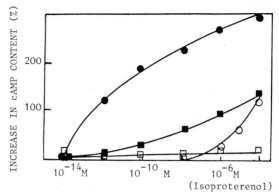

The cAMP content in unelutriated cells (O) or cells of the first (●), second (■) and third (□) fractions of elutriated cells was determined in the presence of papaverine and isoproterenol. The cAMP content is expressed as the percentage of cAMP content measured in the presence of papaverine alone. Four representative curves are shown.

finding might indicate a direct relationship between the volume/surface ratio (number of receptors) for a cell and its inducibility. Unelutriated cells are less responsive to isoproterenol than cells of fraction 2, although at high hormone concentrations the peak of cAMP content corresponds to the value obtained with cells of fraction 2.

4. Conclusion

Centrifugal elutriation has proved useful in separating cells of different size without any loss of viability of the cultures. This method made it possible to obtain a MDCK subculture with adenylate cyclase twice as sensitive to isoproterenol than in the original strain.

5. References

1. Simmons N.L. (1982) Gen. Pharmac. 13, 287-291.
2. Rindler M.J., Chuman L.M., Schaffer L. and Saier M.H. (1979). J. Cell. Biol. 81, 635-648.
3. Handler J.S., Perkins F.M. and Johnson J.P. (1980). Am. J. Physiol. 238, F1-F9.
4. Grantham J.J. and Orloff J. (1968). J. Clin. Invest. 47, 1154-1161.
5. Brown B.L., Albano J.D.M., Ekins R.P., Sgherzi A.M. and Tampion W. (1971). Biochem. J. 121, 561-562.
6. Lowry O.H., Rosebrough N.J., Farr A.L. and Randall R.J. (1951). J. Biol. Chem. 193, 265-275.
7. Rabito C.A., Tchao R., Valentich J. and Leighton J. (1978). J. Membrane Biol. 43, 351-365.
8. Abaza N.A., Leighton J. and Schultz S.G. (1974). In vitro 10, 172-183.
9. Brown C.D.A. and Simmons N.L. (1981). Biochem. Biophys. Acta, 649, 427-435.

The Role of Fetal Calf Serum (FCS) During the First Stages of Hepatocytes Cultures

M. J. Gómez-Lechón and J. V. Castell

Centro de Investigación, Ciudad Sanitaria La Fe, Valencia-9, Spain

ABSTRACT

Fibronectin (FN) from serum of unrelated vertebrates have the same ability as FCS to allow hepatocyte attachment and spreading.FN mediated attachment is an active process selective for viable cells that shows sigmoid kinetics,strong dependence of temperature and divalent cations. The presence of glucagon and albumin in culture was found to be important environmental requirements for complete hepatocyte spreading that involves RNA,protein synthesis and cytoskeleton rearrangement.

1. INTRODUCTION

Studies "in vitro" on cultured cells suggest that attachment and spreading of vertebrate cells to a solid substrate is essential for normal cell physiology and survival (1).It is known that freshly isolated hepatocytes do not attach directly onto polystyrene surfaces in total absence of FCS.However,they readily attach to a variety of substrates containing ligands for which cells have receptors (2,3).In order to replace FCS we have studied its role during early stages of cultures and compared with other attachment-promoting non-serum factors i.e. lectins (LEC) and polylysine (PL).

2. MATERIAL AND METHODS

Hepatocytes were isolated as previously described (4).Culture medium was Ham F-12 with 0.2 % BSA,10^{-8}M insulin and antibiotics.Culture dishes were coated with sera FNs (rat,rabbit,goat,calf and human) enriched fractions (50 % precipitated by $(NH_4)_2SO_4$ and DEAE-column cromatography),or with 0.1 % LEC (concanavalin A and wheat germ lectin) or 0.1 % PL.attachment index was measured according to Ballard and Tomkins (5).Metabolic inhibitors were used at a dose of 10^{-6}M cycloheximide,0.2 μg/ml actinomicin D,2 μg/ml colchicin and 5 μg/ml cytochalasin B.

3. RESULTS AND DISSION

Freshly isolated hepatocytes do not attach to nacked plastic dishes when cultured in serum-free media.However FCS coated dishes readily promote effective cell attachment and spreading (2).This attachment-promoting activity was first isolated by 50 % $(NH_4)_2SO_4$ precipitation.Then purified by DEAE- cellulose column cromatography,electrophoresed in non-denaturating conditions (Fig.1A) and the proteins transferred to Millipore sheets (Fig.1B).When this sheet was incubated with an hepatocyte suspension,cells selectively attached to one protein band (Fig.1C).Data from SDS-mercaptoethanol PAGE gels evidentiated that it is a two subunit protein,molecular weight 220K and was identified as plasma FN (6).Culture dishes coated with FN from phylogenetically unrelated vertebrates serum had the same ability as FCS to allow attachment (Fig.2).No matter which serum was used this activity could be blocked by rabbit IgG against rat serum FN,thus suggesting a close relationship between immunological determinants and biological activity. Hepatocyte adhesion can also be mediated by non-serum factors such as LEC and PL.When compared to that mediated by FN,it became evident that kinetics of FN attachment was sigmoid with an initial lag phase of 10 min while for LEC and PL was hyperbolic (Fig.3).During the lag this process was not affected by metabolic inhibitors.The specific divalent

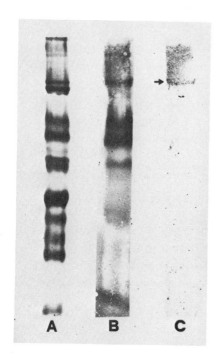

Fig.1 Electrophoretic identification of FN:Biological assay.

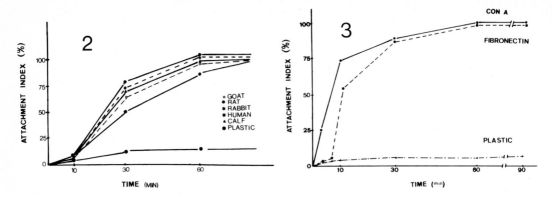

Fig.2 Cell attachment mediated by different sera FNs.
Fig.3 Kinetics of cell attachment to different substrata.

cations requirements (Fig.4) and,in particular,the strong temperature
dependence (Fig.5) clearly distinguish attachment mediated by FN from
other substances (7).Maximal attachment was found at 37ºC when 2.5 mM
Ca^{2+} and Mg^{2+} were present in culture medium.FN was highly selective
for viable cells.A sensible number of dead hepatocytes,which in fact
had lost the capacity for specific binding to FN,were attached on LEC
and PL coated plates.Concerning the effect of the hormones during this
step of the culture,insulin greatly enhanced cell attachment,whereas
dexamethasone that largely improved cell survival,and glucagon did not
play any role during this period.Hepatocytes are very restricted in
their environmental requirements for spreading since during this phase RNA,protein synthesis and cytoskeleton rearrangement are involved.
FN but not LEC and PL coated dishes allowed reproducible and complete spreading during the first few hours after plating.It is possible
that additional conditioning of these substratum by cells is required
for complete extension (2).In this sense,during cell attachment FCS only could be replaced by plasma FN from different animal sources.The
role of FCS during extension of cells,once they are attached on FN,
could be replaced by protein (0.2 % BSA) and 10^{-6}M glucagon supplemented media.This hormone greatly facilitates hepatocyte spreading
(Fig.6) probably due to the increase of specific protein synthesis involved in spreading.Finally,culture medium renewal shortly after cell
plating (1-2 H),is essential to obtain complete hepatocyte spreading.

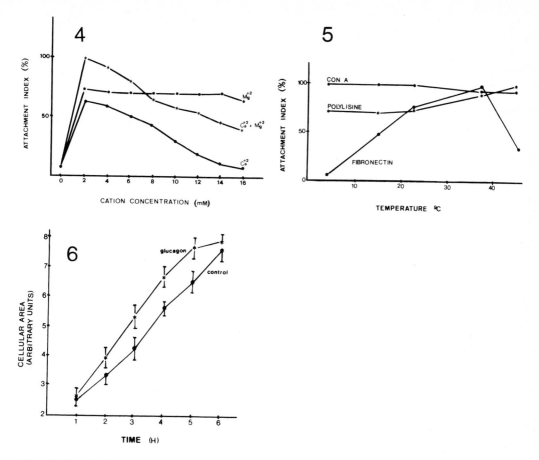

<u>Fig.4</u> Divalent cation concentration effect on hepatocyte attachment.
<u>Fig.5</u> Effect of the temperature on cell attachment.
<u>Fig.6</u> Effect of glucagon on hepatocyte spreading.

<u>4. REFERENCES</u>

(1) Gospodarowicz,D.D.,(1980) Proc.Soc.Acad.Sci.USA 77,4094
(2) Gjessing,R. and Seglen,P.O.,(1980) Exp. Cell Res. 129,239
(3) Johansson,S.,Kjellen,L.,Hook,M. and Timpl,R.,(1981) J.Cell Biol. 90,260
(4) Gómez-Lechón,M.J.,Barberá,E.,Gil,R. and Báguena,J.,(1981) Cel.Mol. Biol. 27,695
(5) Ballard,P.L. and Tomkins,G.M.,(1970) J. Cell Biol. 47,222
(6) Yamada,K.M. and Olden,K.,(1978) Nature 275,179
(7) Seglen,P.O. and Gjessing,J.,(1978) J. Cell Sci. 34,117

Modulation of Specific Functions in Adult and Fetal Hepatocytes Maintained in a Co-Cultured System

C. Guguen-Guillouzo, G. Lescoat, G. Baffet, E. Le Rumeur, B. Clément, D. Glaise, and A. Guillouzo

Unité de Recherches Hépatologiques U 49, INSERM, Hôpital de Pontchaillou, F-35011 Rennes Cedex, France

ABSTRACT

   When co-cultured with another epithelial cell type derived from rat liver, human and rat hepatocytes can survive for several weeks in a serum-free medium. Adult parenchymal cells retained specific functions at high levels, such as albumin secretion whereas fetal cells continued to differentiate. Co-cultured cells appeared to be able to produce their own extracellular matrix. This emphasizes the need for cultured hepatocytes to have a specific reconstructed environment.

1.   INTRODUCTION

   Cells in vivo are influenced by a complex set of nutritional, hormonal and stromal factors, which need to be defined in order to reconstitute an adequate environment for long-term cell survival and functioning in vitro. A defined medium has thus far not been devised for culturing hepatocytes which are highly differentiated cells. Recent emphasis was placed on the role played by the extracellular matrix. However, although complex matrices, particularly the one derived from the liver connective biomatrix, could strongly improve hepatocyte survival, no concomitant quantitative maintenance of functional activities were obtained. This led us to hypothesize that as in vivo, hepatocytes require in vitro specific cell-cell interactions. When hepatocytes were co-cultured in a serum-free medium with undifferentiated liver epithelial cells (LEC), thought to derive from biliary ductular cells, the following points were observed : 1) the cells were able to secrete an abundant and heterogenous extracellular material, 2) adult hepatocytes retained highly differentiated functions, and 3) fetal hepatocytes differentiated.

2.   CELL OBTAINMENT AND CULTURE

   After isolation by collagenase perfusion or dissociation, adult and fetal hepatocytes from rat and human liver were plated in polystyrene flasks in Ham F_{12} medium containing albumin, insulin and 10 % fetal calf serum (FCS) (1,2). Three hours later, the medium was discarded and rat liver epithelial cells (LEC) were added. The medium, with or without FCS, and supplemented with 3.5×10^{-6} M hydrocortisone hemisuccinate, was renewed daily.

3. SURVIVAL RATE AND FUNCTIONING OF CO-CULTURED HEPATOCYTES

In conventional culture conditions as previously described (3,4) adult hepatocytes did not survive for more than a few days and rapidly lost their highly differentiated functions, whereas in co-cultures, they remained viable for at least 6-8 weeks. During this period no significant loss of hepatocytes or proliferation of LEC was shown. Cell viability was not dependent on the presence of FCS while hydrocortisone was required ; in its absence hepatocytes did not survive for more than about 1-2 weeks and hormone-dependent effects were observed (5). At the ultrastructural level, parenchymal cells maintained typical characteristics of in vivo cells, including flattened rough endoplasmic reticulum and numerous glycogen particles. Golgi complexes were located in the vicinity of bile canaliculus-like structures.

Both human and rat adult hepatocytes remained capable of secreting high levels of albumin (1,2). This secretion level was higher when the cells were cultured in the presence of FCS and could be modulated. A decreased albumin production by hepatocytes cultured for a few days in conventional conditions could be reversed by addition of LEC. Active albumin secretion required the establishment of cell-cell contacts between the two cell populations. LEC could not be replaced by a conditioned medium or a cell extract. Cell-cell contacts were followed by a rapid and abundant production of extracellular material (EM) located mainly between the two cell types and in hepatocyte cords. Qualitative and quantitative differences were found in the amounts and the organization of EM in co-cultured human and rat hepatocytes. Preliminary analysis of this material indicated that it was rich in fibronectin and type III collagen. It also contained laminin, type IV collagen and low amounts of type I collagen. Among the other differentiated functions retained were the inducibility of tyrosine aminotransferase by dexamethasone and drug metabolizing enzyme activities. Adult human hepatocytes were capable of conjugating drugs for at least 3 weeks (6).

In co-culture, human and fetal rat hepatocytes also survived for several weeks instead of 1-2 weeks as in conventional conditions (7,8). Moreover, while they initially secreted large amounts of alpha-fetoprotein and low levels of albumin, they quickly began secreting high levels of albumin while in parallel those of alpha-fetoprotein declined. In these co-cultures the secretion of an abundant EM also occurred (manuscript in preparation).

CONCLUSIONS

These observations demonstrate for the first time that adult rat and human hepatocytes might survive for several weeks in a serum-free medium. This was possible by mimicking specific cell-cell interactions normally existing in the intact liver. Indeed it may be assumed that cooperation between hepatocytes and LEC occurred because LEC are presumed to derive from bile ductular cells and therefore are in close contact with parenchymal cells in vivo. This is sustained by the absence of cooperation between hepatocytes and non hepatic cells such as epithelial cells from rat kidney and bovine cristalline lens. In addition LEC could not be replaced by epithelial cells isolated from the human gall bladder. Moreover they had to be untransformed, i.e., used before their progressive spontaneous transformation which occurred around the 50th passage.

If it was clearly demonstrated that cell-cell contacts had to be established between the two cell populations, it remains to elucidate the nature of the signal which induces cell-cell interactions. Hydrocortisone appeared essential and could act by exerting a permissive effect at the plasma membrane level (5). Cell contacts were followed by the rapid secretion of an abundant EM which was heterogenous as is the case of liver extracellular matrix. Its complete characterization as well as the respective participation of the two cell types in the production of the different components are under study. Nevertheless, it is likely that the EM presents a great tissue-specificity and that it plays an important role in long-term survival and functioning of co-cultured hepatocytes. Although the composition of the nutrient medium would need to be more accurately defined it appears that a co-culture system associating hepatocytes with LEC represents a promising tool for various investigations of hepatic functions. Particularly, it could be suitable for long-term studies of drug toxicity and hepatocarcinogenesis as well as hepatic differentiation.

ACKNOWLEDGMENTS

We thank Mrs M. André for typing the manuscript. This work was supported by INSERM grants (CRL 822021 and 827015).

REFERENCES

1. Guguen-Guillouzo C., Clément B., Baffet G., Beaumont C., Morel-Chany E., Glaise D. and Guillouzo A., Exp. Cell Res., 1983, in press.
2. Guguen-Guillouzo C., Baffet G., Clément B., Bégué J.M., Glaise D. and Guillouzo A. in "Isolation, characterization and use of hepatocytes", Harris R.A. and Cornell N.W. Eds, 1983, Elsevier, in press.
3. Guguen C., Guillouzo A., Boisnard M., Le Cam A. and Bourel M., Biol. Gastroenterol., 1975, 8, 223-231.
4. Guguen-Guillouzo C., Campion J.P., Brissot P., Glaise D., Launois B., Bourel M. and Guillouzo A., Cell Biol. Intern. Rep., 1982, 6, 625-628.
5. Baffet G., Clément B., Glaise D., Guillouzo A. and Guguen-Guillouzo C., Biochem. Biophys. Res. Comm., 1982, in press.
6. Bégué J.M., Le Bigot J.F., Guguen-Guillouzo C., Kiechel J.R. and Guillouzo A., submitted for publication.
7. Guguen-Guillouzo C., Tichonicky L., Szajnert M.F. and Kruh J., In Vitro, 1980, 16, 1-10.
8. Guguen-Guillouzo C., Marie J., Cottreau D., Pasdeloup N. and Kahn A., Biochem. Biophys. Res. Comm., 1980, 93, 528-534.

Cell Culture and Differentiated Properties of Nephron Epithelial Cells in Defined Medium

M. Horster, P. D. Wilson, M. Schmolke, and D. Kühner

Physiologisches Institut, Universität München, D-8000 München, FRG

ABSTRACT

A new method for in vitro culture of epithelial cells derived from individual defined nephron segments has been developed. Cell isolation and substratum are decisive for initial anchorage and mitotic activity. These nephron epithelia have differential requirements, depending upon the cell type, for growth and proliferation in serum-free medium supplemented with hormones and growth factors. The cultured nephron epithelia express differentiated characteristics. Activation of adenylate cyclase by hormones is cell-type specific. Cells derived from the cortical collecting tubule (CT) have different mitochondrial fluorescence indicating two cell populations. Na-K-ATPase activity in cultured CT cells was quantitated. These cells also express a transepithelial ouabain-sensitive voltage. The new method for culture of segmental nephron cell populations is suitable for studies on the regulation of functional differentiation.

METHODS

Cell culture. Defined nephron segments were dissected from fresh slices of the rabbit kidney and explanted individually into culture dishes (Petriperm) coated with a substratum of collagen/plasma (100/1,v/v), as described previously (1-4). Microdissection of single nephron segments was done without proteinase or chelating agents, using tweezers only (5). The cell types studied for requirements of proliferation were: cortical collecting tubule (CTc) and thick ascending loop (TALc),medullary collecting tubule (CTm) and thick ascending loop (TALm),the proximal straight tubule (PST) and the embryonic nephron Anlage (Fig.1). A Lucite ring was placed on the substratum to facilitate outgrowth and anchorage of the epithelial cells. The defined nephron culture medium (NCM) and its hormonal supplements for growth in fibroblast-free cultures have been described (2).

^{3}H-thymidine uptake. Monolayer cultures were incubated for 24 h at 37° in medium containing 1 µCi/ml ^{3}H-thymidine; they were coated with a liquid emulsion (L4, Ilford) after fixation and exposed for 6 days as previously reported (6). The number of ^{3}H-thymidine labeled nuclei and the total number of nuclei were counted in each culture.

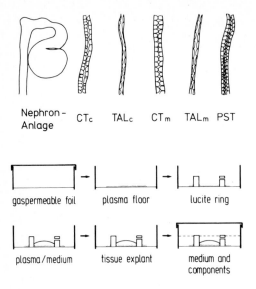

Fig.1. Scheme of method for in vitro culture of renal epithelial cells derived from individual nephron segments.

Nephron-Anlage   CTc   TALc   CTm   TALm   PST

gaspermeable foil   plasma floor   lucite ring

plasma/medium   tissue explant   medium and components

Cytochemistry. A histochemical lead capture technique was used for the localisation of adenylate cyclase activity. Monolayer epithelia were shock frozen and incubated in a buffered medium (Tris maleate 50mM, pH 7.2; MgCl2 4 mM; adenylylimidophosphate 0.3 mM; Pb(NO3) 2 mM). To stimulate basal adenylate cyclase activity, one of the following hormones was added to this medium: arginine vasopressin (25 µU /ml); PTH (10 I.E./ml); isoproterenol (10^{-5}M). The reaction product was converted to black lead sulphide and examined by lightmicroscopy (7).

Mitochondrial fluorescence. Cells derived from TAL and CT were incubated with a specific mitochondrial probe (DASPMI, 100 µg/ml; 30min; 37°) and evaluated in an inverted-type microscope (Zeiss IM35). Fluorescence of single cells was measured using a scanning stage, photometer and multiplier (Zeiss), at 455 to 499 nm excitation. Exposure time was 220 msec per cell, 200 cells of each type were measured as previously described (8).

Quantitation of Na^+-K^+-ATPase activity. The sodium transport enzyme was measured in cell monolayers of CT. Cell numbers were between 900 and 12.000. The new modification of a micromethod measures the labeled phosphate released in the culture by hydrolysis of $\left[\gamma\text{-}^{32}P\right]$ ATP. Total and ouabain-insensitive ATPase activity were obtained in paired cultures of identical cell populations. Enzyme activity was expressed as picomoles of inorganic phosphate per cell per hour (9).

Transepithelial electrical potential difference. Confluent cell monolayers were grown on special membranes manufactured from collagen. They were placed in a Lucite holder and incubated in a culture dish. The holder was removed from the dish in intervals and inserted into a modified miniature Ussing chamber; transepithelial voltage (V_t, mV) was recorded while the cells were examined by lightmicroscopy (1).

RESULTS

Differential growth response. Distal nephron epithelia from TAL and CT grow in confluent monolayers. Cells are anchorage-dependent. Substratum and a thyroid supplement (T_3;T_4) of NCM were essential for initial outgrowth from the donor segment. Cell proliferation of distal nephron cell types (Fig.2A) was sustained in a segment-specific way by hormones and growth factors in serum-free medium(1-4). Dexamethasone, insulin,and prolactin were particularly stimulating for nephron cell growth. Metanephric Anlagen differentiated into convoluted tubules only on semisolid substratum in serum-supplemented medium (1). PST,by contrast, form monolayers in NCM with FCS(3%). Therefore, we conclude that requirements for proliferative growth of nephron epithelia in culture depend on the segmental cell type.

DNA-synthesis. ^{3}H-thymidine incorporation by indirect (autoradiography) and direct (scintillation) measurements revealed that the growth-supporting factors dexamethasone,thyroxine,insulin,prolactin and EGF stimulate nuclear thymidine uptake to different extents (6). By contrast, hormones concerned with renal ion and water transport, such as vasopressin,isoproterenol,db-cAMP and aldosterone, inhibit the incorporation of thymidine to different extents in segmental cell cultures (6).

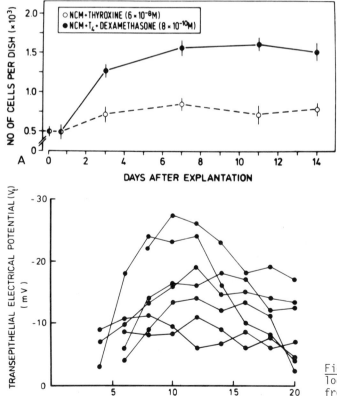

Fig. 2. (A) Growth pattern of loop of Henle cells in serum-free medium. (B) Voltage (mV) across collecting tubule cells.

350

Stimulation of hormone-sensitive adenylate cyclase. The presence and
the amount in response to hormones of the adenylate cyclase in monolayer cultures of
CTc,TALc,CTm and TALm showed that the extent of enzyme activation by hormones is differential according to the epithelium of origin (7).

Quantitation of mitochondrial fluorescence. The quantitation revealed a
normally distributed histogram of medium-range intensity in TAL cell cultures; by
contrast, CT cultures exhibited a two-peak pattern of mitochondrial fluorescence distribution among CT cells suggesting that two populations of differing mitochondrial
content are present in CT cultures (8).

The sodium transport enzyme. The activity of Na-K-ATPase in 10-day cultures
of CT cells (n,18) was 0.79 ± 0.14 pmoles per hour per cell (9), suggesting that a-
bout 70 % of the in vivo activity of the enzyme are expressed in serum-free, partially supplemented medium (10).

Transcellular voltage. V_t was 16.3 ± 9 mV (n,7), negative on upper cell side
facing the medium, in CT cultures incubated in NCM plus dexamethasone(10^{-9}M) for 10
days (Fig. 2B). Values of V_t on day 10 fall within the range of in vivo data (11).

REFERENCES

(1) Horster,M.,Pflügers Archiv 382:209, 1979
(2) Horster,M., Int. J. Biochem. 12:29, 1980
(3) Horster,M.,Wilson,P.D., Cell Biol. Int.Rep. 5:765, 1981
(4) Horster,M.,Wilson,P.D., Proc.VIII.Int.Congr.Nephrol.RH105, 1981
(5) Horster,M.,Am.J.Physiol. 235, F 387, 1978
(6) Wilson,P.D.,Horster,M.,Am.J.Physiol., 1983 (in press)
(7) Wilson,P.D.,Horster,M., J.Histochem.Cytochem., 1983 (in press)
(8) Horster,M., et al., J. Microscopy, 1983 (in press)
(9) Schmolke,M.,Horster,M.,Pflügers Archiv (submitted)
(10) Schmidt,U.,Horster,M.,Am.J.Physiol. 233:F55, 1978
(11) Horster,M.,Zink,H.,Kidney Int. (in the press, 1982)

Multiplication of Adult Rat Hepatocytes in Monolayer Cultures

Dieter Paul and Angelika Piasecki
Department of Toxicology, Hamburg University Medical School, Grindelallee 117,
D-2000 Hamburg 13, FRG

Hepatocytes isolated from fetal or newborn rats have been shown to multiply in monolayer culture in selective arginine-free medium (1). In contrast, adult rat hepatocytes have been difficult to stimlulate to divide although some observations of hepatocytes entering S phase have been published (2-5) and some hormone-dependent proliferative activity has been reported in such cells after 1-2 days adaptation in plastic dishes (6) and on fibronectin-coated dishes (7,8). We report here on the cultivation of adult rat hepatocytes in primary cultures which multiply in response to serum and a hormone mixture in a complex culture medium (MX-76) free of arginine (9).

Materials and Methods

Hepatocytes were isolated by perfusing normal or regenerating livers of adult male or female Wistar rats (180 - 250 gr) with buffered saline, then for 12 min with buffered collagenase solution (2 mg/ml) at a flow rate of 7 ml/min at 37° C essentially as described (10).The liver capsule was then slit and tissue and cells suspended in collagenase solution and stirred magnetically (1) at 37° C for 10 min. Supernatants of one to three such digestions were pooled and centrifuged, the pellet washed and the cells suspended in medium free of arginine and counted (haemocytometer). Cell viability (trypan blue) was usually 40-50 %. Usually 1-2 x 10^8 cells in single cell suspension were obtained from one liver. Cells were incubated in medium free of arginine supplemented with dialyzed fetal calf serum (dFCS) in Falcon plastic dishes in a humidified CO_2-incubator at 37° C.The medium was changed on day 1, the cultures were washed twice and fresh arginine-free medium was added back containing the desired supplement. Determinations of (^{3}H)-thymidine and autoradiography were conducted as described (11).

Results and Discussion

When adult rat hepatocytes prepared as described in Metarials and Methods in arginine-free medium are plated on plastic dishes or on gelatin-coated dishes they do not attach or spread unless serum or plasma is present in the culture medium. Cells cultured in the presence of 15% dFCS in arginine-free medium can be kept for several weeks without sign of mitotic activity. Also, cells do not appear to proceed into S (autoradiography). Up to day 28 cells have been shown to convert (^{3}H)ornithine into (^{3}H)arginine (c.f.ref.1), presumably via the liver-specific urea cycle, indicating that liver-specific functions remain stable during this period. Thus, it

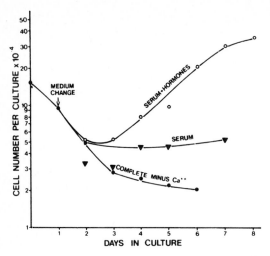

Fig. 1. Growth curves of adult normal
rat liver cells in primary cultures.
Cells were seeded at $2x10^5$ cells per
3 cm dish in arginine-free medium
containing 15% dFCS, insulin, hydrocortisone and glucagon (see text).
After a medium change with two washes
with warm medium, the desired fresh
arginine-free medium was added back
to the cultures. o dFCS plus insulin,
hydrocortisone and glucagon. ▼ dFCS.
● complete medium minus calcium.

seems possible to select for hepatocytes (i.e. arginine-producing cells) in arginine
free medium and thus to suppress growth of non-hepatocytes in the cultures.

When $2x10^5$ cells are plated in 3 cm dishes in arginine-free medium containing
15%dFCS, insulin (1 ug/ml), hydrocortisone (1 ug/ml) and glucagon (10 ug/ml) ("Complete Medium") cells plate out normally. Although the number of attached cells drops
during days 1-3 cell number starts to increase after day 3 and continues rising until
day 8 (Fig.1). Cell multiplication is strictly dependent on the presence of serum,
hormones and calcium (Fig.1). Hepatocytes derived from male or female normal or regenerating liver (24 hrs post partial hepatectomy) display similar growth patterns
as shown in Fig. 1.

Autoradiographic analyses after pulsing cultures with (^{3}H)thymidine for 24 hrs
revealed that hepatocytes start entering S phase at day 1. Although quantitation is
difficult, sparse cultures contain up to 40-60% labeled nuclei (days 2-4) and the
labeling index (LI) of confluent areas in multiplying cultures (day 5) was surprisingly high (about 40%).This pattern is unlike that observed in fibroblasts, where
the LI in confluent areas is usually extremely low (12). The final cell density in
complete medium is proportional to the serum concentration suggesting the presence
of depletable growth factors in serum. Since medium containing hormones and plasma did not appear to support hepatocyte multiplication, platelet growth factors
could be implicated (c.f.ref.13). Platelet-derived growth factor (PDGF) (14) did
not show mitogenic activity in the presence of plasma and hormones suggesting that
other platelet growth factors could be responsible for the mitogenic effect of serum. Mitogenic activity of Epidermal Growth Factor (EGF)(15), which has been implicated in stimulating hepatocyte proliferation in vivo (16), has been observed in
some experiments, but in contrast to findings by others (5,6) the response in our
cultures is variable and requires clarification. When the medium is changed daily,
cells grow significantly slower than in control cultures, suggesting the presence of
conditioning factors in the medium.

The effectiveness of the selective arginine-free medium used for culturing hepatocytes is strongly suggested for the following reasons:(a) the extent of conversion of (^{3}H)ornithine into (^{3}H)arginine increased with growing cell number in multiplying cultures indicating that the bulk of the cells consisted of arginine-producers; (b) 3T3 cell number per culture decreased when incubated in medium conditioned by hepatocytes (day 7) unless supplemented with arginine; (c) prelabeled (^{3}H)3T3 cells co-cultured with unlabeled hepatocytes are eliminated from the cultures during hepatocyte multiplication unless arginine is added to the cultures; (d)cultures incubated in serum do not proliferate unless hormones are added (Fig.1); (e) usually few cells with non-hepatocyte morphology are seen in the cultures; (f) the finding that PDGF did not support cell multiplication in cultures containing plasma and hormones suggest that few PDGF-responsive cells (e.g.fibroblasts (14)) are present as contaminating cell populations.

Although it is clear that hepatocytes in primary cultures display specific functions capable of converting (^{3}H)ornithine into (^{3}H)arginine, we have not been able to subculture hepatocytes in arginine-free medium.The morphology of cells in secondary cultures appears similar to that observed in primary cultures but cells appear to loose at least some liver specific functions upon disruption of cell monolayers by either trypsin, collagenase or EDTA used to detach cells during subcultivation.

It is c ncluded, that adult rat liver cells multiply in cultures when provided with the adequate nutrients and growth factors in the appropriate medium. The significance of these findings for the understanding of the mechanisms underlying liver regeneration are under investigation.

Acknowlegdements

We are indebted to Dr.H.Marquardt for continuous support and constructive criticism.Thos work was supported by the Deutsche Forschungsgemeinschaft (Bonn).

References

1) Leffert, H.L. and Paul,D. J.Cell Biol. 52:559-568 (1972)
2) Richman, R.A. et al. Proc. Nat Acad.Sci.USA 73: 3589-3593 (1976)
3) Sirica, A.E. et al.Proc. Nat. Acad. Sci. USA 76: 283-287 (1979)
4) Laishes,B.A. and Williams, G.M. In Vitro 12: 821-832 (1976)
5) Strain, A.J., McGowan,J.A. and Bucher,N.L.R. In Vitro 18:108-116 (1982)
6) Koch,K.S. and Leffert H.L. Cell 18: 153-163 (1979)
7) Reid,L.M. at al.Ann. New York Acad. Sci. 349: 70-76 (1980)
8) Marceau, N., Noel,M., and Deschenes, J. In Vitro 18: 1-11 (1982)
9) Seglen, P.O. in: Methods in Cell Biology Vol. 13 (ed.D.M.Prescott) pp. 29-83 (1976)
10) Paul, D. This volume
11) Paul, D. and Walter, S. Proc.Soc.Exp.Biol.Med. 145:456-460 (1974)
12) Lipton,A.,Klinger,I.,Paul,D. and Holley,R.W. Proc.Nat.Acad.Sci.USA 68: 2799-2801 (1972)
13) Kohler, N. and Lipton, A. Exp.Cell Res. 87: 297-301(1974)
14) Ross,R. and Vogel, A. Cell 14: 2o3-210 (1978)
15) Savage,C.R. and Cohen, S. J.Biol.Chem. 247: 7609-7611 (1972)
16) Bucher,N.L.R., Patel, U. and Cohen, S. In: CIBA Foundation Symposium No.55,"Hepatotrophic Factors" Elsevier/Exc.Medica/North Holland, New York, pp. 95-107 (1978)

Short-Term Modulation of Glycogenolysis, Glycolysis and Gluconeogenesis in Cultured Hepatocytes by Arterial and Venous Oxygen Concentrations

D. Wölfle, H. Schmidt, and K. Jungermann

Institut für Biochemie, Georg-August-Universität, Humboldtallee 7, D-3400 Göttingen, FRG

ABSTRACT

The influence of different oxygen concentrations on metabolic rates was studied in primary cultures of rat hepatocytes maintained in defined serum-free media with either 10 nM insulin or 10 nM glucagon. Using 4% O_2 (v/v) the rate of lactate formation was 70% higher than under 13% O_2 (v/v), while gluconeogenesis remained constant in the range from 4% O_2 (v/v) to 20% O_2 (v/v). The effects of oxygen on these metabolic rates were similar under the different hormonal conditions tested. The present results are in agreement with the model of "metabolic zonation" of the liver parenchyma: the lower O_2 tensions in the perivenous zone would enhance carbohydrate uptake to a greater extent in this zone.

1. Introduction

Oxygen tension is a critical parameter for survival and metabolism of cells in culture. However, little quantitative data exist on metabolic changes in the range of physiological oxygen tensions (1). The influence of oxygen on enzyme induction in cultured hepatocytes has been studied under various oxygen tensions mimicking the conditions of hepatic blood supply (6% O_2 v/v $\triangleq$ 43 mm Hg, venous concentration; 13% O_2 v/v $\triangleq$ 95 mm Hg, arterial concentration) (2). The aim of the present study was to investigate short-term effects of oxygen on metabolic rates of adult rat hepatocytes in primary culture.

2. Methods

Hepatocytes were maintained for 48 h in serum-free culture on Falcon plastic under 15% O_2 (v/v) with either high (10 nM) or low (0.5 nM) insulin concentrations and addition of glucagon (10 nM) to induce conditions displaying predominantly glycolytic ("perivenous" cells) and gluconeogenic ("periportal" cells) activities respectively. Metabolic rates were determined by incubating the cells for additional

2 h with ^{14}C-labelled substrates as described previously (3) under varying gas atmospheres containing 5% CO_2/0-20% O_2 (v/v) and correspondingly 95-75% N_2 (v/v) as indicated.

3. Results

Glycogenolysis: The rate of glucose and lactate formation from glycogen was 1.6 fold higher under 6% O_2 (v/v) (mimicking venous O_2 tension) and 3.5 fold higher under 4% O_2 (v/v) (mimicking hepatovenous O_2 tension) compared with the rates under arterial oxygen tension (Fig. 1). Using anaerobic conditions glycogen breakdown reached its maximum in cells treated with high insulin concentrations ("perivenous" cells).

Glycolysis: The rates of lactate formation from glucose under 4% O_2 (v/v) were found to be 1.7 fold higher than under 13% O_2 (v/v). The stimulation of glycolysis by reduced oxygen concentrations was similar in insulin and glucagon induced hepatocytes.

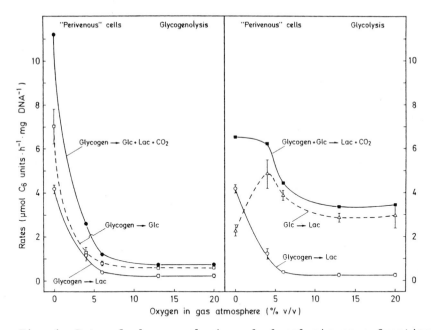

Fig. 1. Rate of glycogenolysis and glycolysis as a function of oxygen concentration. Cells were cultured 48 h with 10 nM insulin ("perivenous" conditions) under 15% O_2 (v/v). Using the indicated O_2 concentrations metabolic rates were determined radiochemically.

Gluconeogenesis: No significant effect on glucose formation from lactate was observed within the physiological range of venous to arterial O_2 concentrations (Fig. 2). Only under anaerobic conditions there was a pronounced decrease of glucose production in cultures maintained in the presence of glucagon ("periportal" cells).

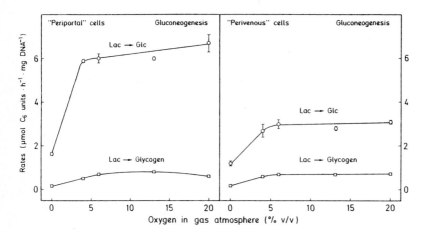

Fig. 2. Rate of gluconeogenesis as a function of oxygen concentration in glucagon ("periportal") and insulin ("perivenous") treated cells.

4.   Conclusions

The present results demonstrate that different physiological oxygen concentrations can modulate glycolysis and glycogenolysis. According to the concept of "metabolic zonation" of the liver parenchyma, glycolysis should be preferentially catalyzed by the perivenous (efferent) zone and gluconeogenesis by the periportal (afferent) zone (4). In agreement with this model the lower O_2 tension in the perivenous zone would further enhance carbohydrate uptake and breakdown already prevalent in that area.

5.   References

(1)   Taylor, W.G. and Camalier, R.F. (1982).
          J. Cell. Physiol. 111, 21-17.
(2)   Nauck, M., Wölfle, D., Katz, N. and Jungermann, K. (1982).
          Eur. J. Biochem. 119, 657-661.
(3)   Probst, I., Schwarz, P. and Jungermann, K. (1982).
          Eur. J. Biochem. 126, 271-278.
(4)   Jungermann, K. and Katz, N. (1982).
          Hepatology 2, 385-395.

Muscle Cells, Epithelial Cells, Fibroadipogenic Cells, Melanocytes and Chondrocytes

Differentiation of Primary Muscle Cells Cultured in a Serum-Free Chemically Defined Medium

P. Dollenmeier[1] and H. M. Eppenberger

Institut für Zellbiologie, CH-8093 Zürich, Switzerland

I. Primary chick myoblasts proliferate and undergo differentiation to multinucleated myotubes 'in vitro' provided embryo extract and horse or calf serum are present in the culture medium. There is increasing evidence that the behaviour of muscle cells 'in vitro' depends also on the condition of the medium, and that changing amounts of medium factors might represent signals which prompt myogenic cells either to proliferate or to terminally differentiate. In order to better control at least the starting conditions of a myogenic cell culture several attempts have been made to either simplify media or to replace the complex medium, containing mammalian serum and embryo extract, by a medium which is composed of entirely defined components.

The use of a completely defined medium has a number of advantages, e.g. is it possible to identify and characterize material which newly appears during cultivation (e.g. by secretion) or to study the effects of a given substance (e.g. growth factors, mitogens, hormones) on the cultivated cells without interference from serum factors. There are, however, also other aspects which have to be considered carefully: first, in the case of myogenic cells neither the overall morphology of fused myotubes nor the time course of survival compares too favourably to cultures grown in serum-containing medium; second, no defined medium stays defined for very long after addition of cells. The medium is modified ("conditioned") continuously by the metabolic activity of the cells and becomes undefined again. This has already been discussed in earlier publications and we came to the conclusion that development of a medium, also fully defined and fully reproducible only at the onset of culture, may nevertheless be of considerable value to solve a number of problems in myogenesis (1,2).

---

[1]Present address: Friedrich Miescher Institut, Ciba-Geigy Ltd., CH-4002 Basel, Switzerland.

II. Myogenic cells in vitro grow normally as a monolayer and subsequently most of the studies on muscle differentiation in culture
have been carried out on cells attached to the substratum. Normal
proliferation of non-transformed myogenic cells seems to depend
on substrate attachment while differentiation goes on independently from anchorage of the cells to the substrate (3). Therefore in order to allow proliferation in a fully defined medium it
is essential to have the factor(s) present which promote attachment. In the course of an earlier investigation in our laboratory
with a simplified but not fully defined, serum-free culture medium,
it could be shown that myogenic cells were easily detached from
the substrate while contaminating fibrogenic cells remained attached (4).

Subsequent experiments demonstrated the need of serum for attachment which, however, could be replaced by the serum component
fibronectin (5). Fibronectin was included in every defined medium
for primary muscle cells in order to keep the cells attached.

In a first attempt for a serum-free medium for primary chicken
muscle cells Ham's F 12 basic medium was supplemented with fibronectin (50 μg/ml), Insulin (5 μg/ml), transferrin (10 μg/ml), and
with antibiotics.

Cells plated out in this medium adhered to the substrate and
survived for at least 3 days. Some myoblasts fused into small
myotubes, but only after addition of serum and embryo extract
before the third day also some large contractile myotubes
appeared. An improvement of proliferation and differentiation
was then achieved by first replacing the Ham's F 12 formulation
with the medium MCDB 201 which had been specifically developed
for non-transformed chicken cells (6). This included also the
change from bicarbonate buffer to HEPES. An even further improvement could be demonstrated by adding fibroblast growth factor
(FGF) to the medium which is believed to make cells competent for
ongoing proliferation and to stimulate DNA-synthesis (7). A number of additional components which were known to either influence
favourably proliferation or differentiation were subsequentially
tested and lead ultimately to the formulation of the so called
"DMN"-medium (Defined medium for Muscle and Nerve cells) as shown
in table I (1,2).

Table I . COMPOSITION OF THE MEDIUM "DMN"

MDCB 201 containing the following components:

Insulin	5	μg/ml
Transferrin	10	μg/ml
Fibronectin	50	μg/ml
FGF	300	ng/ml
Glutamine	5	mM
Penicillin	100	IU/ml
Streptomycin	100	μg/ml
Beta-Hydroxybutyrate	500	μM
Cortisol-21-phosphate	10	μM
Cobalt chloride	100	nM
Glycerol	40	mM
Biotin	1	μg/ml
Oleate	10	μg/ml

III. Primary skeletal muscle cell cultures were prepared according to published standard procedures (1,8). These cells were plated into complete or incomplete DMN-medium and the following parameters were studied: a) DNA-synthesis; b) total protein-synthesis; c) cell behaviour and morphology; d) appearance of differentiated phenotype; and e) specific protein patterns (1,2). As can be seen in figure 1 DNA-synthesis and protein-synthesis largely depend on

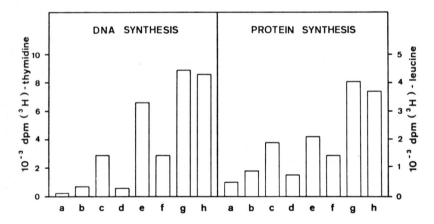

Fig. 1. Effect on DNA and protein synthesis of components included in medium DMN. Cells were plated in MCDB (+) and components included in medium DMN were added at appropriate concentrations. The overall DNA and protein synthesis was measured in cultures after labelling from 18-66 h with (^{3}H) thymidine or (^{3}H) leucine, respectively. Supplements to medium MCDB (+) at concentrations as listed in table I were as follows: a, None; b, FN; c, FN+insulin; d, FN+ transferrin; e, FN+FGF; f, FN+transferrin+insulin; g, FN+trans- ferrin+insulin+FGF; h, complete medium DMN. (From Dollenmeier et al., Exp. Cell Res. 135, p. 48, 1981; with permission).

the components present in the medium DMN. Insulin as well as FGF
exhibit major effects, the data presented even suggest a synergistic operation of the two factors. The morphological appearance
of cells grown in defined medium differs somewhat for cultures
grown in standard medium containing serum and embryo extract.
The spindleshaped appearance of mononucleated myoblasts appears
after 24 h and is indistinguishable from standard cultures; after
72 h, however, fused myotubes are in general very thin and contain less nuclei than comparable cultures in standard medium
(fig. 2). Contractions, on the other hand, can be observed after
42 h, an indication for the existence of functional myofibrils,
and furthermore for the ongoing differentiation towards the specific muscle phenotype.

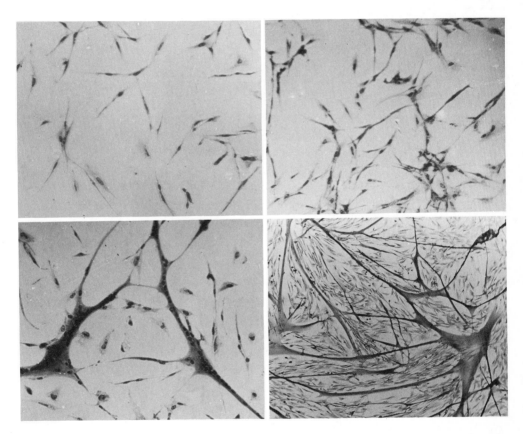

Fig. 2. Myogenic cultures in medium DMN: a, 24 h after plating;
b, 42 h; c, 72 h; d, culture in standard medium (incl. horse
serum and embryo extract) 42 h after plating.

A histochemical confirmation of the presence of myofibrils was obtained by using the indirect immunofluorescence technique. Presence of the M-line proteins myomesin (9) and MM-CK (10), both specific for the differentiated phenotype, could clearly be demonstrated in myotubes grown in DMN medium (fig. 3). During myogenesis frequently an isoprotein transition from an ubiquitous

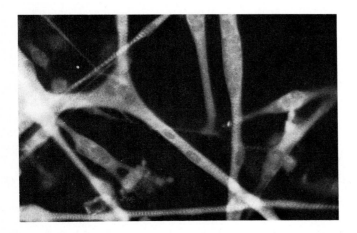

Fig. 3. Culture 42 h after plating. Immunofluorescence staining of myofibrils with antibody against myomesin (see ref. 9).

and/or embryonic isoprotein to a muscle-specific isoprotein type can be observed (11,12). Furthermore, the appearance of proteins typical for the differentiated phenotype but not for the precursor cells (e.g. myomesin) indicate the switching on of genes specific for differentiated muscle cells (9). We have shown that muscle-specific proteins which can be identified to date on 2-D-gel electrophoresis also can be demonstrated for cultures differentiated in DMN-medium (1,2). In the serum-free medium, however, muscle cells also exhibit a set of proteins which is not normally expressed in differentiating cells and which we think represents a modulation of the muscle phenotype due to DMN-medium (13). We believe that these proteins are "stress-proteins" induced by the culture conditions in DMN-medium. These proteins were detected as secreted cellular proteins after labelling the cells with ^{35}S methionine. One of the proteins synthesized and secreted by muscle cells into the medium has a molecular weight of 22'000. Induction of a particular protein synthesis pattern as a response to environmental stress had also been demonstrated earlier after heat shock (14) and after butyrate (15) or arsenate (16) supplementation of the culture medium.

However, synthesis and release into the medium of the particular stress-protein with a M_r of 22'000 is repressed again by supplementing DMN-medium with serum but not with embryo extract (fig. 4). It could well be that lack of one or more components in the DMN-medium, which are present in the serum, is responsible for a not yet defined chemical or nutritional stress situation resulting in the switching on of the particular gene(s).

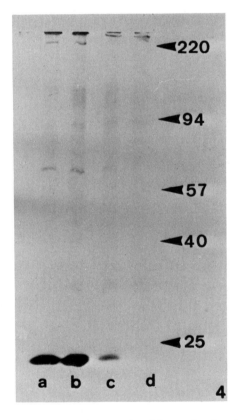

Fig. 4. Polyacrylamide gel electrophoresis of protein released into conditioned medium: The myogenic cultures were labelled from 24 to 72 h in vitro with ^{35}S-methionine, a, DMN-medium; b, DMN and 10 % chick embryo extract; c, DMN and 3 % horse serum; d, DMN and 5 % horse serum.
(Positions of marker proteins in Kd).

IV. DMN-medium represents, despite of the reservations made, a formulation which fullfills major criteria which have to be required for a chemically defined medium. It allows proliferation and differentiation of skeletal muscle cells up to about 2 weeks. An additional advantage is the fact that also heart myocytes and neurons survive in DMN-medium, thus allowing cocultivation of muscle cells and nerve cells (1,2). Several problems occurring during myogenesis may become solvable by employing DMN-medium. We think of the effects of conditioned medium, the relationship of growth factors in proliferation and initiation of terminal differentiation; the study of the influence of exogenous or endogenous toxic components may also become easier amenable. Finally, one may use the defined medium to optimize cell culture conditions since absence of the stress-inducible proteins may be a good criterion to decide on the performance of a serum-free medium.

This research was supported by a predoctoral ETH-fellowship and a grant to HME from the Muscular Dystrophy Assoc. Inc.

References

1. Dollenmeier, P., and Eppenberger, H.M., Exp. cell res. 135 (1981) 47-61.

2. Dollenmeier, P., PhD-Thesis, ETH No.6982 Zürich (1982).

3. Puri, E.C., Caravatti, M., Perriard, J.C., Turner, D.C., Eppenberger, H.M., Proc. Natl. Acad. sci. U.S. 77 (1980) 5297-5301.

4. Puri, E.C., and Turner, D.C., Exp.cell res. 115 (1978) 159-173.

5. Chiquet, M., Puri, E.C., Turner, D.C., J. biol.chem. 254 (1979) 5475-5482.

6. Mc Keehan, W.L., and Ham, R.G., J. cell biol. 71 (1976) 727-734.

7. Linkhart, T.A., Clegg, C.H., Hauschka, S.D., Dev. biol. 86 (1981) 19-30.

8. Turner, D.C., Maier, V., Eppenberger, H.M., Dev. biol. 37 (1974) 63-89.

9. Eppenberger, H.M., Perriard, J.C., Rosenberg, U.B., Strehler, E.E., J. cell biol. 89 (1981) 185-193.

10. Wallimann, T., Turner, D.C., Eppenberger, H.M., J. cell biol. 75 (1977) 297-317.

11. Perriard, J.C., Caravatti, M., Perriard, E., Eppenberger, H.M., Arch. biochem. biophys. 191 (1978) 90-100.

12. Whalen, R.G., Sell, M.S., Butler-Browne, G.S., Schwartz, K., Bouveret, P., Pinset-Härström, I., Nature 292 (1981) 805-809.

13. Dollenmeier, P., and Eppenberger, H.M., Experientia (1982) submitted.

14. Wang, C., Gomer, R.H., Lazarides, E., Proc. natl. acad. sci. U.S. 78 (1981) 3531-3535.

15. Minty, C., Montarras, D., Fiszman, M.Y., Gros, F., Exp. cell res. 133 (1981) 63-72.

16. Johnston, D., Oppermann, H., Jackson, J., Levinson, W., J.biol. chem. (1980) 6975-6980.

Study of a Teratoma-Derived Adipogenic Cell Line 1246 and Isolation of an Insulin-Independent Variant in Serum-Free Medium

Ginette Serrero-Davé

Cancer Center, Q-058, University of California, San Diego, La Jolla, CA 92093, USA

INTRODUCTION

Adipose differentiation has been actively studied since the isolation and establishment in culture of several triglyceride-producing cell lines which provide useful *in vitro* models (1-6). It is now possible to investigate various problems related to the process of differentiation, particularly the determination of the nature and role of extracellular factors controlling the growth and the differentiation of adipocyte-like cells. Since serum-free culture has been successfully done with a number of cell lines for the past few years (7), one possible approach to the latter problem is to cultivate adipocyte-like cells in a serum-free medium. If the identities of the factors supporting adipocyte growth and differentiation are known, understanding their function might be possible. Attempts were made to cultivate, in serum-free medium, three different adipocyte-like cell lines. There were 3T3-L1 (8), Ob17 (Gaillard et al, in preparation) and 1246 (6). 3T3-L1 cell line is derived from Swiss mouse 3T3 fibroblasts (10; Ob17 cell line has been isolated from the epididymal fat pad of C57B16J Ob/Ob mouse (3); 1246 cell line has been clonally derived from a cell line, C17-S1-D-T984, isolated from a teratoma obtained by injecting an embryonal carcinoma cell line C17-S1 into a C3H mouse (6,9). It was found that 3T3-L1 and Ob17 cell lines have the same growth requirements in serum-free medium, i.e., fibronectin, insulin, transferrin, fibroblast growth factor (FGF) and a factor isolated from female rat submaxillary gland extracts (8,10). The 1246 cell line only requires fibronectin, insulin, transferrin and FGF, and does not need the presence of the submaxillary gland factor (6). In order for 3T3-L1 and Ob17 cell lines to undergo adipose conversion, it is necessary to add at least 1% fetal calf serum (FCS) to the medium described above (8), suggesting the existence in the serum of an adipogenic factor. This was also demonstrated by Kuri-Harcuch and Green (11). In contrast, 1246 cells can differentiate in serum-free medium if dexamethasone and 3-isobutyl-1-methyl-xanthine (dex mix) are added to the medium when cells reach confluency (12). The differentiation is accompanied by an increase (a) in the amount of triglycerides accumulated, (b) in enzymatic activities related to lipid metabolism such as triglyceride lipase, diglyceride lipase, monoglyceride lipase, lipoprotein lipase and cholesterol esterase, (c) in the levels of acetate and palmitate incorporated into triglycerides and (d) in the responses to lipolytic hormones (12). Dex mix has been shown to accelerate the differentiation of 3T3-L1 cells in the presence of 10% FCS (13) but does not have any effect when 3T3-L1 are maintained in serum-free medium (Serrero, unpublished observations). Because the 1246 cell line could grow and undergo adipose differentiation in serum-free medium, we chose this cell line as a model for studying the differentiation process. This paper will deal with some recent results obtained.

MATERIAL AND METHODS

Dulbecco's modified Eagle's medium and Ham's nturient mixture, F12, were purchased from Gibco (Grand Island, NY), FCS from REheis Chemicals (Phoenix, AZ), penicillin and streptomycin from Calbiochem-Behring (La Jolla, CA) and ampicillin from Bristol Laboratories, (Detroit, MI). Triple-distilled water was used to prepare all media and solutions for tissue culture. Disposable plasticware (Falcon) was used for all cell culture experiments. The following compounds were obtained from Sigma (St. Louis, MO): trypsin, bovine insulin, human transferrin, bovine heart cAMP-dependent protein kinase, dexamethasone, 3-isobutyl-1-methylxanthine, N-2-hydroxyethylpiperasine-N'-2-ethonesulfonic acid (Hepes), sodium bicarbonate, triglycerides assay kit (UV 305), triethanolamine, dihydroxyacetone phosphate (dimethylketal dicyclohexylamine form), nicotinamide adenine dinucleotide reduced form (NADH) and ethanolamine. Fibroblast growth factor and human fibronectin were purchased from Collaborative Research (Waltham, MA).

Methods

Cell culture:

Cell culture of 1246 in serum-supplemented and serum-free medium was performed as described previously (13).

Differentiation in serum-free medium:

The 1246 cells, inoculated at a density of $0.2-0.5 \times 10^4$ cells/cm^2, were grown for 4 days in the serum-free medium described above. At day 4, when the cells reached confluency, dexamethasone (2×10^{-7} M) and 3-isobutyl-1-methylxanthine (2×10^{-4} M) (dex mix) were added to the serum-free medium for 48 h. The medium was then replaced by fresh serum-free medium without dex mix and changed every 3 days. For the experiments performed in the presence of serum, 1246 cells were grown in serum-free medium for 4 days, and 2% FCS was added at day 4 with the dex mix and was maintained in the culture medium until the cells were harvested.

Biochemical assays:

The cells were harvested as previously described for enzymatic assays (12). Glycerol-3-phosphate dehydrogenase was assayed as described by Wise and Green (14). Triglycerides were assayed as described by Darmon et al (6). Proteins were determined by the method of Lowry (15).

RESULTS

Replacement of residual FCS by Growth Hormone to stimulate adipose differentiation of 1246 cells

Previous work has shown that 1246 cells cultivated in DME-F12 medium supplemented with fibronectin, insulin, transferrin and FGF can grow as well as cells maintained in the presence of 10% FCS (6,16). Moreover, the addition of dexamethasone and 3-isobutyl-1-methylxanthine to confluent cells maintained in this medium resulted; (1) in an appearance of lipid droplets in the cell cytoplasm, (2) in an increase in enzymatic activities related to lipid metabolism, (3) in the incorporation of acetate and palmitate into triglycerides, (4) and in the response to lipolytic hormones such as ACTH, glucagon and epinephrine (12, 16). The activities measured were triglyceride lipase, diglyceride lipase, monoglyceride lipase and cholesterol esterase. Even though differentiation could take place when 1246 cells were treated with dex mix in serum-free medium, we found that the enzymatic activities reached higher levels (2 to 3-fold) if 2% FCS was added with dex mix. Part of the work presented in this paper is an attempt to eliminate the need for the residual serum. We chose to study glycerol-3 phosphate dehydrogenase activity (G3PDH) becuase it undergoes more marked changes during the process of differentiation than the activities studied previously. Wise and Green (14) demonstrated that glycerophosphate dehydrogenase activity was induced in 3T3 cells undergoing adipose differentiation and reached high levels (1000 mUnits/mg of protein) in the differentiated cells, thus appearing as a suitable marker for following adipose differentiation. In the case of 1246 cells, G3PDH activity increased during adipose differentiation in serum-free medium but the G3PDH specific activities found in cells treated with dex mix in the presence of serum was 2-fold higher than in its absence (Table I).

We attempted to substitute the residual 2% FCS with factors known to have an effect on lipid metabolism by testing their ability to further increase G3PDH specific activities. Three factors were found active (Table I). These were: T_3, found to accelerate the adipose conversion of Ob17 cell line in the presence of serum (17); $EtNH_2$, shown to replace FCS in stimulating the growth of a rat mammary carcinoma cell line (68-24 cell line) (18); and h.GH, which is known to bind to adipose cells and to influence their lipid metabolism (19-21). The addition of growth hormone to cells treated with dex mix in 4F medium, resulted in an additional increase in G3PDH specific activity equivalent to the one measured in the presence of 2% FCS (Table I). The simultaneous addition of GH, T_3 and $EtNH_2$ had a positive effect on the increase of G3PDH specific activities whether or not the cells were treated with dex mix (Table I).

Table I

Development of Glycerol-3-Phosphate Dehydrogenase Activity in 1246 Cells

Condition	G3PDH mU/mg protein
4F (day 4)	ND
4F (day 9)	29
+ dex mix	108
+ dex mix + 2% FCS	202
+ dex mix + T_3	141
+ dex mix + $EtNH_2$	134
+ dex mix + h.GH	224
+ dex mix + GH + T_3 + EtHN$_2$	290
+ GH + T_3 + EtNH$_2$ + (-dex mix)	133

Cells were inoculated in DME-F12 supplemented with fibronectin, insulin, transferrin and FGF (12). Dex mix was added at day 4 alone or with 2% fetal calf serum (FCS), triiodothyronine (T_3) 10^{-11} M, ethanolamine ($EtNH_2$) 5×10^{-6} M or human growth hormone (h.GH) 50 ng/ml. Dex mix was removed on day 6 but other factors were maintained until day 15, the time at which cells were harvested and G3PDH assay performed. G3PDH specific activity was expressed in mU/mg of protein. 1 mU (milliunit) of enzymatic activity was defined as the oxidation of 1 nmole of NADH per minute. ND = not detectable.

Effect of the Omission of Insulin and Individual Components of 4F Medium on the Growth and Differentiation of 1246 Cells

Effect on growth:

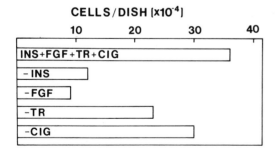

Figure 1. Effect on the growth of 1246 cells of removing individual factors from 4F medium. Cells were grown in DME-F12 under the following conditions: (INS + FGF + TR + CIG) 4F medium containing insulin (10 µg/ml), FGF (100 ng/ml), transferrin (10 µg/ml) and fibronectin (5 µg/ml); (-INS) 4F medium lacking insulin; (-FGF) lacking fibroblast growth factor; (-TR) lacking transferrin; (-CIG) lacking fibronectin. Cells were counted on day 4.

Figure 1 shows the effect of the individual omission of fibronectin, insulin, transferrin and FGF on the cell number, 4 days after inoculation. Omission of insulin and
FGF resulted respectively in a 3-fold and a 4-fold decrease in cell number. Omission
of transferrin and fibronectin reduced cell growth by 37% and 20% respectively.

1246 cell growth was measured at increasing concentrations of insulin. Figure 2
indicates that growth is stimulated by insulin concentrations as low as 1 ng/ml.
The dose response curve reaches a plateau around 100 ng/ml. The growth response to
FGF varies with the quality of the fraction obrained. In the best cases, 1246 cells
respond to FGF concentration of 10 ng/ml. In most cases, the growth is optimally
stimulated by concentrations of 100 ng/ml.

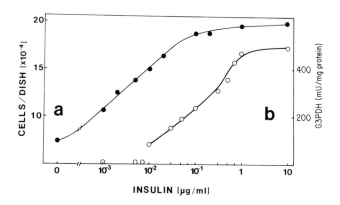

Figure 2. Growth and differentiation of 1246 cells as a function of insulin concentration. In this experiment, the concentrations of transferrin, fibronectin and FGF
were held constant (see legend of Figure 1) whereas the concentration of insulin was
varied over the range indicated. Insulin was added everyday since it had been shown
that it was inactivated under the culture conditions due to the presence of cysteine
in F12 medium. a = Cell number (counted on day 4) as a function of insulin concentration. b = G3PDH specific activity as a function of insulin concentrations (see legend
of Table I).

Effect on differentiation:
The effect of the omission of individual factors on 1246 differentiation was studied
by measuring G3PDH activity in cells maintained for 15 days in 4F medium lacking one
factor. Table II shows that the omission of insulin or transferrin prevents the
appearance of G3PDH activity. In the absence of FGF and fibronectin, the specific
activities measured are equivalent to or slightly smaller than the ones found in cells
maintained in 4F medium (Table II).

Table II

Effect of Removal of Individual Factors on Development of G3PDH Activity

Condition	G3PDH activity (mU/mg protein)
4F	283
-insulin	0
-insulin + 3A	20
-transferrin	0
-FGF	280
-fibronectin	240

Cells were cultivated in the presence or absence of individual factors from day 0. At day 4, dex mix was added, removed on day 6 and cells maintained for an additional 11 days. 3A = 10% of medium conditioned by 1246-3A, was added on day 4. G3PDH activity was measured at day 15. Specific activities were expressed in mU/mg of protein. (See legend of Table I).

No fat accumulation was observed in the cells cultivated in media from which insulin or transferrin has been removed. However, it was possible to observe a few cells that began accumulating triglycerides when they had been maintained more than 15 days in the absence of transferrin. 1246 cell differentiation was measured at increasing concentrations of insulin (1 ng/ml to 10 µg/ml) by assaying G3PDH activity. When insulin was added at a concentration of less than 10 ng/ml, no induction of G3PDH was observed (Figure 2). For insulin concentrations greater than 10 ng/ml, the specific activities increased and reached a plateau at concentrations above 1 µg/ml.

Isolation of Variants of 1246 Cells Independent of Insulin for Their Growth in Serum-free Medium

As previously describe in Figure 1, omission of insulin resulted in an inhibition of 1246 cell growth. Figure 3 indicates that in this condition the cell number reached a plateau 2 days after inoculation of cells and increased very slowly thereafter. However, after maintaining 1246 cells for more than 15 days in the absence of insulin, it was possible to observe groups of cells that began to grow in spite of this absence, thus indicating that there existed certain populations of cells independent of insulin for their growth. These cells were isolated and subsequently cloned in serum-free medium deprived of insulin. Based on differences in morphology and in growth characteristics, 6 cell lines were chosen. In the present paper, only one of them, called 1246-3A, will be analyzed. The growth curves for 1246-3A cells cultivated in the absence and in the presence of insulin are identical (Figure 4), indicating that

1246-3A cells are independent of insulin for their growth. 1246-3A cells grow with a shorter generation time and reach higher cell densities than the parent cell line, 1246 (Figures 3 & 4).

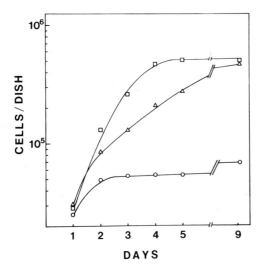

Figure 3. Growth curve for 1246 cells. Cells were grown in either 4F medium (containing insulin) (△), 4F medium lacking insulin (O) and 4F medium lacking insulin but containing 10% of DME-F12 medium conditioned by 1246-3A cell line ([]). Values represent cell number per 35 mm dish.

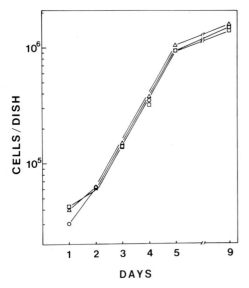

Figure 4. Growth curve for 1246-3A cell line. The conditions were the same as the ones described in the legend of Figure 3.

1246-3A variant has lost the ability to undergo adipose differentiation, since the addition of dex mix in the presence or in the absence of insulin does not induce any increase of G3PDH activity and any triglyceride accumulation (results not shown). So far, we have not found any variant able to differentiate into adipose cells.

1246-3A Cells Produce a Factor Which Stimulates the Growth of 1246 Cells in the Absence of Insulin

As 1246-3A cells can multiply in the absence of insulin, one might assume that they produce a growth factor capable of acting in place of insulin. To test this hypothesis, we collected, every 48 hours, medium conditioned by confluent 1246-3A cells maintained in DME-F12 alone and assayed it for growth promoting activity on 1246 cells maintained in 4F minus insulin conditions. 1246-3A conditioned medium stimulated the growth of 1246 cells in the absence of insulin (Figure 3). In contrast, conditioned medium did not induce additional improvement of the growth of 1246-3A cells maintained in the absence of insulin (Figure 4).

By assaying G3PDH activity, we checked if the activity present in 1246-3A conditioned medium could replace insulin in promoting adipose differentiation of 1246 cells. Table II shows that G3PDH specific activity remains low when 1246 cells are cultured in a medium in which insulin is replaced by 1246-3A conditioned medium. The activity produced by 1246-3A cells is able to substitute for insulin for promoting the growth but not the differentiation of 1246 cells.

We attempted to characterize the activity present in 1246-3A cultures. The activity remained unchanged when conditioned medium was acidified to pH 2.0, alkalinized to pH 11.0 and submitted to a temperature of 85°C. The activity was eluted out of Sephadex G100 with an apparent molecular weight of 20,000 to 30,000 dalton. Purification of the active fraction is underway.

CONCLUSION

The 1246 cell line, derived from a mouse teratoma, has been shown to grow and differentiate in serum-free medium (12,16). We demonstrated previsouly that 1246 cells possessed certain characteristics of adipocyte-like cells such as hormone sensitive lipase activity (12) and that they could be considered as a suitable model to study adipose differentiation *in vitro*. The medium in which 1246 cells grow and differentiate is simple. Growth occurs in a medium supplemented with insulin, transferrin, FGF and fibronectin. Differentiation takes place when dexamethasone and 3-isobutyl-1-methylxanthine are added to the 4F medium.

Experiments in which individual components from the serum-free medium have been omitted showed that they can be classified in three categories:

    (a)   factors that influence both growth and differentiation, such as insulin;

    (b)   factors that influence only growth, such as FGF;

    (c)   factors that influence only differentiation, such as transferrin and dex mix.

Other factors have been shown to stimulate the differentiation of 1246 cells, the most active being human growth hormone (Table I). We found that growth hormone was active on the differentiation of 1246 cells in serum-free medium but that its role was only to accelerate the process of differentiation and to allow higher levels of G3PDH to be reached (Table I). Growth hormone did not have any mitogenic activity on 1246 cells either in the presence or in the absence of insulin. The role of insulin appears to be the most important. In the absence of insulin, 1246 cells can neither grow nor differentiate. No increase in G3PDH activity, in triglyceride accumulation or in triglyceride lipase activity were observed in the absence of insulin (16). If the cells are cultured for 4 days in the presence of insulin and if insulin is removed at confluency at the time of treatment with dex mix, G3PDH activity remains low (results not shown). Conversely, when 1246 cells are cultured in the absence of insulin but are treated with insulin at the time of the addition of dex mix, an increase of G3PDH activity occurs. Thus, insulin appears to regulate the differentiation of 1246 cells. Factors such as dexamethasone, 3-isobutyl-1-methylxanthine, growth hormone, T_3 and ethanolamine, which accelerate the process of differentiation of 1246 cells, are inactive if the medium is deprived of insulin. These results are different from the ones concerning 3T3-L1 and 3T3-F442A cells. Recently, Morikawa, Nixon and Green (22) have found that growth hormone was responsible for the adipose conversion of 3T3-F442A cells. Cells maintained in the presence of 1% calf serum, 1.5% cat serum, biotin, insulin, transferrin, T_3, EGF and sodium ascorbate undergo adipose differentiation only in the presence of growth hormone indicating that growth hormone is indispensable to the induction of differentiation in 3T3-F422A cells. The role of insulin is thought to be enhancing the differentiation of 3T3-L1 and 3T3-F422A cells (23). Thus, it seems that the process of adipose conversion of 1246 cells and 3T3-F442A cells is under the control of different extracellular factors.

The culture of 1246 cells in a serum-free medium supporting their growth and differentiation has allowed us:

    (a) to distinguish between factors that regulate the differentiation and factors that accelerate its process,

    (b) to isolate from 1246 cells cultured in the absence of insulin, cell lines that were independent of insulin for their growth in serum-free medium and were producing a growth factor able to replace insulin for stimulating growth of 1246 cells. This activity is different from insulin since it is not precipitated by anti-insulin antibody (Fong and Serrero, unpublished results). By its molecular weight (20,000 to 30,000 dalton) it appears to be distinct from somatomedin C. Its characterization is underway.

In addition to these findings, the 1246 cell line in serum-free medium can be used as a model to study the effect of growth hormone on adipose differentiation. Growth hormone is constituted by a complex of proteins which have been isolated and purified (21). It is possible to assay these different fractions of growth hormone for their ability to stimulate increases in glycerophosphate dehydrogenase specific activities during the adipose conversion of 1246 cells in order to get information on the relation between growth hormone structure and its function on adipocyte-like cells.

ACKNOWLEDGEMENTS

G.S. thanks Dr. Gordon Sato for the use of laboratory facilities and stimulating comments; Dr. James Lewis and Luciano Frigeri for the gift of growth hormone, Henry Fong for performing insulin radioimmunoassay and Drs. Michel Darmon and Don McClure for helpful discussion. Thanks also go to M. A. Zurbach for the processing of the manuscript. This work was supported by N.I.H. grant CA 19731 and N.S.F. grant PCM82-02797.

REFERENCES

1. Green, H. and Kehinde, O. Sublines of mouse 3T3 cells that accumulate lipid. Cell, 1: 113-116 (1974).
2. Green, H. and Kehinde, O. Spontaneous heritable changes leading to increased adipose conversion in 3T3 cells. Cell, 7: 105-113 (1976).
3. Negrel, R., Grimaldi, P. and Ailhaud, G. Establishment of preadipocyte clonal cell line from epididymal fat pad of Ob/Ob mouse that responds to insulin and lipolytic hormones. Proc. Natl. Acad. Sci. USA: 6054-6058 (1978).
4. Hirogun, A., Sato, M. and Mitsui, H. Establishment of a clonal cell line that differentiates into adipose cells *in vitro*. In Vitro, 16: 685-693 (1980).
5. Van, R. L. R., Bayliss, C. E. and Roncari, D. A. K. Cytological and enzymological characterization of adult human adipocyte precursors in culture. J. Clin. Invest. 58: 699-704 (1976).
6. Darmon, M., Serrero, G., Rizzino, A. and Sato, G. Isolation of myoblastic, fibro-adipogenic and fibroblastic clonal cell lines from a common precursor and study of their requirements for growth and differentiation. Exp. Cell Res. 132: 313-327 (1981).
7. Barnes, D. and Sato, G. Methods for growth of cultured cells in serum-free medium. Anal. Biochem. 102: 255-270 (1980).
8. Serrero, G., McClure, D. and Sato, G. Growth of mouse 3T3 fibroblasts in serum-free, hormone-supplemented media. In: Hormones and Cell Culture. Cold Spring Harbor Conferences on Cell Proliferation, Vol. 6. (G. Sato and R. Ross, eds.) Cold Spring Harbor, NY, pp. 523-530 (1979).
9. Jacob, E., Buckingham, M., Cohen, A., Dupont, L., Fiszman, M. and Jacob, F. A skeletal muscle cell line isolated from a mouse teratocarcinoma undergoes apparently normal terminal differentiation *in vitro*. Exp. Cell Res. 114: 403-408 (1978).
10. McClure, D. B., Ohasa, S. and Sato, G. Factors in the rat submaxillary gland that stimulate growth of cultured glioma cells: Identification and partial characterization. J. Cell. Physiol. 87: 195-207 (1981).

11. Kuri-Harcuch, W. and Green, H. Adipose conversion of 3T3 cells depends on a serum factor. Proc. Natl. Acad. Sci. USA, 75: 6107-6109 (1978).
12. Serrero, G. and Khoo, J. C. An *in vitro* model to study adipose differentiation in serum-free medium. Anal. Biochem. 120: 351-359 (1982).
13. Rubin, C. S., Hirsh, A., Fung, C. and Rosen, O. M. Development of hormone receptors and hormonal responsiveness. J. Biol. Chem. 253: 7570-7578 (1978).
14. Wise, L. S. and Green, H. Participation of one isozyme of cytosolic glycerophosphate dehydrogenase in the adipose conversion of 3T3 cells. J. Biol. Chem. 254: 273-275 (1979).
15. Lowry, O. H., Rosebrough, N. J., Farr, A. L. and Randall, R. J. Protein measurement with the folin phenol reagent. J. Biol. Chem. 193: 265-275 (1951).
16. Serrero, G. and Sato, G. Growth and differentiation of a teratome-derived fibroadipogenic cell line. In: Growth of Cells in Hormonally Defined Media. Cold Spring Harbor Conferences on Cell Proliferation, Vol. 9. (G. Sato, A. Pardee and D. Sirbasku, eds.) Cold Spring Harbor Laboratory, NY, pp. 943-955 (1982).
17. Gharbi-Chihi, J., Grimaldi, R., Torresani, J. and Ailhaud, G. Triiodothyronine and adipose conversion of Ob 17 preadipocytes: Binding to high affinity sites and effect on fatty acid synthesizing and esterifying enzymes. J. Receptor. Res. 2: 153-173 (1981).
18. Kano-Sueoka, T. and Errick, J. E. Effect of phosphoethanolamine and ethanolamine on growth of mammary carcinoma cells in culture. Exp. Cell Res. 136: 137-145 (1981).
19. Gavin, J. R. III, Saltman, R. J. and Tollefsen, S. E. Growth hormone receptors in isolated rat adipocytes. Endocrinology, 110: 637-643 (1982).
20. Goodman, H. M. Growth hormone and the metabolism of carbohydrate and lipid in adipose tissue. A-n. NY Acad. Sci. 148: 419-440 (1968).
21. Lewis, U. J., Singh, R. N. P., Tutwiler, G. F., Sigel, M. B., Vanderlaan, E. F. and Vanderlaan, W. P. Human growth hormone: A complex of proteins. Rec. Progr. Hormone Res. 36: 477-508 (1980).
22. Morikawa, M., Nixon, T. and Green, H. Growth hormone and the adipose conversion of 3T3 cells. Cell, 31: 783-789 (1982).
23. Green, H. and Kehinde, O. An established preadipose cell line and its differentiation in culture, II. Factors affecting the adipose conversion. Cell, 5: 19-27 (1975).

Primary and Secondary Cultures of Rabbit Articular Chondrocytes in a Serum-Free Medium

M. Adolphe, X. Ronot, B. Froger, M. T. Corvol, and N. Forest

Laboratoire de Pharmacologie cellulaire de l'E. P. H. E., Institut Biomédical des Cordemiers, F-75006 Paris, France

Abstract

Cell growth and function is partly under the control of hormones and growth factors. Their effect on cartilaginous tissue was studied by developing a serum free medium in which chondrocytes are able to grow inculture. The defined medium contains various spreading and nutrient factors: BSA, bovine fibronectin, transferrin, thrombin, selenium as well as hormones and growth factors: insulin, hydrocortisone, MSA, BGF or FGF. Growth stimulation in this medium was largely due to the growth factors used. This medium does not affect the specific function of type II collagen synthesis.

1 Introduction

The growth of most of cell culture requires the addition of serum to synthetic media. It has been postulated that serum contains certain hormones and growth factors which are necessary for continuous proliferation. The replacement of serum environmental influences by combinations of hormones, nutrient attachment and growth factors enables studies to be made on the physiology of cartilaginous cells. This study describes the growth of rabbit articular chondrocytes in a synthetic serum free medium. Experiments performed in the absence of serum require the addition of a substance promoting the attachment of cells on culture plates; collagen has been selected as a good spreading factor.

2 Material and Methods

Cells: Chondrocytes were obtained from young rabbit articulations according to the technique of Green (1). Cells were removed from primary culture by a mild trypsinization followed by a trypsin inhibitor step and plated at the concentration of 10^5 cells per 35 mm Petri dishes in defined medium with an adherence step of 24 hr in Ham F 12 medium + 10 % FCS, or directly, when a collagen film is used.

Medium: Ham F 12 was supplemented with various spreading and nutrient factors: bovine albumin (1mg/ml), bovine fibronectin (2µg/ml), transferrin (5µg/ml), thrombin (1µg/ml, 100 NIH), selenium (4ng/ml), as well as hormones and growth factors: insulin (5µg/ml), hydrocortisone (20ng/ml), MSA (0.05ng/ml) and bovine growth factor (BGF: 10µg/ml (2)) or FGF (100ng/ml).

378

Growth measurements: The medium was removed, cells trypsinized and growth measured by counting the total cell number, the growth curve was compared to that obtained with or without 10 % FCS.

Immunofluorescence localization of type II collagen: For extra and intracellular fluorescence labeling of chondrocytes in primary culture, monolayers were fixed with formaldehyde (3.7 %) and ethanol (70 %) exposed to purified antibodies (anti II) for 30 min. at 37°C and subsequently treated with FITC-conjugated goat antibodies to rabbit IgG (3).

3 Results

1) Growth of chondrocytes in secondary culture

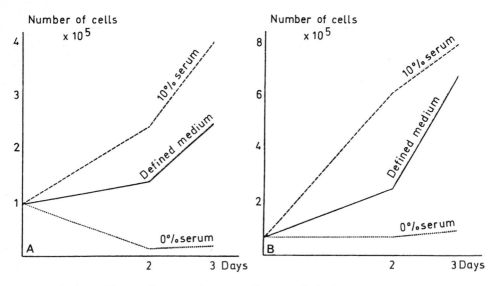

A: experiment with an adherent step on collagen substratum.
   (plastic culture surfaces were precoated with a thin, transparent film of collagen before introduction of the cell suspension and cells were plated in the
   defined medium).

B: experiment with an adherent step of 10 % FCS.
   (after 24 hr seeding in medium supplemented with 10 % FCS, cells were washed
   3 times with serum free Ham F 12 and medium replaced by defined medium).

2) Growth and differentiation of chondrocytes in primary culture

Growth of chondrocytes was measured after an adherent step of 48 hr in Ham F 12 + 10 % FCS; the mean number of cells 7 day after seeding was 8.3×10^5 with a control value of 12.1×10^5.

Chondrocytes seeded as monolayers continue to synthesize type II collagen which is the normal collagen of cartilage.

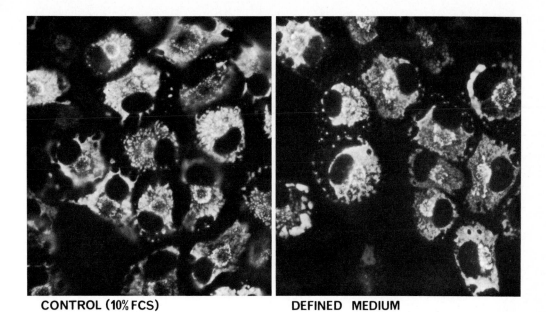

CONTROL (10% FCS)   **DEFINED MEDIUM**

Immunofluorescence micrographs of chondrocytes stained with anti II antibodies.

4 Concluding remarks

Growth:-Growth stimulation in the serum free medium seems to be largely due to the growth factors used. BGF is the most effective mitogen factor and MSA displays an additive stimulatory effect.

-No difference was found between the cells seeded with serum or in Petri dishes precoated with collagen.

Differentiation: Growth of chondrocytes in serum free medium does not affect the specific function of type II collagen synthesis in primary culture.

Acknowledgments
This investigation was supported by grant n° 82 163 from DGRST.

Literature references
1- GREEN W.T. Behaviour of articular chondrocytes in culture ; Clin. Orthop., 1971, 75, 248.
2- BARRITAULT D, PLOUET J., COURTY J. and COURTOIS Y. Purification, characterization and biological properties of the Eye-Derived Growth Factor from retina: analogies with Brain-Derived Growth Factor. J. Neuroscience, 1982, in press.
3- GRIMAUD J.A., DRUGET M., PEYROL S., CHEVALIER O., HERBAGE D. and EL BADRAWY N. Collagen immunotyping in human liver, light and electron microscope study.
J. Histochem. Cytochem., 1980, 28, 1145.

Vanadate Antagonizes Detrimental Effects of Serum Deprivation in Cultured Rat Heart Muscle Cells

G. Bauriedel, K. Werdan, W. Krawietz, and E. Erdmann

Medizinische Klinik I der Universität München, Klinikum Großhadern, Marchioninistr. 15, D-8000 München 70, FRG

INTRODUCTION

Looking for a possible digitalis-like role of vanadium (Na_3VO_4; V) (1,2) we discovered beneficial effects of this essential trace element (3) on cellular function of spontaneously beating rat heart muscle cells, incubated in a serum-free medium. Further investigations revealed that this action was similar to the effects of insulin on the heart muscle cells.

METHODS

Experimental procedures for preparation and cell culture of heart cells as well as measurements concerning beating, (^3H)-2-deoxy-D-glucose-uptake, $^{86}Rb^+$-influx and K^+-content of the cells have been reported elsewhere (4,5).

RESULTS

Long term experiments with spontaneously contracting rat heart muscle cells in culture demonstrate (fig.1) that, within 24 hours, beating frequency and automaticity as well as $(^{86}Rb^+ + K^+)$-uptake rate and intracellular K^+-content stay fairly constant in the presence of complete culture medium (CMRL 1415 ATM + 10% fetal calf seum + 10% horse serum = CCM).

Substitution of this growth medium by a Hepes-buffered salt solution (HeS) leads to a drastic decline in all four parameters within the first 8 hours, the extent varying from experiment to experiment. After this period values adjust to rather stable basal activity levels (fig.1).

Addition of vanadium to the buffered salt solution, however, antagonizes - at least in part - these detrimental effects after serum deprivation (fig.1).

In contrast, addition of V to the CCM does not provoke any stimulation of the $(^{86}Rb^+ + K^+)$-uptake nor marked modification of the intracellular K^+-content. Even a concentration-dependent reduction of automaticity of these cells can be observed - at least in some of our experiments at $(V) \geqslant 10^{-4}$ M (compare fig.1).

A striking similarity exists between the effects of V and insulin (I) on K^+-influx and cellular K^+-content of rat myocardial cells: Both compounds stimulate the $(^{86}Rb^+ + K^+)$-uptake rate in a concentration-dependent manner (I: $SC_{50} \approx$ 0.1 - 1.0 mU/ml, max. stim. 80%; V: $SC_{50} \approx 20$ uM, max. stim. 100%); no additive effect can be provoked by V under an optimal I-induced stimulation and conversely. Concomitantly both compounds increase cellular potassium (control 588 ± 16; 10 mU/ml I 621 ± 20; 3×10^{-4} M V 620 ± 15 (in nmoles/mg protein; n=3)).

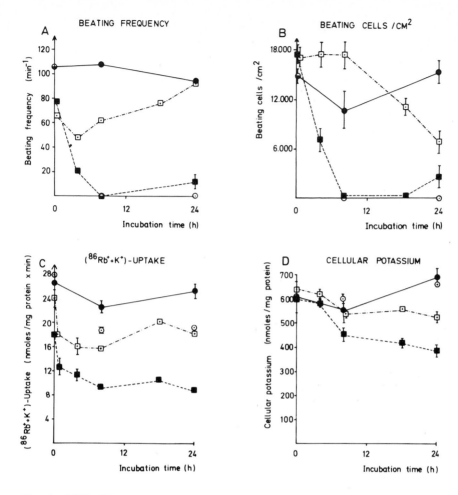

Fig.1. LONG TERM EFFECTS OF Na$_3$VO$_4$ IN BEATING RAT MYOCARDIAL CELLS IN CULTURE: BEATING FREQUENCY, AUTOMATICITY, (^{86}Rb$^+$+ K$^+$)-UPTAKE AND CELLULAR K$^+$. Incubation conditions: CCM (●), HeS (■), HeS + 10^{-4} M V (□) and CCM + 10^{-4} M V (○). Values are m $\pm$ S.E. (beating frequency and beating cells/cm^2, n=8) and m $\pm$ S.D. ((^{86}Rb$^+$+ K$^+$)-uptake and cell-K$^+$, n=3), the st. dev. lie within the symbols used, unless arrows are indicated. 1.39 x 10^6 cpm (^{86}Rb$^+$)/flask; 0.7 mg protein/flask.

Moreover, V as well as insulin enhances (^{3}H)-2-deoxy-D-glucose-uptake in these cells (control (C) 0.21 $\pm$ 0.01; 10 mU/ml I 0.53 $\pm$ 0.06; 3 x 10^{-5} M V 0.42 $\pm$ 0.02 (in nmoles/mg protein x min, n=3)). This parallel stimulation of both parameters, however, is dependent on the examined cell type: In guinea pig heart non-muscle cells, hexose- and (^{86}Rb$^+$+ K$^+$)-uptake are reduced in the presence of V, but enhanced by insulin ((^{3}H)-2-deoxy-D-glucose-uptake: C 0.23 $\pm$ 0.02; 10 mU/ml I 0.52 $\pm$ 0.04; 3 x 10^{-4} M V 0.11 $\pm$ 0.01. (^{86}Rb$^+$+ K$^+$)-influx: C 14.3 $\pm$ 0.2; I 17.8 $\pm$ 0.4; V 11.0 $\pm$ 0.1 (in nmoles/mg protein x min, n=3)).

CONCLUSIONS

Spontaneously beating rat heart muscle cells are very susceptible to new culture conditions: Substitution of CCM by HeS brings about a time-dependent reduction of all examined parameters to basal activity levels (fig.1). Addition of V to the serum-free medium, however, antagonizes - at least in part - the demonstrated detrimental effects of serum deprivation (fig.1).

In contrast to this finding, the combination of V and CCM does not result in any enhancement of K^+-uptake nor cellular K^+-content (fig.1). In this respect V behaves very similarly to insulin: In aggregates of cultured chicken heart cells, Elsas et al. (6) could not find any stimulatory insulin effect on amino acid transport unless the cell material had been preincubated in a balanced salt solution in order to reduce the transport activity to basal levels.

An insulin-like role of V is also found in cultured rat myocardial cells in monolayer form in respect to K^+-influx, cell-K^+ and hexose-uptake. However, this similarity between V and I is a cell type-dependent phenomenon: In cultured guinea pig heart non-muscle cells, insulin enhances hexose- and ($^{86}Rb^+ + K^+$)-uptake, whereas the same parameters are reduced by V. This heterogeneity of V´effects in various heart tissues may be explained by the following hypothesis (7): Depending on the different cellular capacity for reduction of vanadate (V^V) to vanadyl (V^{IV}) attributable to each cell type, vanadium may act more digitalis-like (inhibitory) or more insulin-like (stimulatory).

In cell cultures with serum-free medium, insulin supports growth and viability of cultured rat myocardial cells (8). Our results suggest that vanadium in the 4-valence state is either essential for cultivating these cells or mimics the action of another essential factor - for instance insulin.

REFERENCES

(1) Hackbarth, I., Schmitz, W., Scholz, H., Erdmann, E., Krawietz, W., Philipp, G. (1978) Nature 275, 67
(2) Nechay, B. R. and Saunders, J. P. (1978) J. Environment. Pathol. Toxicol. 2, 247 - 262
(3) Hopkins, P. M. and Mohr, H. E. (1974) Fed. Proc. 33, 1773 - 1775
(4) Werdan, K., Bauriedel, G., Boszik, M., Krawietz, W., Erdmann, E. (1980) Biochim. Biophys. Acta 597, 364 - 383
(5) Werdan, K., Bauriedel, G., Fischer, B., Krawietz, W., Erdmann, E., Schmitz, W., Scholz, H. (1982) Biochim. Biophys. Acta 687, 79 - 93
(6) Elsas, L. J., Wheeler, F. B., Danner, D. J., De Haan, R. L. (1975) J. Biol-Chem. 250, 9381 -9390
(7) Bauriedel, G. (1982) Thesis, University of Munich (in press)
(8) Claycomb, W. C. (1980) Exp. Cell Research 131, 231 - 236

Characterization of Cardiomyocytes Cultured in Serum-Free Medium

Gania Kessler-Icekson[1], Lina Wasserman[1], Ester Yoles[2], and S. R. Sampson[2,3]

[1] The Rogoff-Wellcome, Medical Research Institute, Bar Ilan University, Ramat Gan, Israel
[2] Beilinson Medical Center, Petah-Tikva and the Department of Life Sciences, Bar Ilan University, Ramat Gan, Israel
[3] Department of Experimental Physiology, Bar Ilan University, Ramat Gan, Israel

ABSTRACT

Primary cultures of rat cardiomyocytes were grown in serum-free defined medium. Comparison between these cells and cells grown in the presence of serum has shown that myocytes of both cultures are similar in many aspects and share a number of cardiac specific features. Cardiomyocytes in either medium maintained their beating capacity throughout the culture period (2-3 weeks). Mean transmembrane resting potentials recorded from beating cells grown in defined or complete medium were -77mV and -80mV respectively. Glycogen accumulation and myofibril formation were clearly demonstrated in both types of culture. A cleaner myocytic population was obtained in the defined medium due to reduced proportion of non-myocytes.

Introduction

Primary cultures of cardiac muscle cells (cardiomyocytes) are used by many laboratories as a model for studies of the biology of the myocardial cell (1). Serum of different sources has always been considered an inevitable component of the culture growth medium (2). Nevertheless, as shown already for many other cell types (3), cardiomyocytes were also grown succesfully in serum-free medium for as long as 3 weeks and exhibited normal morphology (4). Since serum-free media have contributed to the knowledge of factors regulating growth and differentiation of various cells (5,6), we further examined the features of cardiomyocytes grown in such a medium. Our results showed a clear expression of cardiac specific functions in these cells, similar to that found in the presence of serum. We therefore suggest the serum-free medium, formulated below, as a valid tool for in vitro studies of the myocardial cell.

Materials and Methods

Medium A contained DMEM:Ham F12 (1:1) (Gibco), glucose 2mg/ml, Hepes 10mM, antibiotics (Biolab, Jerusalem) and horse serum 10% (Biolab). Medium B was the same as A but horse serum was replaced by insulin 25µg/ml, transferrin 25µg/ml, hydrocortisone 0.1µM and fetuin 2mg/ml (all from Sigma). Cell cultures: Hearts were taken from 2 days old Wistar rats (The Laboratory Animal House,Beilinson Med. Centr.). Cardiomyocytes were obtained by repeated dissociations of heart fragments in 0.125% trypsin (Biolab). The cells were collected in medium A and plated at 1.5×10^6/plate (35mm, Nunc) in the same medium. Twenty hours later the cultures were rinsed with PBS and fresh medium A or B was given. Electrophysiological studies: Transmembrane potentials were recorded, as previously described (7), from

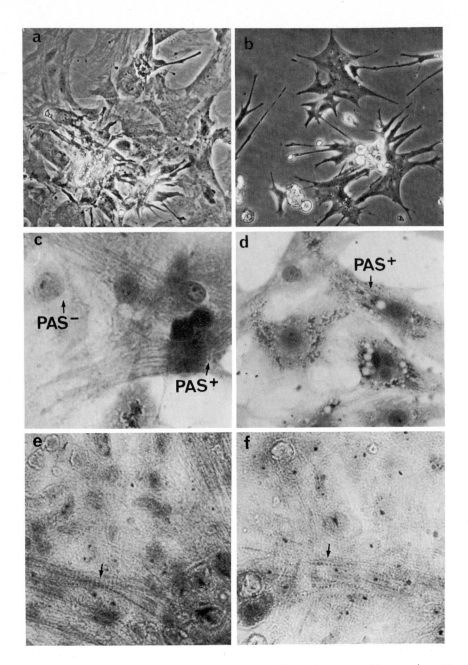

Fig.1. Phase contrast photomicrography of cells 8 days in culture, a) medium A (x100), b) medium B (x200);PAS staining of cells 4 days in culture,c) medium A, d) medium B (x400);PTAH staining for cross striations (arrows) of similar cultures, e) medium A, (f) medium B (x400).

9-16 cells in 1-3 dishes of each medium. Histochemical stainings: The culture dishes (Falcon Film-Line) were rinsed with cold PBS and fixed in cold 4% formalin in 95% alcohol. For PAS staining cultures were treated with 1% aqueous periodic acid, stained with Schiff's reagent and counterstained with Harris hematoxylin (8,9). Mallory's phosphotungstic acid hematoxylin (PTAH) staining (10) was performed on fixed plates treated overnight with 5% mercuric-chloride. All stained cultures were cut out, dehydrated and mounted with Canada balsam on microslides.

Results and Discussion.

On day 2 post plating almost all myocytes (MCs) were beating in medium A and B, although spontaneous beatings could be observed as early as 24 hours. The proportion of non-myocytes (NMCs) in medium A increased gradually and by day 6 they overgrew the MCs, whereas in medium B the number of NMCs remained low, thus no confluency was obtained. The morphology of MCs in both media was much the same, characterized by many extentions adhering to the substrate (Fig.1 a,b). Glycogen deposits, typical for myocardial cells, were clearly detected in MCs by PAS staining. NMCs were PAS negative (Fig.1 c,d). Similarly, only MCs developed striated myofilaments, as demonstrated by PTAH staining (Fig. 1 e,f). When rates of DNA and protein synthesis were examined, the precursor incorporation was lower in medium B than in medium A. However, the changes in rate of incorporation followed a similar pattern in both media, reaching maximal values on day 2 and decreasing gradually to a plateau obtained on day 5 (data not shown).

Transmembrane potentials were recorded from 8 days beating MCs grown in medium A and B (Fig.2). Both cells show a similar configuration of action potential, however, the cell in medium B has no spike and a more pronounced plateau, compared to that in medium A. These differences, as well as the higher overshoot values seen in medium B (Table 1), may originate from differences in ion fluxes and deserve further investigation. Similar mean resting potential values were obtained in medium A and B (Table 1), corresponding to those found in intact heart (1).

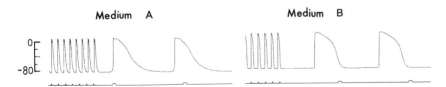

Fig.2. Action potential records of representative cells from 8 days cultures grown in medium A and B. The lower record marks 1 sec. intervals.

Table 1		Medium A	Medium B
Mean values of resting potential (Em),	Em (mV)	80.8 ± 4.7	77.0 ± 5.5
overshoot (OS) and frequency (Freq) obtained	OS (mV)	8.0 ± 6.7	18.6 ± 2.3
from cells 8 days in culture	Freq (Hz)	1.2 ± 0.06	1.1 ± 0.02

Our work confirmed the finding of Claycomb (4) that cardiomyocytes could be cultured in the absence of serum, and further proved that cardiac specific features were expressed under these conditions. The fact that cardiomyocytes are selectively grown in the given defined medium, maintaining their tissue specific functions, permits its application for studies of humoral effects on the myocardial cell.

Acknowledgements : We wish to thank Prof. A. Novogrodsky for his interest and encouragement and Mrs. L. Lipa for her valuable advice in histochemistry.

References

1. Schanne, O. and Bkaily, G (1981) Can.J.Physiol.Pharmacol., 59 : 443 - 467.
2. Frelin, C. (1980) Biol.Cellulaire, 37: 173 - 176.
3. Barnes, D. and Sato, G. (1980) Cell, 22 : 649 - 655.
4. Claycomb, W.C. (1981) Exp.Cell Res. 131 : 231 - 236.
5. Orly, J., Sato, G. and Erickson, G.F. (1980) Cell, 20 : 817 - 827.
6. Florini, J.R. and Ewton, D.Z. (1981), In Vitro, 17 : 763 - 768.
7. Sampson, S.R., Bannet, R. and Shainberg, A. (1982) J.Neurosci.Res.In Press.
8. Nag. A.C., Crandell, T.F. and Cheng, M. (1981) Cytobios, 30 : 189 - 208.
9. McMannus, J.F.A. and Mowry, R.W. In: Staining Methods: histologic and histochemical (1964) Harper and Row, N.Y. pp. 124 - 128.
10. Ibid, pp. 81 - 82.

Serum-Free Cultures of Mouse LM Fibroblasts as a Tool for Biochemical and Genetic Studies in the Cellular Responses to Interferon

P. Milhaud[1], T. Faure[2], J. Chaintreuil[3], and B. Lebleu[2]

[1] Laboratoire de Biologie Moleculaire, ERA CNRS 482, Universite de Montpellier II, F-34000 Montpellier, France
[2] Laboratoire de Biochimie des Proteines, ERA CNRS 482, Universite de Montpellier II, F-34000 Montpellier, France
[3] Laboratoire de Biochimie a Universite de Montpellier I, F-34000 Montpellier, France

ABSTRACT

LM cells continuously growing in the absence of serum and exogenous lipids have been used for studies on the mechanism of action of interferon (IFN). Several of its biological activities, namely the inhibition of virus and cell growth and the increased cytotoxicity to Poly(rI).Poly(rC) (=dsRNA), are shown to be increased in such conditions. None of these three effects of IFN depends on an active prostaglandin biosynthesis, as previously proposed, since cells in our conditions are lacking the necessary precursors.

Variants have been obtained which are resistant to the increased cytotoxicity of IFN-treated cells to Poly(rI).Poly(rC). We believe that this model will be useful for studies on the mechanism of action of IFN through the isolation of variants and the analysis of lipidic and proteic requirements of its activity.

1. INTRODUCTION

There is no need to demonstrate here the usefulness of serum-free cultures to investigate the nutrient, hormonal and substratum requirements of cells undergoing growth or differentiation. However we think it is necessary to emphasize the interest of serum-free cultures for genetic studies as well. We propose the study of the *INTERFERON SYSTEM* as a model. IFN behaves as an hormone : it is an induced molecule acting at very low dose and exhibiting pleiotropic effects : antiviral response, inhibition of the cell division, modifications of the lipid metabolism etc. Studies in serum-free conditions are required because serum interacts with several IFN responses as it does with many hormonal responses.

2. MATERIALS

LM cells (ATCC, CCL 1.2) (mouse fibroblasts derived from L929 cells) are grown in a serum-free medium which consists of RPMI 1640 enriched with Glutamin (2mM), Pyruvate (1mM), Vit B12 (0.8 µg/ml), BSA essentially fatty acid free (Sigma ref. 7511) (100 µg/ml), Penicillin (50 µ/ml) and Streptomycin (50 µg/ml). The generation time is about 20 hours; the cloning efficiency is 30 to 40 % in a fresh medium.

IFN β is a gift from Dr Gresser (IRSC, Villejuif (France)).

3. RESULTS AND DISCUSSION

An increase of cellular responses to a large variety of drugs is usually observed with serum-free cultures. Likewise the removal of serum is currently known to increase several of the cellular responses to IFN, namely : the inhibition of cell division (Gresser et al., 1970 ; Kading et al., 1978), the inhibition of virus development and the rapid cell lysis of IFN-treated cells after exposure to Poly(rI).Poly(rC) (Wallach and Revel, 1979). These experiments were performed on serum-dependent cell lines where the cell growth inhibition was obvious when the serum was removed. On the contrary LM cells will keep growing in the absence of serum. As shown, as an example, the IFN-mediated growth inhibition (Fig.1A) and the cytotoxicity of Poly(rI).Poly(rC) for IFN-treated cells (Fig. 1B) are powerfully enhanced in serum-free conditions.

Double stranded RNA (dsRNA) plays a critical role in the IFN system : it induces IFN production, activates at least two important enzymatic activities (i.e the 2'-5'A synthetase and an IFN induced protein kinase) taking part in the IFN-mediated antiviral activity and increases the IFN-induced inhibition of protein synthesis. We have isolated several variants resistant to the lytic activity of Poly(rI).Poly(rC) (=dsRNA) on IFN-treated cells taking advantage of the increased

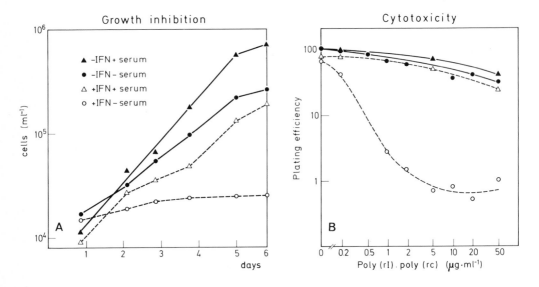

Fig 1A : Cells are plated as indicated (2000 u/ml IFN) and counted every day.

Fig 1B : Cells are plated as indicated (1000 u/ml IFN). 20 hours later Poly(rI). Poly(rC) is added ; 90 mm later the medium is withdrawn and the cells are incubated in their former medium. Colonies are counted 4 days later.

response in serum-free conditions. One of these variants (1022^B) is under investigation : it is a spontaneous low producer of IFN and it responds as its wild type counterpart to treatment with exogenous IFN. We believe that these variants will be useful to unravel the pathway(s) followed by dsRNA to induce the cytotoxicity and the IFN production as well as the presently unknown relationships between these different effects (Burke, 1977).

As early as 1968 LM cells appeared to be one of the best cellular system to allow biochemical and genetic investigations on the lipid metabolism because they grow in a lipid-free medium (Chang and Vagelos, 1976). We took advantage of this asset. Several observations have suggested a role of Prostaglandins (PGs) to mediate the antiviral response to IFN. A L1210 IFN resistant cell line has been reported to lack IFN receptors (Aguet, 1980) and to be deprived of the fatty acid cyclooxygenase activity (Chandrabose et al., 1981). Moreover inhibitors of the fatty acid cyclooxygenase activity inhibit partially the IFN mediated antiviral response on L929 cells (Pottathil et al., 1980). At variance we have confirmed by gas chromatography using a glass capillary column that LM cells do not synthesise PGs for lack of essential lipids although they are very sensitive to IFN in such a medium. Furthermore at non toxic concentration oxyphenbutazone (4 µM) and indomethacin (10 µM) (a more powerful inhibitor) do not inhibit the IFN-mediated antiviral response. These experiments rule out the possibility of a major role of PGs on the IFN-mediated activity and suggest strongly that the fatty acid cyclooxygenase is not involved at least on LM cells.

4.CONCLUSION

LM cells growing in serum-free conditions are a suitable system for
- studies on IFN mechanisms and induction,
- isolation of mutants,
- expression of cloned transfected genes and purification of their products.

5.ACKNOWLEDGMENTS

Supported by grants ATP 82.79.111 and CRL 79.1.112.1 INSERM (FRANCE).

6.REFERENCES

Aguet (1980) Nature, 284, 459-461.
Burke (1977) Trends Biochem. Sci., Nov, 249-251.
Chandrabose et al. (1981) Science, 212, 329-331.
Chang and Vagelos (1976) Proc. Natl. Acad. Sci. USA, 73, 24-28.
Gresser et al. (1970) J. Natl. Cancer Inst., 45, 1145-1153.
Kading et al. (1978) Arch. Virol., 56, 237-242.
Pottathil et al. (1980) Proc. Natl. Acad. Sci. USA, 77, 5437-5440.
Wallach and Revel (1979) FEBS Lett., 101, 364-368.

Separation and Cultivation of Normal Human Melanocytes

H. I. Nielsen[1] and P. Don[2]

[1] The Finsen Laboratory, DK-2100 Copenhagen Ø, Denmark
[2] The Fibiger Laboratory, DK-2100 Copenhagen Ø, Denmark

Normal melanocytes from adult human skin are used at the Finsen Laboratory as controls for studies of the effect of drugs and hormones on the growth, pigmentation and motility of melanoma cells. The experiments reported here were performed in an attempt to optimize the separation and cultivation of melanocytes. Keratinocyte cultures obtained simultaneously are used at the Fibiger Laboratory for studies on carcinogenesis and burn healing.

The most efficient way of producing a suspension of single, viable cells proved to be that of floating keratomed pieces of skin on trypsin (o.25%, Difco) overnight at 4^OC or for one hour at 37^OC. Dermis and epidermis could then easily be separated with tweezers, and alive epidermal cells gently scraped off stratum corneum with a scalpel. A single cell suspension was obtained by pipetting.

Attempts were made to selectively separate the various epidermal cell types. Gradient centrifugation on a preformed, continuous Percoll gradient produced two layers of cells at densities of approximately 1.1oo and 1.o5o, with the majority of melanocytes in the latter. In an attempt to improve the separation, cells were centrifuged in a discontinuous Percoll gradient with densities of 1.o5o and 1.o65. This produced a sediment and two layers of cells that floated on these two respective densities. Although the majority of melanocytes were often found in the second layer of cells and most of the viable keratinocytes usually in the sediment, experience showed this separation technique not to be reliable. An easier and more efficient method proved

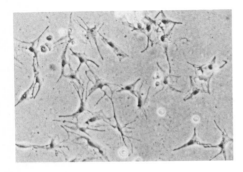

Figure 1. Young culture of melanocytes.

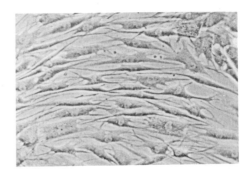

Figure 2. Dense melanocyte culture after 25 days.

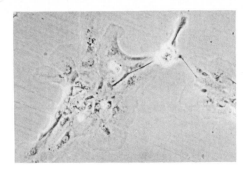

Figure 3. Young culture of
keratinocytes.

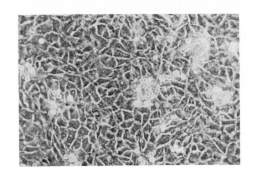

Figure 4. Old confluent
keratinocyte culture.

to be the seeding of non-separated epidermal cells in normal medium (FIB41B)(Don et
al., 198o) with a low content of Mg^{++} and Ca^{++}. This largely inhibited the settling
of keratinocytes - probably due to the absence of sufficient Mg^{++}-ions (Fritsch et al.,
1979).

In an attempt to optimize the culture medium, it was shown that fibroblast conditioned
(24 h) medium was superior to regular medium (FIB41B + lo% FCS) for the growth of melanocytes (4o% increase in successfully established cultures). Replacement of fetal calf
serum by 15% horse serum and addition of polyamines (Roszell et al., 1977) greatly enhanced the growth of melanocytes. Furthermore, cholera toxin ($lo^{-8}M$) improved growth
and dendritic morphology of the melanocytes (Figs. 5 and 6)(Eisinger and Marko, 1982).

From these experiments it can be concluded that the best means of obtaining melanocyte
cultures is to set up epidermal cells in Mg^{++}-free medium for a day or two, then shift
to fibroblast conditioned medium containing horse serum, spermine, spermidine and putrescine. After a few weeks we then shift to normal DME-medium with lo% FCS. In this
way we have kept normal melanocyte lines for 25 weeks (7 passages) to date, and we

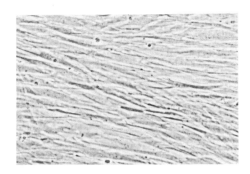

Figure 5. Old culture of
melanocytes growing in
regular FIB41B medium.

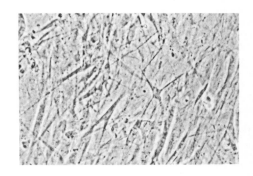

Figure 6. Culture of melanocytes as in fig. 5, but with
cholera toxin in the medium.

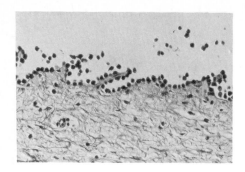

Figure 7. Recent experiments seem to indicate that basal epidermal cells remain loosely attached to the basal lamella (and dermis) after trypsin floating. These cells can be shaken off the dermis and produce especially beautiful and rapidly growing melanocyte cultures when set up in Mg^{++}-free medium.

have been able to freeze and rethaw them. Melanocytes were identified by electron microscopy, by their reaction to cholera toxin (Eisinger and Marko, 1982) and occasionally by their pigment production under the influence of melanocyte stimulating hormone.

Table 1. Percent successfully established cell cultures with ≥ 75% melanocytes after approximately lo days. The cells in A, B and C are separated on a Percoll gradient

Medium	Percent
A. Regular FIB41B medium	14
B. Fibroblast conditioned FIB41B	12
C. Fibroblast conditioned FIB41B + HSSP[o]	78
D. FIB41B, low Mg^{++} and Ca^{++} (no gradient centrifugation)	83

[o] HSSP: horse serum, spermine, spermidine, putrescine

Acknowledgments: The skilled technical assistance of Mrs. M. Bernadotte-Jenny, Mrs. A.M. Madsen and Miss B. Nielsen is greatly acknowledged. The work is supported by a grant to H.I. Nielsen from the Danish Cancer Society.

References: Don, P., J. Kieler & M. Vilien (198o) in M. de Brabander (ed.) Cell Movement and Neoplasia, Pergamon Press, pp. 121-131.

Eisinger, M. & O. Marko (1982) Proc. Natl. Acad. Sci. USA, 79, 2o18-2o22.

Fritsch, P., G. Tappeiner & G. Huspek (1979) Cell Biol. Int. Reports, 3, 593-598.

Roszell, J.A., C.J. Douglas & C.C. Irving (1977) Cancer Res., 37, 239-243.

The Use of Cytodex 3 Microcarriers and Serum-Free Media for the Production of a Nerve Growth Promoter from Chicken Heart Cells

G. Norrgren[1], T. Ebendal[2], H. Wikström[1], and Ch. Gebb[1]

[1] Pharmacia Fine Chemicals AB, Box 175, Uppsala, Sweden
[2] Institute of Zoology, Box 561, Uppsala, Sweden

ABSTRACT

Cytodex 3 microcarriers were used for the production of an active nerve growth promoting factor from chicken heart cells. Such cells release into their culture medium
a substance which stimulates the growth of nerve fibres from explanted ciliary,
spinal and sympathetic neurons. In addition, culture in serum-free medium reduces the
presence of contaminating proteins and facilitates biochemical analysis of this factor.
A mixture of DME/FIO was supplemented with either 10% FCS, or a low molecular weight
fraction of FCS, or different hormones and growth factors. Cells cultured in media
supplemented with insulin, transferrin, human serum albumin and fibronectin in combination with 10% FCS-dialysate or a mixture of FGF, EGF, dexamethasone, calmodulin
and thrombin progressed through the cell cycle with kinetics similar to those obtained
with 10% FCS. Maximum amount of cells in $(S+G_2)$ phase was obtained after 18-20 hrs.
The cells proliferated on Cytodex 3 at a rate similar to cells grown on cell culture
plastic. The results confirm the potential of microcarrier cell culture in serum-free
media for scaling up the high yield production of a specific cell product.

Microcarrier techniques provide a large culture surface area to volume ratio and make
it possible to obtain high yields of anchorage-dependent cells (7). Furthermore,
microcarrier culture has been used for the production of cell-derived material such
as interferon (3,5), insulin (2) and interleukin (8). In this study, we examined the
growth of chicken embryo primary heart cells on Cytodex 3 microcarriers for the production of a factor which stimulates neurite outgrowth from chicken embryo ciliary,
sympathetic and spinal ganglia (1,6). In order to facilitate future biochemical analysis and purification of this factor we have combined the microcarrier technique
with growth of cells in serum-free media. The use of serum-free media provides a way
of reducing the concentration of contaminating proteins and we report here formulations which successfully supported the growth of chicken heart cells.

Primary chicken heart cells were prepared as described earlier (9) and cultured in
80:20 (v/v) DME:F10 containing non essential amino acids (1%,v/v) 2 mM glutamine and
various supplements. Supplements included either 10% (v/v) FCS, a low molecular weight
fraction of FCS (tube dialysis, cut off MW 10 000, against base medium, volume ratio
1:10 at +4°C for 10 days) or different hormones and growth factors i.e. insulin (I,
1 µg/ml), transferrin (T, 25 µg/ml), human serum albumin (A, 1 mg/ml), fibronectin

(F, 10 μg/ml), dexamethasone (200 ng/ml), EGF (20 ng/ml), FGF (20 ng/ml), calmodulin (20 ng/ml) and thrombin (90 ng/ml). Preliminary growth tests were conducted in Petri dishes. When a certain combination of supplements resulted in growth, cell cycle kinetics were determined by flow cytometry. The preparation for flow cytometry was performed as previously reported (9). Formulations resulting in kinetics similar to those obtained with 10% FCS were then tested in microcarrier cultures with Cytodex 3 (Pharmacia). The methods for microcarrier culture have been described (7,9). 100 ml conditioned medium was collected after 12, 24, 36 and 48 hrs, concentrated by pressure dialysis through a Diaflo membrane (cut off MW 10 000) and assayed for nerve growth promoting activity (4,9). Titre was determined from the degree of neurite outgrowth after 24 and 48 hrs using an arbitrary scale from 0 to 1.0 (biological units (BU), zero indicating absence of neurites, 1.0 indicating a dense circular outgrowth). The distribution of relative DNA content among the cells was examined by flow cytometric analyses of synchronous populations grown in different media (Fig. I). When compared with medium containing 10% FCS the kinetics of the cell cycle were only slightly altered in media supplemented with insulin, transferrin, albumin and fibronectin (ITAF) and 10% FCS-Dialysate or a mixture of FGF, EGF, dexamethasone, calmodulin and thrombin. The growth rate of heart cells in microcarrier culture under

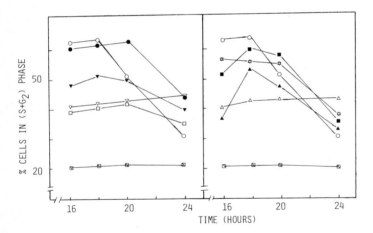

Fig. 1. The presentages of cells in the (S+G$_2$) phases of the cells cycle, as a function of time following synchronization. o--o 10% FCS, ●-● ITAF+10% FCS-dialysate, ▽-▽ ITAF+EGF, ▼-▼ ITAF+EGF, calmodulin, ▲-▲ ITAF+dexamethasone, ▵-▵ ITAF+thrombin, ✫-✫ ITAF+FGF, ■-■ ITAF+FGF, calmodulin, dexamethasone and thrombin, □-□ ITAF, ⬢-⬢ Base medium.

different experimental conditions is shown in Fig. 2. Serum-free media could support the growth of cells on Cytodex 3. The cells cultured on Cytodex 3 proliferated at a rate similar to cells grown in monolayer. Conditioned media were collected from

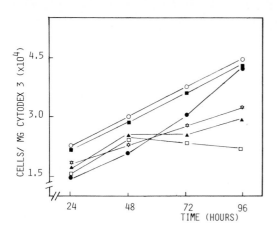

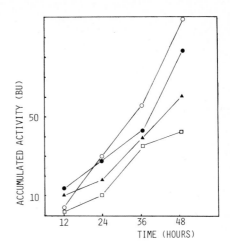

Fig. 2. The effect of the various types of media on the growth of chicken heart cells in microcarrier culture. Symbols as in Fig. 1.

Fig. 3. Production of the chick nerve growth factor determined in a ganglionic bioassay. Symbols as in Fig. 1.

heart cell populations in exponential growth and nerve growth promoting activity was found to be released at a constant rate during the active phase of growth. Medium harvested from cells cultured in ITAF medium with 10% FCS-dialysate contained only slightly less nerve growth promoting activity than media harvested from cells grown in medium containing 10% FCS. Therefore, we conclude that a nerve growth promoting activity can be satisfactorily produced from chicken heart cells growing on Cytodex 3 microcarriers in the presence of serum-free media. Such a system exploits the advantages of microcarriers cell culture and would enable scaling up the production of the factor for further biochemical purification.

References

1) Adler, R., Manthorpe, M., Skaper, S.D. and Varon, S. (1981) Brain Research 206, 129-144.
2) Bone, A.I. and Swenne, I. (1982) In Vitro 18, 141-148.
3) Clark, J.M., Gebb, Ch. and Hirtenstein, M.D. (1981) Developments Biological Standardization, 50, 81-91.
4) Ebendal, T. (1979) Developmental Biology, 72, 276-290.
5) Giard, D.J., Loeb, D.H. and Thilly, W.G. (1979) Biotechnology Bioengineering 21, 433-442.
6) Helfand, S.L., Riopelle, R.J. and Wessels, N.K. (1978) Experimental Cell Research 113, 39-45.
7) Pharmacia Fine Chemicals AB. (1981) Microcarrier cell culture: principles and methods. Technical Booklet series, Uppsala, Sweden.
8) Prestidge, R.L., Sandlin, G.M., Koopman, W.J. and Bennett, J.C. (1981) Journal for Immunological Methods 46, 197-207.
9) Norrgren, G., Ebendal, T., Gebb, Ch. and Wikström, H. (1982) Developments Biological Standardization (in press).

Control of Cell Proliferation and Differentiation in the Myogenic Cell Line L6 by Manipulation of Culture Conditions

Christian Pinset and Robert G. Whalen

Département de Biologie moléculaire, Institut Pasteur, 25, rue du Dr. Roux, F-75724 Paris, France

ABSTRACT

We have found culture conditions which produce a population of und-ifferentiated L6 myoblast cells arrested in the G1 phase of the cell cycle. Morphological and biochemical differentiation can be induced in this population by simple changing media to a serum-free medium contain-ing insulin. About 30% of the cells fuse and differentiate without pass-ing through another S phase. In various serum-free media we can demons-trate the importance of native collagen for attachment, growth and diff-erentiation of L6 cells.

1. INTRODUCTION

L6 myoblasts grown in tissue culture will carry out certain steps of terminal muscle differentiation. In this culture system, two principal stages exist. Mononucleate myoblasts undergo repeated cycles of cell division. Eventually, these myoblasts cease dividing and fuse to form multinucleate myotubes which synthesize some of the contractile proteins specific to muscle tissue (1,2). We have investigated the effect of diff-erent culture techniques on the rate of proliferation and the expression of differentiation in order to control the various steps of myogenesis.

2. NON-PERMISSIVE CULTURE CONDITIONS FOR EXPRESSION OF MYOGENESIS IN THE L6 CELL LINE

In Dulbecco's Modified Eagle (DME) medium plus 10% fetal calf serum (FCS), L6 myoblasts proliferate, attain confluence and they fuse to form myotubes which synthesize α-actin, tropomyosin and embryonic myosin (1, 2). In Ham's F12 medium plus 10% FCS, cells also grow to confluence (Fig. 1A). In this medium however, the cells never fuse to form myotubes. This absence of morphological differentiation was associated with a low level of synthesis of muscle-specific proteins (not shown). F12 was supplemen-ted with several components (Ca^{++}, isoleucine, leucine, glutamine, gluc-ose, sodium bicarbonate and Fe^{+++}) to give the same levels as in DME; fusion was still not observed. Cytofluorometric analysis of nuclei after labeling with ethidium bromide demonstrated that 80-90% of the cell had a diploïd (G1) DNA content. Autoradiography after continuous incorpor-ation of 3H-thymidine for 4 days revealed that no more than 10% of the

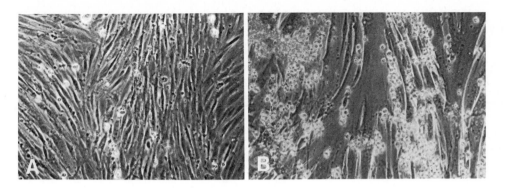

Figure 1. (A) Cells were seeded at 10^4 per cm^2 in F12 plus 10% FCS.
Phase contrast photographs were taken after seven days of culture.
(B) Cells were grown in F12+FCS for six days, were changed to DME plus
10 µg/ml bovine insulin. Photo taken six days later.

cells in the confluent cultures synthesized DNA during this time. We
conclude therefore that growth in F12+FCS produces a confluent population
of myoblasts arrested in G1 which does not express the myogenic program (3).

3. INDUCTION OF MYOGENIC DIFFERENTIATION IN SERUM-FREE MEDIUM

The absence of differentiation in F12+FCS is not due to an irreversible loss of myogenic potency. These myoblasts will fuse to normal levels
if returned to DME+FCS. We can also induce the expression of the myogenic program in serum-free medium composed of DME plus 10 µg/ml of bovine
insulin. Figure 1B shows L6 cells grown for 6 days in F12+FCS and then
changed to DME+insulin. Many myotubes are seen, and the percent of cells
fused was ca.80%. Under these conditions, a fraction of the cells fuse
without passing through another S phase. If the cells were continuously
exposed to 3H-thymidine during the induction of fusion with DME+insulin,
ca. 30% of the nuclei in fusion are not labeled. In contrast, all cells
remaining monunucleate have incorporated thymidine. These results were
confirmed by inducing fusion in the presence of cytosine arabinoside,
an inhibitor of DNA synthesis. Fusions were observed and muscle-specific
proteins were synthesized even in the presence of this drug (not shown).
Thus, about one third of the quiescent L6 population arrested in G1 can
be induced to express the myogenic program in a serum-free medium without
having to pass through an additional cell cycle.

4. ATTACHMENT FACTORS AND SERUM-FREE MEDIUM

In serum-free media, many cell types require some attachment factor
to undergo cell proliferation and the full expression of differentiation

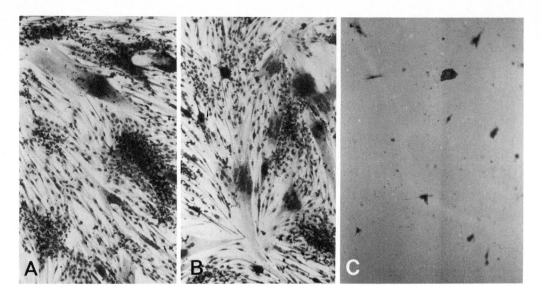

Figure 2. In all 3 panels, cells were seeded at 10^4 per cm^2 in serum-free medium composed of DME:F12 (1:1) plus 200 ng/ml FGF, 10 μg/ml bovine insulin and 5 μg/ml human transferrin. (A) cells seeded into dishes pretreated with DME plus 10% FCS for 24 hrs and then washed with serum-free medium. Dishes pretreated with (B) native collagen and (C) gelatin.

(4). Florini and coll.(5) have used a serum-free medium for L6 cells but it was necessary to grow the cells for 24-48 hrs in serum-containing medium before changing to serum free medium. To study the role of attachment factors in serum-free medium, we have used some purified proteins and a serum-free medium lacking fetuin. In DME:F12 (1:1) plus FGF, insulin and transferrin, L6 cells will proliferate and fuse in dishes pretreated with serum (Fig.2A). If the dishes are pretreated with human fibronectin, laminin, or serum spreading factor (kindly provided by Dr. D. Barnes) the cells will attach and begin to proliferate. The cells detach progressively from the dish, and by 8 days of culture only a few cells remain. If however the dishes are pretreated with native rat tail collagen the cells attach, proliferate and form myotubes after about 3-4 days. Figure 2B shows the cells obtained after 8 days in these conditions. When gelatin is used to pretreat the dish, cells are unable to proliferate (Fig.2C). Thus, in our serum-free medium L6 cells are dependent on native collagen for growth and differentiation. Although cells can adhere to other substrates, they do not remain attached. One possibility is that the cells produce some factor which can bind to collagen but not to gelatin, fibronectin, laminin or serum spreading factor.

References

1. Whalen,R.G., Butler-Browne,G.S. & Gros,F. (1978) J. Mol. Biol. <u>126</u>, 415-431

2. Garrels,J.I. (1979) Develop. Biol. <u>73</u>, 134-152

3. Pinset,C. & Whalen,R.G. (1982) submitted

4. Barnes,D. & Sato,G. (1980) Cell <u>22</u>, 649-655

5. Florini,J.R. & Roberts,S.B. (1979) In Vitro <u>15</u>, 983-992

Serum-Free Culture of Adult Rat Cardiac Myocytes

H. M. Piper[1], I. Probst[2], P. Schwartz[1], J. F. Hütter[1], and P. G. Spieckermann[1]

[1] Zentrum Physiologie und Pathophysiologie, Abt. Herzstoffwechsel, Universität Göttingen, Humboldtallee 7, D-3400 Göttingen, FRG
[2] Zentrum Biochemie, Abt. Biochemie I, Universität Göttingen, Humboldtallee 7, D-3400 Göttingen, FRG

Abstract

An almost intact population of adult cardiac myocytes was kept in culture for a week. For this period the cells maintained morphological, energetical and functional characteristics as in intact tissue.

Keywords: Adult cardiac myocytes, energetical state, stimulatability.

1. Introduction

Isolated adult cardiac myocytes represent a useful tool for studying biochemical, morphological, and functional problems of the ventricular myocardium free from the influence of vascular supply conditions and of pacemaker activity. Up to now biochemical studies were limited due to a short survival time of isolated cells and a large percentage of damaged cells in the final material. Earlier attemps to keep adult cardiocytes in culture resulted in fast cell dedifferentiation (e.g. Schwarzfeld and Jacobsen, 1981). With the method described a population of almost 100 percent viable cells could be kept in culture for at least 6 days.

2. Materials and Methods

Adult cardiac myocytes were isolated as described elsewhere (Piper et al., 1982) from 11 weeks old Sprague Dawley rats. Cells were suspended in M 199 medium, supplemented with 4 % fetal calf serum, 10^{-8}M insulin with or without 5 mM creatine, and plated on Falcon dishes which had been pretreated with the above medium for 12 hours. Three hours after plating only the intact rod shaped cells adhered to the dish, dead cells could be easily washed off. Serum was then omitted from the culture medium. Cells were stimulated electrically via 2 platinum electrodes immersed in the fluid of dishes filled with Tyrode solution instead of M 199.

3. Results and Discussion

Among many procedures tested (including additions of collagen and polyaminoacids) the procedure described was the only one which allowed selective attachment of intact cells. When serum was kept in the incubation medium after cells had attached the number of viable cells was significantly lower than without serum after one day. Irrespective of the initial portion of intact cells after the first wash at 3 hours more than 95 % of the remaining cells were morphologically intact, non-muscle cells were not present. Contents of creatine phosphate and ATP are 10-20 % higher than what is found in whole myocardium - probably due to the portion of about 20 % of weight of non-muscle cells in the whole tissue. These high levels of energy rich phosphates are maintained in culture if creatine is included in the medium (Fig.1).During one week in culture these cells maintain their ultrastructure (Fig.3), but their contours are rounding off (Fig.4) and many develop pseudopodia (Fig.5) which are coated by a ruthenium red stainable "glycocalix" surface layer (Fig.6) as the whole cell. As in whole tissue isolated adult myocytes do not replicate under culture conditions. In culture they are mechanically at rest. However, by application of a varying electrical field, they can be stimulated to synchronous contractions. As shown in Fig.2 the maximum possible contraction frequency (f_m) depends on temperature (T): lowering the temperature by 10°C lowers the maximum possible contraction frequency by a factor of 3 to 4. The relation between f_m and T closely follows the Arrhenius equation (r=0.99). At 37°C f_m is about 3 times higher than the resting heart rate of the rat. It was shown by Trube et al. (1982) that resting potentials and -stimulated- action potentials are as in normal myocardium. These results indicate that isolated ventricular myocytes in culture represent a reliable model for the ventricular myocardium.

Acknowledgement: This study was supported by the DFG, SFB 89 Göttingen

References

Piper, H.M., I. Probst, P. Schwartz, J.F. Hütter, P.G. Spieckermann (1982). J. Mol. Cell. Cardiol. 14, 397-412

Schwarzfeld, T.A., S.L. Jacobsen (1981). J. Mol. Cell. Cardiol. 13, 563-575

Trube G., D. Pelzer, H.M. Piper (1982) Pflügers Archiv, suppl. 394, R 12

Fig.1 : Energy rich phosphates in culture, with and without creatine.
Fig.2 : Maximum contraction frequency at different temperatures.
Fig.3 : 100 h in culture: ultrastructure. Fig.4 : 100 h: single myocytes. Fig.5 : 100 h: myocyte with pseudopodium. Fig.6 : 100 h: ultracut through pseudopodium, surface stained with ruthenium red.

402

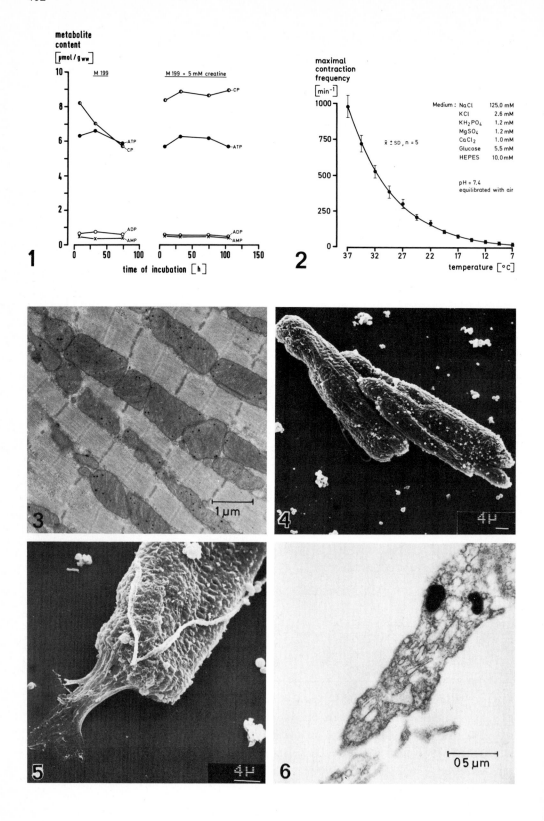

Secretion of α-MSH-Like Molecules in a Human Melanoma Cell Line

N. Van Tieghem, M. Fooij, P.-E. Henry, F. Legros, and J.-M. Prevost

Faculté de Médecine, Université Libre de Bruxelles

ABSTRACT

Receptors for exogenous ^{125}I-α-MSH were detected, at passage 54, on the human melanoma 809 cell line, using a specific hormone receptor assay. Thereafter (at pass. 80-90), receptors were consistently absent. To test the hypothetic blockade by MSH-like molecules, secreted by the non receptive cells themselves, a protein A immunoassay was devised to detect the presence of cross-reacting polypeptides on the cell surface. When receptivity for the hormone disappeared, α-MSH immunoreactivity was present at the cell surface. Moreover, hormone receptive cells (at pass. < 60) were able to interract with serum-free conditioned medium obtained from non receptive cells (at pass. 94). These results suggest that 809 melanoma cells bear on their surface α-MSH-like peptides, which are recognized by highly specific α-MSH antibodies, and release into supernatant medium α-MSH-like molecules, able to interact with specific α-MSH receptors.

INTRODUCTION

α-melanocyte stimulating hormone (α-MSH), a polypeptide containing 13 amino-acids secreted by the pituitary pars intermedia regulates pigmentation in lower vertebrates.

The effect of MSH on melanoma cell biology in culture has been extensively studied in rodent models (2). α-MSH binds to human melanoma cells as well, inhibits cell proliferation and stimulates differentiation (3). Inhibition of DNA replication and production of retroviral markers in human melanoma cultures depends on hormonal stimulation (4). In the 809 human melanoma cell line there was a loss of receptivity to ^{125}I-α-MSH during subculture.

MATERIALS AND METHODS

The 809 pigmented cell line was cultured in HAM-F10 medium supplemented with 15% FCS.

Specific binding tests for α-MSH receptors were performed as described (3). Briefly, cells were incubated in BSA enriched serum-free medium containing 10^{-9}M ^{125}I-α-MSH, with and without a 10^{-4}M excess of unlabelled α-MSH. Radioactivity associated to cell pellets reflects the receptivity of the cells.

Protein A immunoassay: 8.10^{4} cells plated in microtest wells and washed with binding buffer (serum-free BSA enriched medium) were exposed to i) 3 concentrations of α-MSH

(10^{-4}, 10^{-6} and 10^{-8}M) for 1hr, or ii) serum free supernatants of non receptive 809 cells and iii) control medium. After washing, cells were incubated with highly specific anti-α-MSH serum (U.C.B. Bioproducts) (final dilution 1:380.000 and 1:190.000) for 2 hrs. Then they were washed and reacted with iodinated Staphylococcus protein A for 1/2 hr. After 2 last washes, cells were harvested by trypsinization and cell associated radioactivity was counted. In each experiment a set of controls included serum, cell and specificity controls.

Serum-free conditioned medium was obtained as follows : cells were grown to confluency in HAM-F10 medium plus FCS and washed twice with serum-free medium, once for 8 hrs and once for 16 hrs, to eliminate serum proteins. Subsequent 48 hrs collections were taken as "conditioned medium" (5).

Growth curves : cells were grown with constant addition of 10^{-6}M α-MSH in the medium i) at the time of subculture and ii) 2 days after each subculture. Trypsinized cells were counted in a hemocytometer.

RESULTS AND DISCUSSION

At passage 54, 809 melanoma cells exhibited specific receptivity to α-MSH (specific binding ratio: 0,90%); binding of ^{125}I-α-MSH 10^{-9}M was completely displaced by a 10^{-4}M excess of unlabelled hormone. By contrast, on later subcultures the same cell line was consistently negative for hormone receptors (binding ratio at passage 90: 0,17%). One of the most attractive hypothesis to explain this discrepancy was the blockade of cell receptors by products secreted by the cells themselves. In a protein A immunoassay, using an α-MSH highly specific antiserum, we were able to demonstrate what follows :

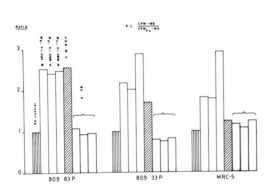 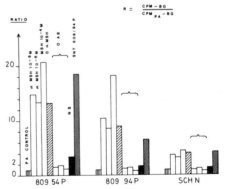

Fig. 1. Protein A α-MSH binding assay to 809 cells at passage 33 and 83 expressed by the ratio CPM-BG/CPM.PA-BG in the presence of α-MSH 10^{-8}, 10^{-6} and 10^{-4}M. Antiserum diluted 1:380.000. MRC5: normal human fibroblasts.

Fig. 2. Protein A α-MSH binding assay to 809 cells at passage 54 and 94. Antiserum diluted 1:190.000. SCHN: human melanoma cell line unreceptive to ^{125}I-α-MSH. NS: normal rabbit serum. SNT 809/94P: serum-free conditioned medium of 809 cells unreceptive to exogenous ^{125}I-α-MSH.

1. receptors for α-MSH were detected on 809 cells using various hormonal concentrations, but most consistently with 10^{-4}M of α-MSH. Receptivity at passage 33, 54,
83 and 94 was different (fig. 1 & 2). At high MSH concentrations (10^{-4}M), normal
fibroblasts showed some receptivity (fig. 1). Another melanoma cell line (SCHN) was
unreceptive in this assay (fig. 2) as well as in specific binding tests.

2. omitting α-MSH on 809 cells at passage 94 does not influence the "spontaneous"
receptivity of the α-MSH antibody with the cells. Normal fibroblasts (fig. 1) or other
human melanoma cells (fig. 2) were not reacting significantly, as compared to protein A
alone or non immune rabbit control serum, in the same assay.

3. using α-MSH receptive 809 cells (P54), conditioned medium from 809 cells (P94),
or control medium, were tested for the presence of α-MSH like molecules. As shown in
fig. 2, 809 receptive cells fix more radioactivity after reaction with 809 (P94) supernatant than with control medium or α-MSH antibody alone.

In conclusion, these results suggest that 809 MSH non receptive cells (P94) bear on
their surface α-MSH like molecules, most probably associated with specific receptors,
and secrete them into supernatant medium; these molecules mimic enough the hormone in
cross-reacting immunologically and interacting at the receptor level. The biological
activity of this product is still inknown. These cells might be expected to have a
survival advantage when they acquire the ability to produce factors that mimic the hormone in occupying the specific receptors (escape mechanism against normal control of
differentiation). This speculation may be true in view of previous results (4) showing
that α-MSH induced inhibition of DNA synthesis as well as melanocyte differentiation
leading to cell death in various melanoma cell lines (2) (3) (4). Consequently, we
tried to cultivate 809 cells in the presence of 10^{-6}M α-MSH (fig. 3).

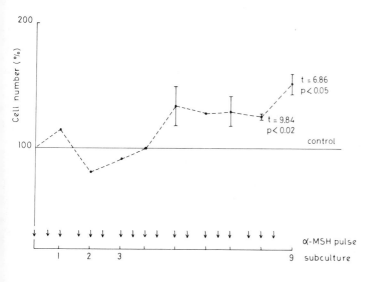

Fig. 3. 809 cells grown
in the presence of 10^{-6}M
α-MSH during 9 subcultures.
Cell number is expressed
in % as compared to control
809 cells grown without
α-MSH (100%).

As compared to control cultures without addition, we selected cells which grow better in the presence of 10^{-6}M α-MSH. This suggests that some cells from the 809 line are able to escape from MSH toxic effects.

ACKNOWLEDGMENT : this work is supported by the Fonds de la Recherche Scientifique Medicale, Brussels (Grant n° 3.4513.81).

REFERENCES
1. PAWELEK, J.M., WONG, G., SAUSONE, M. & MOROWITZ, J. (1973) Yale J. Biol. & Med. 46, 430-443.
2. LEGROS, F., COEL, J., DOYEN, A., VAN TIEGHEM, N., VERCAMMEN-GRANDJEAN, A., FRUHLING, J. & LEJEUNE, F.J. (1981) Cancer Res. 41, 1539-1544.
3. VAN TIEGHEM, N., VERCAMMEN-GRANDJEAN, A., FOOIJ, M., TEMMERMAN, A. & LEJEUNE, F.J. (1982) in "Protides of the Biological Fluids" (PEETERS, H. ed.) 29, 559-562.
4. TODARO, G.J., FRYLING, D. & DE LARCO, J.E. (1980) Proc. Natl. Acad. Sci. USA 77 (9), 5258-5262.

Growth and Differentiation of Human Muscle Cells in Defined Medium

Rose Yasin and Gisela van Beers

Institute of Neurology, Queen Square, London, England

Previous studies on myogenesis have used muscle cells that were grown in a complex undefined medium. Because of this only limited detailed analyses of the influence of environmental factors on muscle differentiation, changes in membrane components and identification of components secreted by cells during different stages of development could be carried out. To overcome these limitations several investigators have described defined media which support both growth and differentiation of primary rat and L6[1] and avian[2,3] muscle cells. A similar system for human cells could provide some insight into the pathogenesis of muscle disease.

In this study we describe growth and differentiation of fetal (NN) and adult (AD) human skeletal muscle in defined medium previously used for growing rat[1] and chick[2] myoblasts.

Materials and Methods

NN and AD muscle cells were isolated from dissociated biopsies as previously described[4] and were grown on gelatin coated Lux dishes in GM medium containing Dulbecco's modified Eagle's medium (DME; Gibco Biocult H21), 16% fetal calf serum (Flow), 1.8% chicken embryo extract (CEE, Flow). To expand the cell numbers the cultures were passaged 3-4 times prior to myoblast fusion and stored in liquid N_2 until used. Two different defined media (SFM) were tested: SFM I consisted of DME, 0.5mg/ml fetuin (Sigma type IV), 10^{-6}M insulin (Sigma), 10^{-7}M dexamethazone (Sigma); SFM II consisted of DME, 10^{-6}M insulin , 0.1mg/ml L-thyroxine (Sigma). Transferrin (0.5, 5.0µg/ml; Sigma) and fibroblast growth factor (FGF; .1, .2, .5µg/ml; CR) were tested for stimulation of growth. Control cultures were grown in SCM containing DME, 8% horse serum (Flow), 1.8% CEE. Cultures were initiated by plating 80,000 cells onto gelatin coated Lux 35 mm dishes containing 1.5ml medium.

Two plating schedules were used. 1) Cells were seeded directly in SFM medium onto dishes which had been additionally coated with fibronectin by preincubation with GM medium for 2 hrs; 2) Cells were seeded first in GM medium and then transferred to SFM I after 48 hrs or SFM II after 24 hrs growth. Experimental cultures were transferred to SCM. Growth was estimated from their protein content as measured by the Lowry method. Creatine kinase (CK) activity and isoenzyme distribution, indicators of muscle differentiation, were measured as described[5]. Myotube specific components were identified by incubating differentiated cultures for 4 hrs with 10µCi/ml ^{35}S-methionine. The labelled components analysed by one dimensional polyacrylamide gel electrophoresis and were then compared to those obtained for myotubes of a human muscle clonal culture.

Results and Discussion

Cells seeded directly into SFM medium showed similar attachment after 24 hrs to control cultures in SCM but failed to proliferate and died after 2-3 days. Transferrin or FGF did not stimulate growth. Proliferation was observed only when the cells were first grown in GM medium, but compared to the control cultures the final growth attained was low. Both NN and AD cultures yielded 50-60% less protein than the control SCM cultures (Table 1). Although NN and AD myoblasts fused to form multinucleated myotubes at day 3 and day 5 respectively, in both SFM and SCM media, the myotubes appeared more differentiated in SFM medium. Fig. 1 illustrates the morphology of these cultures.

In particular AD cultures grown in SFM displayed long branched myotubes which unlike the controls did not become overgrown by mononucleate cells, thus allowing these cells to be maintained in culture for a longer period. Analysis of proteins

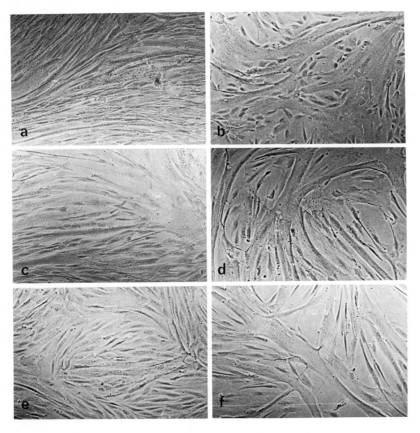

__Fig. 1.__ Representative phase contrast views (x75) of NN (a,c,e) cultures at day 7 and AD cultures (b,d,f) at day 10 grown in SCM (a,b); SFM I (c,d); SFM II (e,f).

Table 1. % Fusion, protein and CK synthesis of NN and AD muscle cell cultures grown in SCM, SFM I or SFM II media.

Medium	% Fusion[1]	Protein mg/plate	CK[2]/mg protein	% Isoenzymes BB	MB	MM
NN						
SCM	38.1	0.39	1.0	43.3	30.5	26.2
SFM I	32.4	0.17	1.2	55.3	37.6	7.1
SCM	54.4	0.49	0.8	-	-	-
SFM II	34.2	0.14	0.6	-	-	-
AD						
SCM	71.4	0.38	1.1	51.7	31.6	16.7
SFM I	55.9	0.17	3.5	25.2	46.8	28.0
SCM	-	0.56	0.9	-	-	-
SFM II	-	0.14	2.0	27.6	44.9	27.5

NN cells were analysed at 8 days in vitro (DIV) and AD cells at DIV 10.
1. Number of nuclei in myotube:total number nuclei x100
2. μmoles of creatine formed/min at 30°C

synthesised by these myotubes revealed that AD and NN muscle cells responded differently to defined medium (Table 1, Fig. 2).   NN muscle cells grown in SFM and SCM media yielded similar CK specific activities and isoenzyme pattern.   Compared to the controls, AD cultures at DIV 10 exhibited a 2-3 fold higher CK specific activity and an increase in the synthesis of the M-CK subunit (Table 1).   These cultures also manifested an enhanced synthesis of the 38K and 23.5K myotube specific proteins (Fig. 2I, track b and c) compared to cells grown in SCM (Fig. 2II, track a).   Protein profile transitions during myogenesis of clonal myoblast cultures clearly show that these components are myotube specific (Fig. 2III, track 3).   NN muscle grown under similar conditions did not show this enhancement in CK specific activity (Table 1) or in the expression of myotube specific proteins (Fig. 2II).

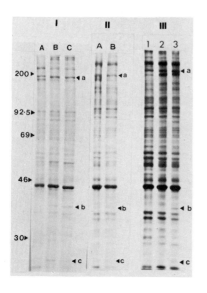

Fig. 2. Fluorography of AD (I), NN (II) differentiated cultures, and a human clonal myoblast culture (III) labelled with ^{35}S-methionine. (A) SCM; (B) SFM I; (C) SFM I plus transferrin (5μg/ml). Clonal myoblast culture was grown in GM first and then transferred to SCM. 1 represents prefusion, 2 - midfusion and 3 - postfusion. Band a - 195K, band b - 38K and band c - 23.5K proteins.

In conclusion our results clearly illustrate that human muscle cells can differentiate and synthesise muscle specific proteins in defined medium but that serum is required for proliferation. We have also observed that NN and AD muscle cells respond differently to defined medium with respect to expression of muscle specific proteins.

This work was supported by the Muscular Dystrophy Group of Great Britain.

References

1. Florini, J.R. and Roberts, S.B. (1979) In vitro 15, 983.
2. Kumegawa, M., Ikeda, E., Hosoda, S. and Takuma, T. (1980) Dev. Biol 79, 493-499.
3. Dollenmeier, P., Turner, D.C. and Eppenberger, H.M. (1981) Exp. Cell Res. 135, 47-61.
4. Yasin, R., van Beers, G., Nurse, K., Landon, D.N. and Thompson, E.J. (1977) J. Neurol. Sci. 32, 347-360.
5. Yasin, R., Kundu, D. and Thompson, E.J. (1982) Exp. Cell Res. 138, 419-422.

Tumor Cells

Tissue Culture of Human Colon Carcinomas.
Therapy Experiments in Vitro

Jürgen van der Bosch

Diabetes-Forschungsinstitut an der Universität Düsseldorf, Auf'm Hennekamp 65,
D-4000 Düsseldorf, FRG

Individual human tumors, even if derived from the same tissue of
origin, differ from each other in many respects. Most importantly
for cancer therapy, they differ in their responsiveness to the various
treatments, which are available at present and chances are high that
they will differ with respect to treatments to be developed in the
future. Therefore, it is highly important to work out in vitro-
systems, which allow the quantitative investigation of the effects of
additives like hormones, lectins, interferons, monoclonal antibodies
and anti-cancer drugs as well as of cytotoxic cells of the immune
system on the population development in primary cultures of individual
tumors and to correlate these in vitro results with the in vivo-be-
haviour (especially the drug responsiveness) of these tumors.

For this purpose the tumor-derived cultures should fulfill the
following demands:

1. Cell types, not belonging to the tumor should be excluded.
2. The culture conditions should support the net growth of the
   tumor under investigation.
3. The cultured material should be representative of the viable
   portion of the tumor and not only of minor subpopulations.
4. Culture preparation procedures should yield sufficient material
   for multiple cultures.
5. Seeding procedures should yield identical replicate cultures for
   use in quantitative investigations on a per cell basis.
6. It should be possible to control the cellular environment easily
   by quantitative medium changes. This is especially important for
   investigations concerning the dependence of population developments
   in such cultures on drug concentrations and drug application
   schedules.
7. Detachment and recollection of cells from primary cultures should
   be practicable in order to re-use these cells for secondary
   purposes (e.g. implantations in test animals or secondary
   cultures).

8. A cell counting method should allow quantitative measurements
    of population changes in such cultures. For this purpose it should
    be also possible to record the cell cycle phase distributions in
    such cultures.

Working with 11 individual human colon carcinomas, which were serially
transplanted in the athymic nude mouse, we have elaborated conditions,
which fullfill these demands for seven of these tumors completely,
whereas for the remaining four tumors not all of the demands are
fullfilled (1, 2, 3). Especially, two of the tumors ceased growing
after about one doubling in vitro and developed pronounced multi-
nucleation. This latter observation shows, that the culture conditions
used were not unfavourable for DNA replication even in these cases,
but mitosis was not performed correctly. Up to now we were not able
to improve this situation by any variation of the culture conditions.

The medium used in these experiments with primary cultures was a modification of the serum-free medium developed by Murakami and Masui (4)
for a colon tumor cell line. It consists of a (1:1)-mixture of
Dulbeccos modification of Eagle's medium (DMEM) and Ham's F12 medium
(F12) containing in addition insulin, transferrin, epidermal growth
factor, trijodothyronine and sodium selenite.

Growth curves of primary cultures of all 11 tumors in this serum-
free medium have been reported (1). In all cases maximum growth rates
were observed during the first days after seeding, indicating high
percentages of viable stem cells in these explants. Minimal population
doubling times varied among the 11 tumors between 2 and 7 days,
demonstrating the individuality of these tumors in vitro. Also the
density dependent saturation kinetics varied from tumor to tumor.
All tumors shed dead cells in varying quantities into the culture
medium, as this is a characteristic of colon tumors and normal colonic
mucosa in vivo.

The individuality of these tumors was also expressed in chemotherapy
experiments. Pronounced differences in the sensitivity of four tumors
against a doxorubicin-derivative (4-deoxy-doxorubicin = deo DX)
were detected (2). The sensitivity ranking derived from these in
vitro experiments for the four tumors was in good aggreement with
the ranking deduced from chemotherapy experiments with transplants
of the same tumors in the athymic nude mouse (2, 5, 6).

The development of resistance against deo-DX in vitro was investigated with the most sensitive of the four tumors. Resistance developed very much like in tumor transplants following deo-DX treatment in the athymic nude mouse (2).

In another set of experiments the responses of a tumor to a preparation of human leukocyte interferon and to deo-DX was investigated as they depended on the growth state of this tumor in vitro (3). Nearly stationary and fast growing populations of the same tumor could be produced by seeding very high- and low- density cultures respectively. Such populations can occur in vivo in the same tumor as actively growing and so called dormant domains in close proximity to each other. For a better understanding of the growth and drug response behaviour of tumors in vivo it is very important to analyse the reactions of these two population states separately and to reconstruct the behaviour of the complete tumor from these contributions. The present experiment yielded the following results. Whereas a stationary population could be completely extinguished by an interferon treatment, a fast growing population was only reversibly growth-inhibited by the same treatment. These results were further corroborated, when both populations were injected into athymic nude mice after the in vitro treatment with interferon: the stationary population did not develop any sign of a tumor within 8 weeks, whereas the fast growing population developed tumors within 2 weeks following subcutaneous injection. In both cases untreated control cultures produced palpable tumors within 1 week after inocculation. Deo-DX on the other hand had a strong diminishing effect on fast growing populations, whereas stationary populations were barely affected. This result, too, was corroborated by the course of tumor development after injection into the nude mouse following in vitro treatment.

A striking observation was made, when deo-DX and interferon were applied together to a fast growing tumor population. No additivity of the effects detected in separate treatments could be detected. Instead, interferon antagonized the deo-DX-effect on such populations. An explanation for this antagonism was found, taking in account that the DNA intercalating drug deo-DX is only active with fast growing populations (high S-phase content), whereas interferon reversibly transforms such a population in a non-growing population (low S-phase content), thus preventing deo-DX-action (3).

The procedures and the medium used for primary cultures from nude-
mouse-transplants of colon tumors can also be used for preparing
primary cultures directly from patient's tumorbiopsies. This is shown
in fig. 1. The tumor biopsy was treated according to the procedures
published (3), yielding a suspension of small tumor cell aggregates.
These aggregates were seeded as replicate cultures on day O in serum-
free (A) and serum-supplemented (B) medium.

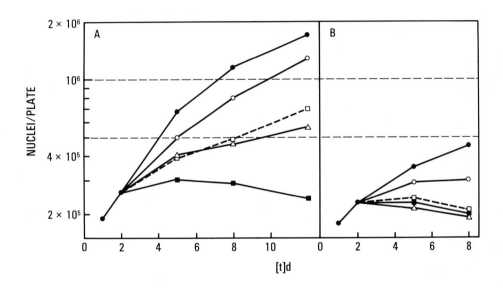

Fig. 1   Development and drug responses of primary cultures derived
          from a patient's colon carcinoma biopsy.
          A) In serum-free DMEM/F12, containing insulin (2 ug/ml),
          transferrin (2 ug/ml), trijodothyronine (200 pM), epidermal
          growth factor (20 ng/ml) and sodium selenite (5 nM).
          B) In the same medium as under A), containing additionally
          2,5 % horse serum and 2,5 % fetal bovine serum. ● control;
          O 1,8 µg/ml 1,3-bis-(2-chloroethyl)-1-nitrosuvea (BCNU);
          □   500 ng/ml 4'-O-methyldoxorubicin (O-DX); Δ 250 ng/ml
          4' deoxydoxorubicin (deo-DX); ■ 160 µg/ml 5-fluorouracil
          (5-FU). The medium was changed in all cultures every two
          days. Details of the seeding and drug treatment are described
          in the text. Cell nuclei were prepared and counted as report-
          ed earlier (1).

On day 2 after seeding both sets of cultures (A) and (B) were sub-
divided in 5 subsets. Each subset was treated for 1h with one of the
four drugs listed in the legend of fig. 1 in serum-free (A) or serum-
supplemented (B) medium, whereas the controls received drug-free
media. As can be seen, this tumor grows much better in serum-free
medium than in serum-supplemented medium and the responses to chemo-
therapy-drugs are changed in the presence of serum. A growth inhibiting effect of serum has been observed with several colon tumors
and a more detailed investigation of the effect of serum and other
additives, like hormones, on drug activity and tumor responsiveness
is certainly warranted.

In conclusion, procedures and media have been developed, which allow
a detailed investigation of a range of human colon carcinomas in
vitro. Up to now predominantly nude mouse-transplants of such tumors
were investigated. Research should be extended now to include more
investigations of cultures, directly from patients' tumor biopsies.
This has been shown to be practicable with biopsies from small cell
carcinomas of the lung by Carney et al. (7), using a serum free
medium selective for this kind of tumor. It is now possible to
investigate in vitro several problems associated with the therapy of
human tumors. For example, the emergence of drug-resistant tumor cell
populations can be followed in vitro and experiments aimed at the
prevention of drug resistance can be performed. The sensitivity of
tumor cell populations against various treatments can be investigated
as it depends on cell cycle phases and population growth states.
This may contribute to the development of more effective therapy
schedules. The tumorigenicity of cell populations treated in vitro
can be compared in the athymic nude mouse with the tumorigenicity of
the untreated control. Also, changes due to in vivo-treatments can be
analysed in vitro now. Furthermore, tumor tissue cultures can be
used as a first step in drug screening programs and in clinical drug-
sensitivity tests for individual tumor patients.

Acknowledgement
The experimental work, on which this article is based, has been
performed in Prof. Gordon Sato's laboratory at the University of
California, San Diego, during 1979-1981. The collaboration of Drs.
Hideo Masui and Krim Zirvi is gratefully acknowledged. The author
was supported by a Habilitantenstipendium (Bo 500/3) of the Deutsche
Forschungsgemeinschaft.

References

1. van der Bosch, J., Masui, H. and Sato, G. Growth characteristics of primary tissue cultures from heterotransplanted human colorectal carcinomas in serum-free medium.Cancer Res., 41: 611-618, 1981.

2. Zirvi, K., van der Bosch, J. and Kaplan, N.O. In vitro responses of nude mouse-xenografted human colon carcinomas exposed to doxorubicin derivatives in tissue culture and in the mouse. Cancer Res. 42: 3793-3797, 1982.

3. van der Bosch, J. and Zirvi, K. Growth state-specific responsiveness of primary cultures of a nude mouse-xenografted human colon carcinoma to 4'deoxydoxorubicin and a crude human leukocyte -Interferon preparation. Cancer Res., 42: 3789-3792, 1982.

4. Murakami, H. and Masui, H. Hormonal control of human colon carcinoma cell growth in serum-free medium. Proc. Natl. Acad. Sci. U.S.A. 77: 3464-3468, 1980.

5. Giuliani, F. and Kaplan, N.O. New doxorubicin analogs active against doxorubicin resistant colon tumor xenografts in the nude mouse. Cancer Res.,40: 4682-4687, 1980.

6. Giuliani, F., Zirvi, K., Kaplan, N.O. and Goldin, A. Chemotherapy of human colorectal tumor xenografts in athymic nude mice with clinicallly active drugs. Int. J. Cancer, 27: 5-13, 1981.

7. Carney, D., Bunn, P., Gazdar, A., Pagan, J. and Minna, J. Selective growth in serum-free medium of tumor cells obtained by biopsy from patients with small cell carcinoma of the lung. Proc. Natl. Acad. Sci. U.S.A. 78: 3185-3189, 1981.

Human Prostatic Cells in Serum-Free Medium

M. E. Kaighn

Laboratory of Experimental Pathology, National Cancer Institute, Frederick Cancer Research Facility, Frederick, MD 21701, USA

The importance of developing serum-free media for cultured cells can hardly be overemphasized (1-3). Perennial problems associated with the use of serum such as lot-to-lot variability in growth-promoting activity, toxicity, interference with specialized cellular functions, and contamination by adventitious agents such as mycoplasma, viruses, bacteria, bacteriophage and other organisms can be eliminated. The high cost of serum, the scarcity of suitable serum lots, and the time and expense incurred in serum evaluation provide additional motivation to develop serum-free media.

Our efforts to develop media and culture procedures for human prostatic cells began in 1974. At that time, no human prostatic epithelium had survived beyond primary culture. By using our standard medium, F12K, and a selected lot of fetal bovine serum, we were able to isolate a number of clonal strains from a benign prostatic adenoma (4). The same approach was unsuccessful with either normal prostatic epithelium or prostatic carcinoma tissue. In an attempt to overcome this problem, we adapted the approach of Ham (5). This involved titration of individual media components in a basal medium containing a growth-limiting level of serum. All of the media components tested were found to be at optimal levels in F12K (6). However, we observed that variability in the growth-promoting activity of serum was important, especially for normal cells. For this reason, we concentrated on addition of growth factors and hormones as advocated by Sato and associates (2).

In this paper I would like to describe the development of PFMR-4 and its use for human prostatic cell culture.

Isolation of Prostatic Cell Lines

Development of PFMR-4 resulted from efforts to isolate human prostatic cells. The earliest success was with the carcinoma line, PC-3 (7). Metastatic tumor tissue was dissociated and cultured in PFMR-1 with 20% selected fetal calf serum (FCS). This specimen gave

rise to an established cell line that has been extensively characterized (8). In order to culture normal prostatic epithelium a
non-enzymatic method was developed to dissociate the cells (9).
In connection with isolation of the line NP-2s, nutrient medium
PFMR-4 was developed (9). Subsequently, the NP-2s line has been
transformed by treatment with SV40 virus (10). Characteristics of
four prostate lines are summarized in Table 1.

Development of PFMR-4

PFMR-4 evolved from Ham's F12 (11). The initial modification
(mF12), used for several avian and mammalian cell types, was described
by Coon (12). Major changes in mF12 included doubling the concentration of amino acids and pyruvate and increasing calcium and bicarbonate levels (Table 2). Other minor alterations resulted from the use
of Konigsberg's modification of Hanks' saline as diluent (13). The
slightly modified formulation of Coon's mF12, which had been in use in
the author's laboratory since 1968, was referred to as F12K in a 1973
publication (6). After addition of HEPES buffer (Table 2), it was
designated PFMR-1 (14). The initials refer to the Pasadena Foundation
for Medical Research. This was done to avoid further confusion as a
result of proliferating modifications of F12. Addition of HEPES and
decrease in the level of $NaHCO_3$ as suggested by Dr. Ham greatly
improved F12K for prostatic cells.

Clonal titrations of selected components of PFMR-1 were carried
out in PFMR-1 supplemented with "stripped" 1 to 2% fetal calf serum
(s-FCS). The serum had been passed through a Sephadex G10 column at
45°C as previously reported (9) to remove steroids and other compounds of less than MW 700. The growth responses of NP-2s and PC-3
to selected nutrients is summarized in Table 3.

The stripped serum was included at a growth-limiting level
(1-2%) because no clonal growth could be obtained without it. The
growth responses of PC-3 and NP-2s were substantially the same; the
compounds tested were either at their optima in PFMR-1 or had no
effect. Folinate (16) had no greater growth-promoting activity than
folate and was not included in PFMR-4. Cystine, the oxidized form of
cysteine, was substituted for cysteine to avoid possible reduction of
the disulfide bonds in insulin and other factors (17). Calcium and
magnesium ions were also titrated (18) and the levels of both in
PFMR-1 were optimal for both PC-3 and NP-2s. However, maximal growth
is attained with PC-3 at about 3.0E-5M/1 calcium whereas the NP-2s

Table 1. Characteristics of human prostatic cell lines.

Characteristic	NP-2s (Ref. #8,9)	PC3 (ref. #7,8)	NP-2s/T1 (ref. #10)	NP-2s/T2 (ref. #10)
Origin	Neonatal prostate	Bone	SV40-treated NP-2s	SV40-treated NP-2s
Morphology	Epithelial-like	Epithelial-like	Epithelial-like	Epithelial-like
Ultrastructure	Smooth surface, normal organelles	Abundant microvilli, blebs, ruffles, loose cell clusters, extensive organelle changes	Microvilli in some cells, abnormal nuclei and organelles	Abnormal nuclei Abnormal organelles
Chromosomes				
Ploidy	Diploid	Aneuploid	87% "diploid"	Pseudodiploid
Chromosome number	46	55-62	44 (38-87)	46
Markers	None	11+	6-7	1-4
Y-chromosome	Present	Not seen	Present	Present
Growth				
Lifespan	35 P.D.	>350 P.D.	85 P.D.	90 P.D.
Doubling time	18 hr	29 hr	28 hr	25 hr
Anchorage-independence	−	+	+	+
Tumorigenicity (nude mice)	−	+	−	−
Factor response (K_m)				
Serum (FBSP)	2,240 g/ml	10 g/ml	8.90 g/ml	11.6 g/ml
EGF	0.24 ng/ml	no effect	0.23 ng/ml	0.10 ng/ml
FGF	6.76 ng/ml	no effect	6.59 ng/ml	no effect
ECGS	7.40 ng/ml	no effect	no effect	17.6 g/ml
HC	Synergistic with EGF or FGF	no effect	no effect	
Other				
5α-reductase	++	+	N.T.	N.T.
Acid phosphatase	+	+	N.T.	N.T.

Table 2. Modification of medium F12 for human prostatic cells.[1]

	F12	mF12	F12K	PFMR-1	PFMR-4	DME/F12
Essential amino acids						
Arginine	1.0E-3	2.0E-3	2.0E-3	2.0E-3	2.0E-3	7.0E-4
Cysteine	2.0E-4	4.0E-4	4.0E-4	4.0E-4	-	1.0E-4
Half-cystine	-	-	-	-	3.0E-4	2.0E-4
Glutamine	1.0E-3	2.0E-3	2.0E-3	2.0E-3	2.0E-3	2.5E-3
Histidine	1.0E-4	2.0E-4	2.0E-4	2.0E-4	2.0E-4	1.5E-4
Isoleucine	3.0E-5	6.0E-5	6.0E-5	6.0E-5	6.0E-5	4.2E-4
Leucine	1.0E-4	2.0E-4	2.0E-4	2.0E-4	2.0E-4	4.5E-4
Lysine	2.0E-4	4.0E-4	4.0E-4	4.0E-4	4.0E-4	5.0E-4
Methionine	3.0E-5	6.0E-5	6.0E-5	6.0E-5	6.0E-5	1.2E-4
Phenylalanine	3.0E-5	6.0E-5	6.0E-5	6.0E-5	6.0E-5	2.2E-4
Threonine	1.0E-4	2.0E-4	2.0E-4	2.0E-4	2.0E-4	4.5E-4
Tryptophan	1.0E-5	2.0E-5	2.0E-5	2.0E-5	2.0E-5	4.5E-5
Tyrosine	3.0E-5	6.0E-5	6.0E-5	6.0E-5	6.0E-5	2.2E-4
Valine	1.0E-4	2.0E-4	2.0E-4	2.0E-4	2.0E-4	4.5E-4
Nonessential amino acids						
Alanine	1.0E-4	2.0E-4	2.0E-4	2.0E-4	2.0E-4	5.0E-5
Asparagine	1.0E-4	2.0E-4	2.0E-4	2.0E-4	2.0E-4	5.0E-5
Aspartate	1.0E-4	2.0E-4	2.0E-4	2.0E-4	2.0E-4	5.0E-5
Glutamate	1.0E-4	2.0E-4	2.0E-4	2.0E-4	2.0E-4	5.0E-5
Glycine	1.0E-4	2.0E-4	2.0E-4	2.0E-4	2.0E-4	2.5E-4
Proline	3.0E-4	6.0E-4	6.0E-4	6.0E-4	6.0E-4	1.4E-4
Serine	1.0E-4	2.0E-4	2.0E-4	2.0E-4	2.0E-4	2.5E-4
Vitamins						
Biotin	3.0E-8	3.0E-8	3.0E-7	3.0E-7	3.0E-7	1.5E-8
Folate	3.0E-6	3.0E-6	3.0E-6	3.0E-6	3.0E-6	6.0E-6
Lipoate	1.0E-6	1.0E-6	1.0E-6	1.0E-6	1.0E-6	5.0E-7
Niacinamide	3.0E-7	3.0E-7	3.0E-7	3.0E-7	3.0E-7	1.7E-5
Pantothenate	1.0E-6	1.0E-6	1.0E-6	1.0E-6	1.0E-6	9.0E-6
Pyridoxine	3.0E-7	3.0E-7	3.0E-7	3.0E-7	3.0E-7	1.7E-5
Riboflavin	1.0E-7	1.0E-7	1.0E-7	1.0E-7	1.0E-7	5.5E-7
Thiamin	1.0E-6	1.0E-6	1.0E-6	1.0E-6	1.0E-6	6.5E-6
Vitamin B_{12}	1.0E-6	1.0E-6	1.0E-6	1.0E-6	1.0E-6	5.0E-7

[1]The composition of media leading to PFMR-4 are listed. All concentrations are in moles per liter except for CO_2. The letter E is used to designate a power of 10. Thus 1.5E-4 means 1.5×10^{-4} moles per liter. This notation (as used by Dr. Ham) was adopted to facilitate media comparisons. References to the different media are given in the text. DME/F12 (1:1) values were calculated from Ham's paper (11) and from a Tissue Culture Association publication (15).

Table 2 (continued)

	F12	mF12	F12K	PFMR-1	PFMR-4	DME/F12
Purines and Pyrimidines						
Hypoxanthine	3.0E-5	3.0E-5	3.0E-5	3.0E-5	3.0E-5	1.5E-5
Thymidine	3.0E-6	3.0E-6	3.0E-6	3.0E-6	3.0E-6	1.5E-6
Other Organic Compounds						
Ascorbate	--	8.5E-5	--	--	--	--
Choline	1.0E-4	1.0E-4	1.0E-4	1.0E-4	1.0E-4	6.5E-5
Glucose	1.0E-2	7.0E-3	7.0E-3	7.0E-3	7.0E-3	7.8E-3
I-inositol	1.0E-4	1.0E-4	1.0E-4	1.0E-4	1.0E-4	7.0E-5
Linoleate	3.0E-7	3.0E-7	--	--	--	1.5E-7
Putrescine	1.0E-6	1.0E-6	2.0E-6	2.0E-6	2.0E-6	5.0E-7
Pyruvate	1.0E-3	2.0E-3	2.0E-3	2.0E-3	2.0E-3	1.0E-3
Inorganic ions						
Calcium	3.0E-4	9.0E-4	9.2E-4	9.2E-4	9.2E-4	1.1E-3
Magnesium	6.0E-4	6.8E-4	2.1E-3	2.1E-3	6.8E-4	7.0E-4
Potassium	3.0E-4	4.3E-4	4.2E-3	4.2E-3	4.2E-3	9.5E-4
Sodium	1.5E-1	1.5E-1	1.6E-1	1.6E-1	1.3E-1	1.5E-1
Chloride	1.5E-1	1.4E-1	1.4E-1	1.4E-1	1.1E-1	1.3E-1
Phosphate	1.0E-3	1.4E-3	1.2E-3	1.2E-3	1.2E-3	1.5E-1
Sulfate	--	1.6E-4	1.6E-3	1.6E-3	1.6E-4	--
Trace elements						
Copper	1.0E-8	1.0E-8	1.0E-8	1.0E-8	1.0E-8	5.0E-9
Iron	3.0E-6	3.0E-6	3.0E-6	3.0E-6	3.0E-6	1.6E-6
Manganese	--	--	--	--	1.0E-9	--
Molybdenum	--	--	--	--	7.0E-9	--
Nickel	--	--	--	--	5.0E-10	--
Selenium	--	--	--	--	3.0E-8	--
Silicon	--	--	--	--	5.0E-7	--
Tin	--	--	--	--	5.0E-10	--
Vanadium	--	--	--	--	5.0E-9	--
Zinc	3.0E-6	3.0E-6	5.0E-7	5.0E-7	5.0E-7	1.5E-6
Buffers and Indicators						
Bicarbonate	1.4E-2	3.3E-2	3.0E-2	1.4E-2	1.4E-2	2.9E-2
CO_2	5%	5%	5%	5%	2-3%	5%
HEPES	--	--	--	5.0E-2	3.0E-2	--
Phenol red	3.3E-6	3.3E-6	8.3E-6	8.3E-6	6.0E-6	2.2E-5

Table 3. Clonal titrations of various nutrients in PFMR-4
          supplemented with stripped serum.

Compound tested	Result
Amino acids	
Arginine, cyteine, cystine, glutamine, histidine, leucine	Optimum as in PFMR-1
Vitamins	
Niacinamide, folate	Optimum as in PFMR-1
Folinate	No benefit over folate
Retinol, ascorbate	No effect
Other organics	
Glucose, choline, pyruvate, putrescine	Optimum as in PFMR-1
Acetate, glycerol, linoleate	No effect
Glyoxylate	Toxic at high levels

line requires 1.0E-3M/l or more (18). Several other compounds were
tested including hydrocortisone, dexamethasone, and 17-β estradiol
and were found to have no effect on the growth of either cell line.
The pH of PFMR-4 was 7.5 when equilibrated with 3% CO_2. Its osmolality was measured as 280 mOsm compared to 333 mOsm for F12 and
323 mOsm for DME/F12 (Table 2). Finally, the trace element stock L
of Ham's MCDB 104 (19) was included in PFMR-4.

As a result of this work, it appeared that PFMR-4 was adequate
and it was decided to emphasize the approach of Sato and co-workers
of replacing serum with growth factors (2). This approach was
successful with NP-2s and made possible an overall reduction of
27.5-fold in serum required by inclusion of hydrocortisione,
1.0E-6M/l and epidermal growth factor, 5ng/ml (18). On the other
hand, no effective factors were found for PC-3 by this approach.

Growth of Prostatic Cells in Serum-Free Medium

Following the reports by Sato and coworkers (20-22) that the
PC-3 line could be grown in serum-free medium supplemented with
growth factors, we attempted to replace serum with the reported
effective factors. Addition of the factors listed in Table 4 singly
and in selected combinations failed to stimulate growth in the clonal
assay (23).

Table 4. Factors tested in the clonal assay

_____

Single factors

Bovine serum albumin	100 µg/ml
Dihydrotestosterone	1.0 E-7 M/l
Endothelial cell growth supplement	200 µg/ml
Epidermal growth factor	5 ng/ml
Fibroblast growth factor	1 ng/ml
Hydrocortisone	1.0 E-7 M/l
Insulin	5 µg/ml
Luteinizing hormone	1 µg/ml
Multiplication stimulating activity	150 ng/ml
Platelet-derived growth factor	3 µg/ml
Thyroid hormone releasing factor	1.0 E-9 M/l
Transferrin	5 µg/ml
Triiodothyronine	1.0 E-11 M/l

Combined factors

Insulin and transferrin
Insulin, transferrin and triiodothyronine
Insulin, transferrin and luteinizing hormone extract
Insulin, transferrin and thyroid hormone releasing factor
Insulin, transferrin and fibroblast growth factor

_____

No growth was observed with DME/F12 even with 0.05% serum (20).
However, when the basal medium was PFMR-4, both BSA and serum permitted clonal growth (Table 5). In order to clarify our apparent
contradictory results, the assay was repeated with the high density
cultures used by Sato and co-workers rather than clonal cultures (23).
Cells were plated at 10^5 per 60 mm culture dish (5,100 cells/cm^2) in
the experimental media. Floating and attached cells were pooled and

Table 5. Clonal growth of PC-3 SF12 in the presence and absence
          of serum and growth factors.[1]

Basal medium	Serum-free			Fetal calf serum		
	None	+Factors	+BSA	None	+Factors	+BSA
DME/F12	--	--	--	--	--	--
PFMR-4	--	--	4.2(0.42)[2]	1-2(0.40)	1-2(0.40)	5.9(0.47)

[1]Culture dishes (50mm) containing 4 ml medium and the various
factors listed in Table 3 were inoculated with 500 cells (SF-12).
They were fixed, stained and counted after 12 days' incubation. FCS
at 0.05% contained 19.5 µg/ml fetal bovine serum protein (FBSP).
[2]Values are clonal plating efficiency (population doublings/day).

Table 6. Growth stimulation by factors in high-density cultures
          (PC-3 SH12).

| Factor(s) | Fold increase in cell number (SEM) | |
	PFMR-4	DME/F12
None	4.25 (0.43)	1.55 (0.13)
Insulin (I)	6.16 (0.16)	2.37 (0.40)
Transferrin (T)	4.49 (0.25)	2.22 (0.10)
Insulin, transferrin	5.67 (0.46)	2.85 (0.08)
I + T + Triiodothyronine	6.07 (0.38)	3.15 (0.31)
I + T + Thyroid releasing factor	5.13 (0.41)	3.84 (0.23)
I + T + Luteinizing hormone release factor	5.09 (0.03)	3.51 (0.18)
I + T + Luteinizing hormone extract	5.92 (0.24)	3.94 (0.25)
I + T + Fibroblast growth factor	5.52 (0.01)	2.94 (0.10)

counted 12 days later (Table 6). Under these conditions, the population increased 4.2-fold in 12 days (0.35 PD/day) in PFMR-4 as compared
to 1.55-fold (0.13 PD/day) in DME/F12. Growth in PFMR-4 alone was
greater than the maximal level in hormone-supplemented DME/F12
(0.33 PD/day). Insulin provided the greatest stimulation with PFMR-4
as the basal medium (0.51 PD/day). When DME/F12 was used, the
combinations of insulin and transferrin with triiodothyronine,
luteinizing hormone extract and fibroblast growth factor, thyroid
hormone releasing factor all stimulated growth as reported by Sato,
Reid and associates (22).

The discrepancy between the results with clonal vs. high density
cultures was clarified by a further experiment in which clonal growth
of PC-3 and another prostatic carcinoma line, DU 145, were both shown
to be population-dependent (23). This population-dependence was
abolished by conditioned medium or by co-cultivation with mitomycin-C
inactivated homologous cells (23).

The reason for the greater growth response in PFMR-4 than in
DME/F12 is unknown. The composition of these two media are listed
in Table 2. The DME/F12 used in my laboratory had been modified by
addition of HEPES (3.0E-2M/l) and reduction of bicarbonate to
1.4E-2M/l to maintain the same pH as in PFMR-4 (24).

Differences in the composition of the two basal media are summarized in Table 7. Only differences of 2-fold or greater are listed.
Eight amino acids, five vitamins and zinc are higher in DME/F12; and
five amino acids and eight other compounds are lower. Lineolate is

Table 7. Differences in the composition of PFMR-4 and DME/F12.

Concentration in DME/F12 > PFMR-4

Isoleucine, 7.0x   Threonine, 2.3x
Phenylalanine, 3.7x   Tryptophan, 2.3x
Tyrosine, 3.7x   Valine, 2.3x
Leucine, 2.3x   Methionine, 2.0X

Niacinamide, 56.6x   Folate, 2.0x
Pantothenate, 9x   Zinc, 3.0x
Thiamin, 6.5x
Riboflavin, 5.5x

Concentration in DME/F12 < PFMR-4

Biotin, 20x   Pyruvate, 2x
Alanine, 4x   Lipoate, 2x
Arginine, 4x   Putrescine, 4x
Aspartate, 4x   Hypoxanthine, 2x
Glutamate, 4x   Thymidine, 2x
Proline, 4x   Copper, 2x
                                      Iron, 2x

Present in DME/F12 only: Lineolate

Present in PFMR-4 only: sulfate, manganese, molybdenum, nickel,
                         selenium, tin, vanadium

Other parameters: pH 7.4-7.5 in both
                   Osmolality - PFMR-4, 280 mOsm/kg
                               DME/F12, 320 mOsm/kg

---

present only in DME/F12, whereas sulfate and six trace elements are
present only in PFMR-4. DME/F12 has a higher osmolality than PFMR-4
(Table 7). Niacinamide is very high in DME/F12 (cf. Table 3) and
biotin quite low. The significance of these differences is unknown.
Based upon our experience, the higher osmolality and lack of trace
elements might be important. In addition, the DME/F12 used was
prepared from commercially obtained powdered medium. It is conceivable that the ferrous iron might have been oxidized and reduced in
concentration and then removed during filtration (Ham, personal
communication).

In summary: (1) growth of prostatic carcinoma cells in serum-
free medium is population-dependent. (2) Response to specific growth
factors is not the same as a "requirement;" it depends on population
density as well as on the composition of the nutrient medium. (3) At
high density PC-3 and DU 145 respond to insulin and several other
factors as previously reported (20-22).

Prostatic Acid Phosphatase Activity in Serum-Free Medium

The availability of a serum-free system made it possible to investigate the influence of serum on a specific cellular function. Serum acid phosphatase (AP) has been viewed as a marker for cell cultures derived from the prostate (25). We previously found low but measurable AP activity in cultured prostatic cells (7,8). Recently, we described the effects of serum on the expression of AP in two prostatic carcinoma lines (26). In this work, acid phosphatase was measured biochemically with thymolphthalein monophosphate as substrate and histochemically by the Burstone method. Acid phosphatase activity was 7-fold higher in cells maintained in PFMR-4 without serum. When cells (PE3/SF12) were switched to serum-supplemented medium for five days, AP specific activity decreased by 60% or more. Further, without serum the fraction of AP inhibited by tartrate nearly doubled (80 vs 54%). Scanning electron micrographs also revealed marked changes in the cell surface in the presence of serum (26). The changes induced by serum in PC-3 and DU 145 are reversible. This is not necessarily true in other cell types. Ambesi-Impiombato et al. (27) were able to isolate and maintain hormone-dependent rat thyroid cells with medium containing low serum and hormone supplement. In high serum, the functional epithelial cells cells were selectively lost (27). Suppression of hormonally induced functions have also been observed in granulosa cells (28) and colon carcinoma cells (29). Recently, Lechner et al. (30) reported clonal growth of normal human bronchial epithelial cells in a serum-free hormone-supplemented medium. In this system, serum actually inhibited growth of the epithelial cells. Thus, serum can suppress specialized functions, inhibit cell growth by encouraging differentiation, or prevent isolation of functional cell lines altogether.

Summary and Perspectives

A nutrient medium, PFMR-4, has been developed by sequential modifications of Ham's F12 that will support multiplication of two human prostatic carcinoma lines (PC-3 and DU 145). Serum, hormones and growth factors are not required. Growth under these conditions is population-dependent. Clonal growth requires either reproductively-inactivated feeder cells or conditioned medium. Although PC-3 requires no hormones for survival and growth, its growth rate is increased by insulin and several other factors when challenged at high cell density. Normal prostatic epithelial cells (NP-2s) also grow in PFMR-4 but require hydrocortisone, epidermal growth factor and a low level of serum.

Growth of cells without serum simplifies studies on hormonal response. However, it is important to remember that the behavior of cells under these conditions may be considerably different. Serum has been reported to suppress or stimulate differentiation and to suppress or stimulate growth. The result depends on the system used, the cell line and the nutrient medium. In the prostatic cell lines PC-3 and DU 145, serum suppresses acid phosphatase activity.

The availability of defined media tailored for specific cell types and purposes will make possible isolation of new cell types difficult or impossible to culture previously and facilitate standardization of culture systems for studies of carcinogenesis, differentiation and hormone action.

Acknowledgements

I thank Drs. John F. Lechner, David Kirk and K. Shankar Narayan for their major contributions to the work reviewed in this chapter, Dr. Hayden G. Coon for making available his modification of F12 (mF12) before publication and for many stimulating discussions, Drs. Richard G. Ham, Gordon Sato and Lola Reid for advice, Merrill Babcock, Maureen Marnell and Marika Szalay for outstanding technical assistance, Mary Ann Thompson for her work on the acid phosphatase assay, Dr. Lawrence W. Jones and the Pasadena Foundation for Medical Research for their support, and Mary Jo Elsasser for preparation of the manuscript.

References

1. Ham, R.G. In Vitro 10:119-129 (1974).
2. Rizzino, A., H. Rizzino and G. Sato. Nutr. Rev. 37:379-378 (1979).
3. Kaighn, M.E. J. Natl. Cancer Inst. 53:1437-1442 (1974).
4. Kaighn, M.E. and M.S. Babcock. Cancer Chemother. Rep. 59:59-63 (1975).
5. Ham, R.G. and W.L. McKeehan. In Nutritional requirements of cultured cells (Katsuta, H., ed.) Tokyo: Japan Scientific Societies Press, 1978, pp. 63-115.
6. Kaighn, M.E. In Tissue culture: Methods and applications (Kruse, P.F. Jr. and M.K. Patterson, Jr., eds.) New York, Academic Press, 1973, pp. 54-57.
7. Kaighn, M.E., K.S. Narayan, Y. Ohnuki, J.F. Lechner and L.W. Jones. Invest. Urol 17:16-23 (1979).
8. Kaighn, M.E., J.F. Lechner, M.S. Babcock, M. Marnell, Y. Ohnuki and K.S. Narayan. In Models for prostate cancer (Murphy, G.P., ed.) New York: Alan R. Liss, 1980, pp. 85-109.

9. Lechner, J.F., M.S. Babcock, M. Marnell, K.S. Narayan and M.E. Kaighn. _In_ Methods in cell biology, vol. 21B (Harris, C.C., B.F. Trump and G.D. Stoner, eds.) New York: Academic Press (1980) pp. 195-225.

10. Kaighn, M.E., K.S. Narayan, Y. Ohnuki, L.W. Jones and J.F. Lechner. Carcinogenesis 1:635-645 (1980).

11. Ham, R.G. Proc. Natl. Acad. Sci. USA 53:288-293 (1965).

12. Coon, H.G. and M.C. Weiss. Proc Natl. Acad. Sci. USA 62:853 (1969).

13. Konigsberg, I.R. Science 140:1273 (1963).

14. Kaighn, M.E. Cancer Treatment Rep. 61:147-151 (1977).

15. Morton, H.J. In Vitro 6:89-108 (1970).

16. McKeehan, W.L., D.P. Genereax and R.G. Ham. Biochem. Biophys. Res. Comm. 80:1013-1021 (1978).

17. Hayashi, I., J. Larner and G. Sato. In Vitro 14:22-30 (1978).

18. Lechner, J.F. and M.E. Kaighn. _In_ Models for Prostate Cancer (Murphy, G.P., ed.) New York: Alan R. Liss (1980), pp. 217-232.

19. McKeehan, W.L., K.A. McKeehan, S.L. Hammond and R.G. Ham. In Vitro 13:399-415 (1977).

20. Barnes, D. and G. Sato. Anal. Biochem. 102:255-270 (1980).

21. Sato, G. and L. Reid. _In_ Biochemistry and Mode of Action of Hormones, II (Rickenberg, H.V., ed.) Baltimore: University Park Press, Vol. 20 (1978) pp. 219-251.

22. Reid, L., N. Minato and M. Rojkind. _In_ Male Accessory Sex Glands (Spring-Mills, E. and E.S.E. Hafez, eds.) Amsterdam: Elsevier/North-Holland (1980) pp. 617-640.

23. Kaighn, M.E., D, Kirk, M. Szalay and J.F. Lechner. Proc. Natl. Acad. Sci. USA 78:5673-5676 (1981).

24. Shipley, G.D. and R.G. Ham. In Vitro 17:656-670 (1981).

25. Stonington, O.G., N. Szweg and M. Webber. J. Urol. 114:903-908 (1975).

26. Kirk, D., K.S. Narayan, G. Vener and M.E. Kaighn. Ann. N.Y. Acad. Sci. 390:62-72 (1982).

27. Ambesi-Impiombato, F.S., A.M. Parks and H.G. Coon. Proc. Natl. Acad. Sci. USA 77:3455-3459 (1980).

28. Orly, J., G. Sato and G.F. Erikson. Cell 20:817-827 (1980).

29. Murakami, H. and H. Masui. Proc. Natl. Acad. Sci. USA 77:3464-3468 (1980).

30. Lechner, J.F., A. Haugen, I.A. McClendon and E.W. Pettis. In Vitro 18:633-642 (1982).

Culture of Human Lung Carcinoma Cells in Serum-Free Media

Hideo Masui, Kaoru Miyazaki, and Gordon H. Sato

Cancer Center, Q-058, University of California, San Diego, La Jolla, CA 92093, USA

INTRODUCTION

In this article, we describe methods for serum-free culture of human lung carcinoma cells. The original tumors were obtained from surgery and the tumors have been successively transplanted into nude mice. We have studied the growth requirements of these tumor cells in primary cultures and of established cell lines. Each tumor type can be grown as transplantable tumors, either in nude mice or in culture, allowing *in vivo* and *in vitro* experiments. We have developed serum-free media for these cell lines, which allow us to examine the biological effects of many substances.

Human lung epidermoid carcinoma cells (T222):

The culture medium used for lung epidermoid carcinoma cells is a 1:1 mixture of F12 and DME supplemented with insulin (5 μg/ml), glucagon (0.2 μg/ml), selenium (2.5 x 10^{-8} M) and T_3 (5 x 10^{-10} M).

A transplantable human lung epidermoid carcinoma (T222) was established by injecting tumor specimens obtained from a 70 year old male patient. Histological examination showed prominent keratin pearls in the original tumor from the patient. Although the pearl formation was not apparent in the histology of tumors transplanted in nude mice, a large number of cornified cells were always evident when the tumor tissue was minced. This indicates that keratinization occurs in the heterotransplanted T222 tumors.

Preparation of primary cultures: Tumor tissue was minced, washed with serum-free F12/DME medium and then treated with collagenase (1 mg/ml) at 37°C for 2 to 4 hours. After incubation, big clumps of tumor cells which rapidly settled to the bottom of a test tube were removed and small clumps consisting of less than several hundred tumor cells were collected by allowing to sediment by gravity. The cells were washed with serum-free F12/DME, suspended in serum-supplemented F12/DME and plated into Falcon culture flasks. After incubating at 37°C for 40 hours, the serum-supplemented medium was removed, cultures washed with serum-free F12/DME and experimental media added. The cell growth was assayed by counting cell number. We have found that keratinized epidermoid carcinoma cells are insoluble in 1% sodium dodecyl sulfate (SDS), as reported by Sun and Green (1) for human epidermal cells. Furthermore, keratinized cells can be separated into single cells by sonication. The number of keratinized cells was counted as follows: cultures were trypsinized, suspended in 1% SDS - 10 mM Tris buffer (pH 7.5), and sonicated. The details of the methods has been described elsewhere (2).

Cell growth in serum-free medium: When primary cultures of T222 human lung epidermoid carcinoma cells were maintained in serum-supplemented medium, the tumor cells grew poorly and eventually were overgrown by fibroblasts. When the tumor cells were plated in serum-supplemented medium, and then cultivated in serum-free F12/DME without any supplement, the tumor cells divided faster than in serum-supplemented medium. Under this culture condition, there was little growth of fibroblasts. The cell growth of T222 lung epidermoid cells in serum-free F12/DME is strongly dependent on the cell density; the growth of tumor cells was seen only when the cells were plated at a high density.

Hormones and factors, which have been shown to promote the growth of various types of cultured cells (3), were screened for the stimulation of growth of T222 tumor cells in primary culture. Four substances, insulin, selenium, glucagon and T_3, showed significant growth stimulating effects. Selenium was the most important factor for the growth of T222 cells, and the growth stimulatory effects of other substances were seen only in the presence of selenium. Transferrin, epidermal growth factor, fibroblast growth factor and hydrocortisone, common supplements in serum-free media for many types of cell lines (3), were not effective for cell growth. The growth of T222 tumor cells in a serum-free medium supplemented with insulin, selenium and glucagon are shown in Figure 1.

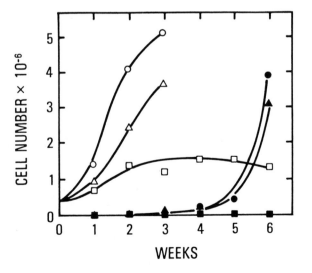

Figure 1. The total cells and keratinized cells were counted as described in the text. After culture in serum supplemented medium, fibroblasts were removed by brief trypsinization. The total cell number of the cultures in serum-free media could not be determined after 3 weeks. F12/DME supplemented with insulin, selenium and glucagon; total cells (O), keratinized cells (●). Serum-free F12/DME; total cells (Δ), keratinized cells (▲). Serum-supplemented medium; total cells (□), keratinized cells (■).

The growth of the tumor cells in this medium was better than in serum-free F12/DME. The addition of T_3 to this medium increased the cell growth slightly, but it affected profoundly the keratinization of these tumor cells as described in the following section.

Keratinization of T222 lung epidermoid carcinoma cells: We have found that these tumor cells underwent keratinization in serum-free F12/DME. Because keratinization is terminal differentiation and thus affects the growth of T222 tumors, we have studied this phenomenon. We have found that the addition of serum, retinoic acid or T_3 inhibited keratinization of these cells (Fig. 1). When primary cultures of T222 tumor cells were maintained in hormone-supplemented F12/DME and subcultured in this medium, the cell growth gradually decreased upon repeated subculture. A permanent line of the T222 tumor cells has not been established in serum-free medium, but a cell line has been established when 0.5% serum was added to the hormone-supplemented F12/DME.

Growth and keratinization of T222 lung epidermoid cell line: The growth requirements and keratinization of the established T222 cell line were studied. The growth requirements are shown in Table 1. Although the T222 cells in primary culture grew faster in serum-free medium than in serum-supplemented medium, the established cells grew faster in serum-supplemented medium than in serum-free, hormone-supplemented medium. Also, the inhibition of keratinization of the established cell line required higher concentrations (at least 100-fold) of retinoic acid or T_3 compared to T222 tumor cells in primary culture. The concentration of serum had to be increased to 10-fold to inhibit the keratinization of T222 cell line (Table 2). These results suggest that subpopulations of T222 tumor cells were selected furing establishment of the cell line.

Table 1

Growth of Human Lung Epidermoid Carcinoma Cell Line (T222)

Supplements	Cell No. x 10^{-5} per dish
None	<0.6
3F	1.69
3F + retinoic acid (10^{-8} M)	1.96
3F + T_3 (10^{-7} M)	1.55
Newborn calf serum (7.5%)	4.16

T222 tumor cells were plated at a density of 0.6 x 10^5 cells per 35 mm culture dishes in serum-supplemented medium. On the following day, cultures were washed with serum-free medium, and the experimental media were added. After an incubation for 11 days, the cell number was counted. The number represents the average of duplicate dishes. 3F: 5 µg/ml insulin, 2.5 x 10^{-8} M selenium and 0.2 µg/ml glucagon.

Table 2

Effects of Serum, Retinoic Acid and T_3 on Keratinization

of Lung Epidermoid Carcinoma Cell Line (T222)

Supplements	Keratinized Cells x 10^{-6}/dish	% of Keratinized Cells
3F	3.17	100
3F + retinoic acid (10^{-8} M)	1.93	61
3F + T_3 (10^{-7} M)	0.76	24
Newborn calf serum (7.5%)	0.12	4

Cultures were prepared as described in the legend of Table 1, except that the cells were incubated in the experimental media for 5 weeks.

Lung Adenocarcinoma Cells (T291):

The culture medium used for lung adenocarcinoma cells (T291) is a 1:1 mixture of F12 and DME medium supplemented with insulin (10 µg/ml), transferrin (10 µg/ml), EGF (2 ng/ml), hydrocortisone (5 x 10^{-8} M), selenium (2.5 x 10^{-8} M) and fatty acid-free albumin (0.5 mg/ml).

Preparation of primary culture: Human lung adenocarcinoma (T291) was maintained by transplanting successively in Balb/C nude mice. The tumor tissue was minced, washed with serum-free F12/DME and treated with collagenase (1 mg/ml) at 37°C for 1 to 2 hr. The tumor cells were collected by centrifugation. When the primary cultures were maintained and passed in serum-supplemented medium, these tumor cells can be established in culture.

Growth requirements of lung adenocarcinoma cells: Using the established lung adenocarcinoma cell line, the growth requirements were tested and a serum-free medium has been developed. Its composition is described above. These cells can be propagated in this serum-free medium, when cells were plated into serum-coated culture dishes. The cells did not attach to the plastic culture dishes without serum-coating. Although cells attached to fibronectin-coated culture dishes, they subsequently detached from the dishes.

The growth curves of the lung adenocarcinoma cells in serum-supplemented medium and in serum-free medium supplemented with insulin, transferrin, EGF, selenium and fatty acid-free albumin are shown in Figure 2. There was only a little cell growth in serum-free F12/DME medium, but the addition of five factors resulted in a significant stimulation of cell growth (90% of that in serum-supplemented medium). The addition of hydrocortisone caused a slight decrease in cell growth, but the cells stayed healthy during a long-term culture.

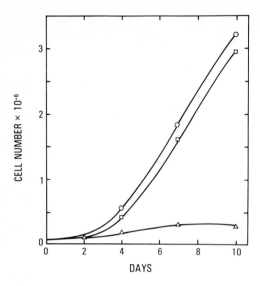

Figure 2. Serum-supplemented medium (O), hormone-supplemented medium (□) and serum-free F12/DME (Δ).

This serum-free medium can be applied for primary cultures of T291 lung adenocarcinoma cells. In this medium, the cells in primary cultures grew at almost the same rate as in serum-supplemented medium. This medium did not support the growth of fibroblasts, whereas the overgrowth of fibroblasts was a serious problem in primary cultures with serum-supplemented medium. The lung adenocarcinoma cells showed essentially the same hormone requirements as the established cell line. Thus far, cell lines have not been established from cells cultured exclusively in this serum-free, hormone-supplemented medium. When 0.5% serum was added to this medium, the cell line was able to establish from T291 lung adenocarcinoma. Presumably, additional factors must be found which will improve the ability of this serum-free medium to support a long-term growth of the lung adenocarcinoma cells in primary culture.

Human Oat Cell Carcinoma Cells (T293):

The culture medium used for T293 tumors was the same as used for the T291 lung adenocarcinoma cells. The tumor tissue was obtained from a patient with lung oat cell carcinoma, injected into nude mice, and thereafter the tumors were transplanted serially.

The primary cultures were prepared by mincing the tumor tissues, treating with collagenase, and plating into serum-coated culture dishes. When a low concentration of serum (0.5%) was added to the hormone-supplemented medium, the T293 tumor cells were able to be propagated and established in culture. The growth rate of the established T293 cells in serum-free, hormone-supplemented medium was 80% of that in serum-supplemented medium.

ACKNOWLEDGEMENTS

This work was supported by N.I.H. grants CA 23052 and CA 19731.

REFERENCES

1. Sun, T-T. and Green, H. Differentiation of the epidermal keratinocyte in cell culture: formation of the cornified envelope. Cell, 9: 511-521 (1976).
2. Miyazaki, K., Masui, H. and Sato, G. Control of keratinization of human broncogenic epidermoid carcinoma cells in primary culture with serum-free medium. Proc. Natl. Acad. Sci. USA, in press (1982).
3. Barnes, D. and Sato, G. Methods for growth of cultured cells in serum-free medium. Anal. Biochem. 102: 255-270 (1980).

Continuous Growth of a Human Breast Cancer Cell Line (MCF-7) in Serum-Free Medium*

P. Briand and A. E. Lykkesfeldt

The Fibiger Laboratory, Ndr. Frihavnsgade 70, DK-2100 Copenhagen, Denmark

ABSTRACT. The MCF-7 cell line has been adapted to growth in serum-free medium by a gradual decrease in the content of serum in the medium. The serum-free medium was composed of DMEM/F12 + glutamine + selenite + insulin + transferrin + EGF, and the culture flasks were coated with collagen IV to increase cell attachment. The doubling time for cells cultivated in serum-free medium for 3 months was 70 hrs. The cells contained free cytoplasmic but not filled nuclear estrogen receptors and formed carcinomas when inoculated subcutaneously into nude mice treated with estrone.

1. Introduction. A serum-free medium for the growth of MCF-7 cells has been described by Barnes and Sato (1). They transferred the cells from a conventional medium with 10% fetal bovine serum (FBS) directly to a serum-free medium consisting of DMEM/F12 (1:1) + insulin (250 ng/ml) + transferrin (25 µg/ml) + epidermal growth factor (100 ng/ml) + prostaglandin-$F_{2\alpha}$ (100 ng/ml) + fibronectin = CIg (7.5 µg/ml) + Na-selenite (10^{-8}M) + Holmes α-1 protein (1 µg/ml). They obtained growth over the following 1-2 weeks equal to that in serum-containing medium and the cells were carried for more than 3 months.

This work presents long-term growth of MCF-7 cells in a more simple serum-free medium with the maintenance of estrogen receptors and tumorgenicity.

2. Cell Growth. MCF-7 cells have been adapted to growth at 0.05% FBS by a stepwise decrease in serum concentration from 5% to 0.5% and from 0.5% to 0.05% over a period of several months. Cells cultivated at 0.05% FBS were transferred to plastic T-flasks coated with collagen IV and grown in a serum-free medium composed of DMEM/F12 + glutamine 2mM + insulin + transferrin + epidermal growth factor + selenite in the concentrations mentioned in the introduction. The collagen coating was found to be essential for cell attachment (Fig. 1).

---

*Sponsored by the Danish Cancer Society.

- collagen coating   + collagen coating

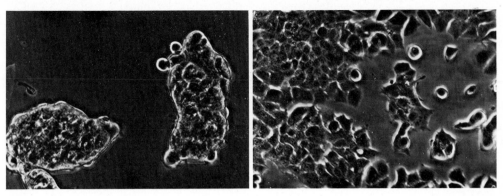

Figure 1.   Effect of collagen IV coating on cell spreading.   (180 x).
Human placental collagen (Sigma, USA), collagen IV, was sterilized by
irradiation and dissolved in 0.5M acetic acid at a concentration of
5 mg/ml.   The collagen solution was treated as described by Schor and
Court (2) for preparation of gels of native collagen fibers except that
equal volumes of 2 x concentrated medium were added to the collagen
solution.

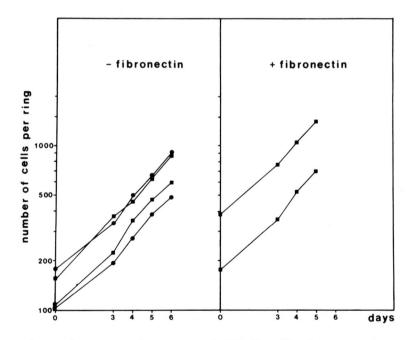

Figure 2.   Growth curves of MCF-7 cells in serum-free medium without
and with fibronectin.
    Each curve represents cell counts in one glass ring.   Cells were
seeded at day -2.

Every one or two weeks, cells were subcultured using trypsin (Difco) 0.1% + EDTA, 0.4 mM, and 5-10 x 10^3 cells per cm^2 were seeded in collagen IV coated T-flasks. The cells have been carried for more than 5 months with a growth ratio (number of cells after 7 days/number of cells seeded) of about 3.

The growth rate was determined by counting the number of cells in 2 mm glass rings fixed on the inner surface of the flask with the use of silicone grease. This in situ counting was preferred to the use of microwell plates to avoid an open system which introduces problems with variations in CO_2 and pH as well as risk of evaporation from the medium. Furthermore, microwell plates tend to form water drops under the lid disturbing cell counting by microscopy. Based on this method very reproducible growth curves were obtained. The doubling time was approximately 3 days and no effect of fibronectin was found (Fig. 2).

3. Estrogen Receptor. Estrogen receptor content was determined by the single saturating dose hydroxylapatite method by Garola and McGuire (3). MCF-7 cells grown in serum-free medium contained estrogen receptor (Table 1) at a level equal to that found in MCF-7 cells grown at 5% FBS.

Table 1. Estrogen receptor content in MCF-7 cells grown in serum-free medium

Weeks in serum-free medium	fmol estrogen receptor per mg cytosol protein ($\bar{x}$ ± s.d.)
1 week	48 ± 7
6 weeks	107 ± 7
14 weeks	67 ± 5

4. Tumorgenicity. MCF-7 cells grown in serum-free medium for 6 weeks were shifted to 0.5% FBS in order to propagate sufficient number of cells for transplantation studies. One week later, the cells were inoculated s.c. into 4 female nude mice treated with estrone 5 µg per ml drinking water. In all animals carcinomas were produced.

5. References

1. Barnes D and Sato G: Nature 1979, 281: 388-389.
2. Schor SL and Court J: J Cell Sci 1979, 38 : 267-281.
3. Garola RE and McGuire WL: Cancer Res 1977, 37 : 3333-3337.

Regulation of Oestrogen Responsiveness of MCF-7 Human Breast Cancer Cell Growth by Serum Concentration in the Culture Medium*

T. C. Dembinski and C. D. Green

Department of Biochemistry, University of Liverpool, P. O. Box 147, Liverpool, L69 3BX, U. K.

ABSTRACT

During the last 5 years we have maintained in serum media two sublines of MCF-7 cells, only one of which retains a significant growth response to oestradiol, as assessed by 'Coulter' counting. The responsiveness to oestradiol can be regulated by the serum concentration in the medium. Cells in the absence of or in low serum (0.5-1%) whilst growing normally, are unresponsive to oestrogen whereas cells in high serum (15%) respond to the hormone with an increased growth rate and macromolecular synthesis. This transition between oestrogen-responsive and unresponsive growth states can also be regulated by dialyzing or charcoal-treating the serum. There appears to be in serum (both calf and human) a "factor" which the cells require to respond to oestrogen. We suggest that this factor (molecular weight 400-1200 daltons) influences the expression of a growth response to oestradiol.

INTRODUCTION

The MCF-7 line of human breast cancer cells has been characterized extensively (1) and the growth and macromolecular synthesis of these cells reported to be stimulated by oestradiol (2-5). Therefore they have been proposed as an in vitro system for studying oestrogen-responsive breast cancer (6). However other studies have shown a lack of responsiveness of these cells to oestrogens (7-10).

This paper describes new conditions under which MCF-7 cells respond to oestradiol and presents evidence in support of a serum factor which interacts with the oestrogen response mechanism.

MATERIALS AND METHODS

Cells and tissue culture - the MCF-7 cell line (1) was kindly provided by Dr. M.E. Lippman. Cells were grown in DMEM (Gibco) supplemented with glutamine (0.6 g/l) and 10% newborn calf serum, NBCS (Gibco) in a humidified incubator in 5% CO_2 at 37° C (11).
Cell growth experiments - The cells were plated into 24-well tissue culture dishes (Linbro Scientific) with 10% NBCS-DMEM. Following 'spreading' of cells (20-30 h), the medium was changed to DMEM with test sera concentrations $\pm$ 10^{-9} M oestradiol. Cells were refed daily.
Thymidine incorporation - ^{3}H thymidine (5 uCi/ml of medium) was added for the last two hours of 48 h incubations $\pm$ oestradiol. TCA-insoluble counts were obtained as previously described (11). Cell number was determined using a Coulter counter method (12).

---

* Supported by M.R.C. grant No. G80/0240/0CA

Preparation of "charcoal-stripped" serum - NBCS was stirred for 24 h at 4° C with 0.25% activated charcoal (Norit A, Sigma) and 0.0025% dextran T-70 (Pharmacia). Charcoal was removed by centrifugation at 10,000 g and the serum filter-sterilized. Dialysis of serum - NBCS was dialyzed against PBS at a vol:vol ratio of 1:100 for 48 h at 4° C and filter-sterilized.

RESULTS AND DISCUSSION

The serum content of the culture medium has a profound effect on the oestrogen-responsiveness of 'our' MCF-7 cells (11). Further, we have observed that whilst addition of oestradiol at low concentrations of NBCS had little effect on growth rate, a significant increase was seen at higher concentrations (Fig. 1). Similar results were obtained with human serum (11), but not with FCS. The transition between oestrogen-responsive and -unresponsive growth states is also affected by the processes of dialyzing (Table 1) or "charcoal-stripping" (CS) serum (Fig. 2). The latter process enhanced cell growth, as compared to native serum, although an oestradiol-induced growth response was no longer observed with concentrations of 1-20% CS-NBCS (data not shown). Similar results were obtained from thymidine incorporation experiments (Fig. 2). Apparently charcoal-treatment removes a bio-molecule(s) which affects both growth "suppression" and hormone responsiveness. Figure 3 shows the effect of oestradiol on cell growth in 'serum-free' medium. A short term exposure to 10% NBCS sensitized the cells to mitogenic effects of oestradiol. Other studies with Human breast cancer cells, namely MCF-7 (13) and ZR-75-1 (14), in 'serum-free' media also support the hypothesis that an undefined biomolecule(s) can influence oestrogen-responsive growth. Our recent gel filtration experiments indicate that the serum "factor" has a molecular weight of 400-1200 daltons (Table 1); its identity is under investigation. A biomolecule with similar properties - mammary growth factor (MGF), presumably phosphoethanolamine (15),

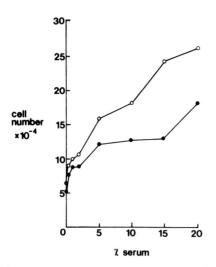

Fig. 1. Effect of increasing serum concentrations on the growth of MCF-7 cells. 1 x 10^4 cells were plated in the presence of 10% NBCS in DMEM. After 2 days the medium was replaced by DMEM containing indicated concentrations of NBCS plus (o) or minus (●) 10^{-9}M oestradiol. Results are 7 day growth points.

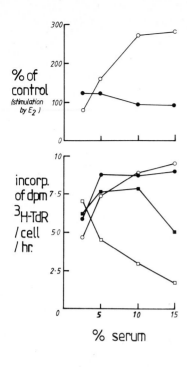

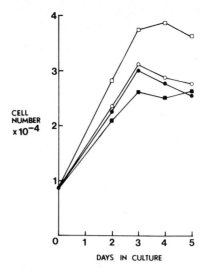

Fig. 3. Growth responses of MCF-7 cells in 'serum-free' medium. 7 x 10³ cells were plated in the presence (□,■) or absence (O,●) of 10% NBCS in DMEM. After 24 h the media was removed and DMEM added with (□,O) or without (■,●) 10⁻⁹M oestradiol.

Fig. 2. Effect of increasing serum concentrations on [³H]thymidine incorporation in MCF-7 cells. 2 x 10⁴ cells were plated in 10% NBCS-DMEM. After 2 days, the medium was replaced by DMEM, containing the indicated concentrations of either charcoal-stripped (CS) NBCS (O,●) or untreated NBCS (■,□), with (●,■) or without (O,□) 10⁻⁹M oestradiol (bottom). Thymidine incorporation rates were determined at 48 h, following addition of oestradiol (Methods).

Table 1. Effect of different treatments of NBCS on oestradiol-induced stimulation of [³H]thymidine incorporation in MCF-7 cells

Treatment	Excluded Mol. wt. size (daltons)	Ratio of rates of thymidine incorporation in E₂-treated dishes: control dishes
NBCS	-	2.0
Dial-NBCS	-	1.1
Void fraction G-10	400	2.5
Void fraction G-15	1,200	1.2
Void fraction G-25	3,000	1.5
Void fraction G-50	13,000	1.3
Void fraction G-75	40,000	1.4
Void fraction G-100	90,000	1.2

2 x 10⁴ cells were plated in 10% NBCS-DMEM. After 24 h the medium was replaced, by DMEM, containing 15% concentrations of untreated NBCS, dialyzed NBCS or NBCS excluded volumes from Sephadex gel filtration columns ± 10⁻⁸M oestradiol. Thymidine incorporation rates were determined at 48 h (Methods).

442

promotes the growth of rat mammary tumour cells in the presence of growth stimulatory hormones (16). The existence of specific tumour growth factors, under oestrogen control and, which are responsible for the growth of hormone-responsive tumours in vivo has also been demonstrated (17). The relationship of these factors to 'our' serum factor is presently under investigation. The existence of such a biomolecule in human serum, which interacts with the oestrogen response mechanism, may have important implications for endocrine therapy of breast tumours.

REFERENCES

1. Soule, H.D., Vasquez, J., Long, A., Albert, S. and Brennan, M.J. (1973) J. Nat. Cancer Inst. 51, 1409-1415.

2. Lippman, M.E. and Bolan, G. (1975) Nature 256, 592-593

3. Lippman, M.E., Bolan, G. and Huff, K. (1976) Cancer Res. 36, 4595-4601

4. Aitken, S.C. and Lippman, M.E. "Control Mechanisms in Animal Cells," (Jimenez de Asua, L., ed.) pp. 133-155, Raven Press, New York, 1980

5. Nawata, H., Bronzert, D. and Lippman, M.E. (1981) J. Biol. Chem. 256, 5016-5021

6. Lippman, M.E., Bolan, G. Monaco, M.E., Pinkus, L. and Engel, L. (1976) J. Steroid Biochem. 7, 1045-1051

7. Stoll, B.A. "Secondary spread in Breast Cancer," (B.A. Stoll, Ed.) pp. 169-191, Heinemann, London, 1977

8. Edwards,D.P., Murthy, S.R. and McGuire, W.L. (1978) Cancer Res. 40, 1722-1726

9. Horwitz, K.B., Koseki, Y. and McGuire, W.L. (1978) Endocrinology 103, 1742-1751

10. Jozan, S. Moure, C., Gillois, M. and Bayard, F. (1979) J. Steroid Biochem. 10, 341-342

11. Page, M.J., Field, J.K., Everett, N.P. and Green, C.D. (1982) Cancer Res. in press

12. Butler, W.B., Kelsey, W.H. and Goran, N. (1981) Cancer Res. 41, 82-88

13. Barnes, D. and Sato, G. (1979) Nature 388-389

14. Allegra, J.C. and Lippman, M.E. (1980) Europ. J. Cancer 16, 1007-1015

15. Kano-Sueoka, T., Cohen, D.M., Yamaizumi, A., Nishimura, S., Mori, M. and Fujiki, H. (1979) Proc. Nat. Acad. Sci. USA 76, 5741-5744

16. Kano-Sueoka, T., Errick, J.E. and Cohen, D.M. (1979) "Hormones and cell culture," (Sato, G. and Ross, R. Eds.) pp. 499-512, Cold Spring Harbour Laboratory.

17. Sirbasku, D.A. (1978) Proc. Nat. Acad. Sci. USA 75, 3786-3790

Induction of Differentiation in Human Solid Tumor Cells by Anti-Tumor Agents in Serum Depleted Medium

A. Rey, D. Cupissol, E. Ursule, and B. Serrou

Laboratoire d'Immunopoharmacologie des Tumeurs, INSERM U236 ERA-CNRS 844, CRLC, BP 5054, F-34033 Montpellier, France

ABSTRACT

In vitro pharmacological and immunological studies of human solid tumors often use cell cultures to study inhibition of cell growth and/or cell differentiation induced by anti-tumor agents such as retinoic acid (RA). The capacity to form colonies in semi-solid agar (SSA) is considered a characteristic phenotypic expression of tumor cells. We investigated some of the factors which play an important role during this expression in primary human cancer and human tumor cells lines (myeloma and ovarian carcinoma). We found major changes in cloning efficiency depending on the serum batch employed, therefore necessitating replacement of this serum by a chemically defined medium. Addition of transferrin, insulin and epithelial growth factor allowed us to culture a human ovarian carcinoma cell line in 1 % serum. Our results show that RA impeded CAL-9 cells colony formation in SSA but enhanced thymidine uptake in liquid cultures (LC)

INTRODUCTION

Tumor cells generally exhibit an altered response to factors that normally control their growth and/or differentiation. The development and use of chemically defined media for cultured cells (1-2) offers a better understanding of factors which play a role in regulating events in cancer cells. Little is known about the requirements of human tumor cells for hormones and other potential growth enhancing or inhibiting factors. There is evidence that retinoid compounds can modify pattern of animal cell proliferation in vitro (3). Recently, human studies (4) have shown that retinoid can induce regression of bronchial metaplasia. In the present study we used semi-solid agar cultures (SSA ; 5) and analysis of human tumor cell growth in LC to show that the loss of the ability to form colonies due to a given factor or drug does not necessarly translate a cytolytic event.

MATERIAL AND METHODS

Cells. The CAL-9 cell line (donated by Prof. C.M. Lalanne, Nice, France) originates from a 44 year old woman ascites on a mucinous cystadenocarcinoma of the ovary. This line was routinely cultured in RPMI, supplemented with 10 % fetal calf serum (FCS).

Cell proliferation. 1) cells were plated at 1×10^4 and 5×10^4 per 35 mm petri dish in 0.3 % agar using medium enriched as described by Pike and Robinson (6). Colonies (more than 40 cells) were counted on day 14. 2) Cells were cultured in liquid medium in micro-wells at 10^4 cells in 200 µl/well. Cultures were evaluated each day for morphology and tritiated thymidine (^{3}H-TdR) uptake 4 hr. (incubation with 1.25 µCi/well) over a seven day period.

Factors, hormones and drugs. Our study evaluated the effects of : insulin (INS), transferin (TF), hydrocortisone (HC), human chorionic gonadotropin (HCG) and epithelial growth factor (EGF). Each were evaluated at 3 different concentrations which were added to the medium at the time of plating.

We also studied in partially defined medium the effects of RA (Tretinoin, a gift from Hoffman-La Roche & Co., Basel) in the same manner as described above.

The last two drugs which we studied were cis-dichloro diammine platinum (CDDP) and adriamycin (ADM). For both of these drugs, the cell were only incubated for one hour with the drug before washing and plating.

RESULTS

Serum depletion. EGF (10 ng/ml), TF (10 µg/ml) and INS (1 µg/ml) gave rise to a marked increase in SSA cloning efficiency (Table 1). We therefore chose these three factors as additives for our serum-free medium. However, we were unable to eliminate serum altogether and established a minimal concentration at 1 % serum. This led to a CAL-9 cell proliferation which was 70 % that obtained with 10 % inactivated FCS.

We found that HC inhibited cell proliferation at a concentration of 100 nM. HCG lad no effect up to concentrations of 100 mIU/ml.

Pharmacological studies. In presence of our partially defined medium we observed an inhibition of SSA colony proliferation with 10^{-8} M RA. This effect disappeared at 10^{-12}M. However, a study of ^{3}H-TdR uptake over 7 days did not show a parallel inhibition and even increased on day 3. This was observed with different cell density cultures (10^3, 5 x 10^3 and 10^4 cells/well ; culture surface : 0.325 sqcm).

SSA and LC studies of CDDP and ADM yielded correlated results from 0.02 to 2 µg/ml concentrations. ADM was more toxic (0 % survival at 2 µg/ml) than CDDP for the same concentrations.

Table 1. Modification of day 3 ^{3}HTdR uptake (cpm) in LC and of cloning efficiency (CE) in SSA of CAL-9 cells. (Percent of control). For abreviations see text. nd = not done.

	CE		CE	cpm
EGF (10 ng/ml)	2091	HC (100 nM)	5	nd
TF (10 µg/ml)	192	RA (10^{-8}M)	12	143
INS (1 µg/ml)	212	ADM (2 µg/ml)	0	20
HCG (100 mUI/ml)	100	CDDP (2 µg/ml)	69	72

DISCUSSION

The present study describes a medium containing EGF, INS and TF which allowed us to culture ovarian cells in medium containing only 1 % serum. Using this serum-poor medium we were able to demonstrate the cytotoxic action of drugs such as ADM or CDDP. We also show that retinoic acid inhibits colony formation on semi-solid medium while CAL-9 ovarian cells were still actively proliferating (^{3}H-TdR uptake and cell counts). Previous work has already established that retinoid substances inhibit colony formation in SSA (7). The liquid medium culture study provides an important finding because it shows that tumor cells were not destroyed but only lost their capacity to proliferate in agar. This reflects an evolution of the tumor cell to a less transformed state (differentiation). Other authors have reported using retinoid substances to inhibit "initiated" cells from evolving to a transformed state (8). These drugs are obviously different than classical cytolytic agents. Anthracyclines appear to belong to both categories of drugs (9).

REFERENCES

1. D. Barnes & G. Sato (1980) Anal. Biochem. 102, 255-270.
2. R.G. Ham (1981) Handbook of Experimental Pharmacology (Springer, Berlin), Vol 57, pp 13-88
3. E.W. Schroder, E. Rapaport, A. Kastan Kabcenel & P.H. Black (1982) Proc. Natl. Acad. Sci USA, 79, 1549-1552.
4. J. Gouveia, G. Mathe, T. Hercend et al. (1982) Lancet 1, 710-712.
5. I. Macpherson & L. Montagnier (1964) Virology 23, 291-294.
6. B.L. Pike & W.A. Robinson (1970) J. Cell. Physiol. 76, 77-84.
7. F.L. Meyskens & S.E. Salmon (1981) Ann. N.Y. Acad. Sci. 359, 414
8. L.J. Mordan, L.M. Bergin, J.E. Budnick, R.R. Meegan & J.S. Bertrams (1982) Carcinogenesis 3, 279-285.
9. A. Raz (1982) JNCI 68, 629-638.

Hormonal Requirements of in Vitro Growth in Human Mammary and Ovarian Carcinoma Cell Cultures

W. E. Simon, F. Hölzel, and M. Albrecht

Universitäts-Frauenklinik, Martinistr. 52, D-2000 Hamburg 20, FRG

ABSTRACT

The in vitro proliferation of tumor cell lines derived from patients with recurrent mammary carcinoma revealed individuality of the response to steroid hormones
and prolactin. The growth response patterns were largely concurring with the endocrine situation of the patients or with the result of endocrine therapy prior to the
cell sampling. Cells derived from ovarian carcinomas of higher histological differentiation reacted to gonadotropic hormone concentrations equivalent to physiological
serum levels.

1. Introduction

Epithelial cellular components of breast or ovary are known as targets for
steroid hormones, prolactin or gonadotropic hormones. Therefore, organotropic hormones are possible candidates for supporting the proliferation of carcinomatous
cells in vivo and in vitro. Evidence for endocrine mechanisms mediating the growth
of human mammary carcinomas in vivo is deductible from tumor regression observed
in about 1/3 of patients under endocrine therapy (1). The present investigation is
aimed at establishing correlations between the hormone responsiveness of carcinoma
cells in serum-free culture and the clinical conditions of patients with mammary or
ovarian carcinoma.

2. Materials and Methods

For the determinations of the hormonal influence on cell growth, a number of
tumor cell strains were established from pleural effusions, ascitic fluids or solid
metastases of patients with recurrent carcinomas. The culture medium was based on
Earle's salts, 2x MEM essential and non-essential amino acids, MEM vitamins, supplemented with 10 nM T_4, 80 mIU/ml insulin, 5 µg/ml fetuin, 2.5 µg/ml transferrin,
0.1 µg/ml glycyl-L-histidyl-L-lysine (2). For the primary cultures, and during the
early passages of cultivation, the presence of 10% fetal calf serum (FCS) was essential; in higher passages a decreasing serum dependence of cell growth was noted. In
early passages, the epitheloid tumor cell cultures were freed of contaminating
fibroblasts or mesothelial cells by differential trypsinization (3), and by incubation periods in serum-free medium. The hormone responsiveness was determined by
cell counts after 5-day incubation periods with hormonal factors in concentrations
corresponsing to physiological serum levels or to serum levels observed during
endocrine therapy. Controls were kept in basal medium (BM) or in BM with 10% FCS.

3. Results

In growth experiments in serum-free BM, optimum concentrations of the hormonal factors applied were determined. Although the cell lines in passage 1-4 of the cultivation showed highly individual reaction patterns, the growth of 5 of 7 lines derived from mammary tumors of postmenopausal patients was enhanced by testosterone (T) which was uneffective on tumor cell lines from premenopausal patients in which androgens have a minor functional role (4). 6 of 10 cell lines compared were stimulated by physiological concentrations of cortisol (C), suggesting an enhancing effect of corticosteroids on the in vivo growth of the corresponding mammary tumors. Cell lines which were stimulated by progesterone (P) or the antiestrogenic compound tamoxifen (TAM) were derived from patients who had been treated unsuccessfully with medroxyprogesterone acetate or TAM prior to the cell sampling. Apparently, the in vitro growth properties of these cell lines reflect resistance or even partial dependence on P or TAM, which developed during the preceding therapy with the compounds (5).

Individual reaction patterns were also evident when the growth rates of the 10 mammary carcinoma cell lines in the presence of the most stimulating or inhibiting hormone concentrations were compared with the capacity to grow in BM or in BM supplemented with 10% FCS (Fig. 1). 6 cell lines (No 1,2,3,5,9 and 10) did not proliferate in BM and required either C (No 1,3,5 and 9), P or T (No 2), estradiol-17ß (No 5 and 10) or prolactin (No 3 and 5) for optimum growth in BM. In the lines 1

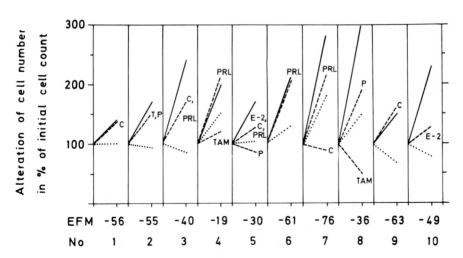

Fig. 1. Growth requirements of 10 different mammary carcinoma cell lines and replacement of FCS by hormonal factors, determined in 5-day incubation periods. ――― BM plus 10% FCS, ----- BM plus maximum stimulating or inhibiting hormone, ····· BM. In reference to the corresponding controls in BM, significantly different effects on the cell growth are shown (p < 0.01 by Student's t-test). C = cortisol, E-2 = estradiol-17ß, P = progesterone, PRL = prolactin, T = testosterone, TAM = tamoxifen.

and 9, the sole application of C was substitute for the growth promoting effect of FCS. The remaining 4 cell lines (No 4,6,7 and 8) were able to proliferate in the absence of steroid hormones, prolactin or FCS, although their growth rates in BM were enhanced significantly in the presence of prolactin (No 4,6 and 7) or P (No 8).

The in vitro growth of most of the ovarian tumor cell lines examined was unresponsive to steroid hormones. Exceptions were cells of a line derived from a cystadenocarcinoma of a postmenopausal patient which were stimulated by 10 nM T, and cell cultures of a clear cell carcinoma in which 100 nM C enhanced the growth rates in BM 3-fold compared to the controls. Individual reaction patterns were observed when the responses of cell proliferation after the application of human follicle stimulating hormone (hFSH) and human chorionic gonadotropin (hCG) were compared among the different ovarian tumor cell lines. hFSH and hCG enhanced the proliferation of cell lines derived from well-differentiated tumors of postmenopausal patients in a dose range corresponding to the physiological serum levels of hFSH and human luteinizing hormone determined in postmenopausal women (6). Cells obtained from a carcinoma with undifferentiated histology did not react to gonadotropin doses equivalent to physiological serum levels. This cell line and the clear cell carcinoma line were able to grow in BM in the absence of gonadotropic hormones or FCS (7).

4.   Conclusions

The results provide evidence that organotropic hormones are potential factors for the in vitro growth of human mammary and ovarian carcinoma cells in serum-free medium. The individual reaction patterns observed for the dose-dependent hormone sensitivity of the cell lines are consistent with the endocrine status of the corresponding patients at the time of cell sampling, or with the results of endocrine therapy regimens applied before.

5.   Literature references

(1) Manni A, Trujillo JE, Marshall JS, Brodkey J, Pearson CH. Cancer 43, 444-450, 1979.
(2) Simon WE, Hölzel F. J Cancer Res Clin Oncol 94, 307-323, 1979.
(3) Owens RB, Smith HS, Nelson-Rees WA, Springer EC. J Natl Cancer Inst 56, 843-849, 1976.
(4) Nordin BEC, Crilly RG, Marshall DH. J Endocrin 89, 131-143, 1981.
(5) Simon WE, Albrecht M, Trams G, Dietel M, Hölzel F. Eur J Cancer Clin Oncol (in press).
(6) Mahesh VB. In: Consensus on Menopause Research. Van Keep PA, Greenblatt RB, Albeaux-Fernet M (eds). Lancaster UK, MTP Press, pp 11-18, 1976.
(7) Simon WE, Albrecht M, Hänsel M, Dietel M, Hölzel F. J Natl Cancer Inst (in press).

Subject Index

International Cell Biology 1980–1981

Papers Presented at the Second International Congress on Cell Biology, Berlin (West), August 31–September 5, 1980
Editor: **H.G.Schweiger**
1981. 595 figures. XVIII, 1033 pages. ISBN 3-540-10475-5

Contents: Opening Lecture. – Genomes and Gene Expression. – Cytoskeleton. – Pathology and Pathogenicity. – Differentiation and Development. – Membrane and Cell Surfaces. – Functional Organization. – Subject Index.

Intrernational Cell Biology 1980–1981 contains contributions presented at the Second International Congress on Cell Biology held in West Berlin, August 31–September 5, 1980. The authors of the contributions were selected as speakers for the Congress for their leading role in their respective fields. The topics cover a uniquely broad range of research areas, providing an excellent reflection of the present status of cell biology. This book will remain a useful source of information to biologists, medical researchers and biochemists for years to come.

Results and Problems in Cell Differentiation
A Series of Topical Volumes in Development Biology
Editors: W.Beermann, W.J.Gehring, J.B.Gurdon, F.C.Katafos, J.Reinert

Volume 11
Differentiation and Neoplasia

Editors: **R.G.McKinnell, M.A.Diberardino, M.Blumenfeld, R.D.Bergad**
1980. 77 figures, 33 tables. XV, 310 pages. ISBN 3-540-10177-2

From the Contents: Cell Differentiation Yesterday and Today. – Gene Injections into Amphibian Docytes. – Differential Histone Phosphorylation During Drosophila Development. – The Current Status of Cloning and Nuclear Reprogramming in Amphibian Eggs. – Genetic Manipulation of the Early Mouse Embryo. – The Effects of Temperature-Sensitive Rous Sarcoma Virus and Phorbol Diester Tumor Promoters on Cell Lineages. – Drug Induced Differentiation of Human Neuroplastoma: Transformation into Ganglion Cells with Mitomycin-C.

Volume 10
Chloroplasts

Editor: **J.Reinert**
With contributions by numerous experts
1980. 40 figures, 11 tables. XI, 240 pages. ISBN 3-540-10082-2

Contents: Types of Plastids: Their Development and Interconversions. – The Continuity of Plastids and the Differentiation of Plastid Populations. – Plastid DNA – The Plastome. – RNA and Protein Synthesis in Plastid Differentiation. – Biosynthesis of Thylakoids and the Membrane-Bound Enzyme Systems of Photosynthesis. – Fraction I Protein. – Factors in Chloroplast Differentiation. – The Survival, Division and Differentiation of Higher Plant Plastids Outside the Leaf Cell. – Subject Index.

Volume 9
Genetic Mosaics and Cell Differentiation

Editor: **W.J.Gehring**
With contributions by numerous experts
1978. 75 figures, 19 tables. XI, 315 pages. ISBN 3-540-08882-2

Contents: Gynandromorph Fate Maps in Drosophila. – Mitotic Recombination and Position Effect Variegation. – Drosophila Chimeras and the Problem of Determination – Estimating Primordial Cell Numbers in Drosophila Imaginal Discs and Histoblasts. Cell Lineage Relationships in the Drosophila Embryo.– Cell Lineage and Differentiation in Drosophila. – Genetic Mosaic Studies of Pattern Formation in Drosophila melanogaster, with Special Reference to the Prepattern Hypothesis. – The Relationship Between Cell Lineage and Differentiation in the Early Mouse Embryo. – Sexual Differentiation in Mammalian Chimaeras and Mosaics. – Behavioral Analysis in Drosophila Mosaics.

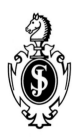

Springer-Verlag
Berlin
Heidelberg
New York
Tokyo